Atlas of Wide-Field Retinal Angiography and Imaging

Igor Kozak • J. Fernando Arevalo
Editors

Atlas of Wide-Field Retinal Angiography and Imaging

Springer

Editors
Igor Kozak, MD, PhD
Senior Academic Consultant
Vitreoretinal Division
King Khaled Eye Specialist Hospital
Riyadh
Saudi Arabia

J. Fernando Arevalo, MD, FACS
Edmund F. and Virginia B. Ball
Professor of Ophthalmology
Chairman, Department of Ophthalmology
Johns Hopkins Bayview Medical Center
Retina Division, Wilmer Eye Institute
The Johns Hopkins University School of Medicine
Baltimore, MD
USA

ISBN 978-3-319-79240-8 ISBN 978-3-319-17864-6 (eBook)
DOI 10.1007/978-3-319-17864-6

Softcover reprint of the hardcover 1st edition 2016

Printed on acid-free paper

This Springer imprint is published by Springer Nature
The registered company is Springer International Publishing AG Switzerland

To my parents, Bozena and Peter, and brother Peter for their endless support; to my friends, mentors, and colleagues, and to all our patients for inspiring us.

Igor Kozak

To my family for their patience and support, to Wilmer Eye Institute, Johns Hopkins University, and King Khaled Eye Specialist Hospital for the privilege to lead the Vitreoretinal Division to the next level, and to God for 4 wonderful and fulfilling years of my life.

J. Fernando Arevalo

Foreword

The eye may act as a window to many systemic conditions. Some retinal imaging techniques provide noninvasive methods for detecting and monitoring such pathologies, with high resolution and sensitivity to allow an ophthalmologist to make the correct diagnosis. Fortunately, clinical research and imaging developments have made notable advances in identifying retinal pathology and have been incorporated in *Atlas of Wide-Field Retinal Angiography and Imaging* to enhance the educational value of this extraordinary text. The desire to view larger areas of the retina that extend to the retinal periphery has always been there, and over the last 20 years, new imaging devices capable of obtaining ultra-wide-field images, fluorescein and indocyanine green (ICG) angiograms, as well as autofluorescence, have emerged to help us diagnose, understand, and treat retinal disease.

Beginning with improvements in photographic, ultrasonographic, and fluorescein as well as ICG angiographic technology in the 1960s, several comprehensive textbooks and atlases have been written to compile advances in imaging of retinal conditions. Even with the recent popularity of **wide-field retinal angiography and imaging**, this is one of the first books to cover the subject comprehensively. The editors, Dr. Igor Kozak and Dr. Fernando Arevalo, and the contributing authors of this text have provided by far the best documentation of **wide-field retinal angiography and imaging** for its readers. Indisputably, the co-authors are all leaders in this field with notable original and lasting contributions to one of more of the principal selected subjects covered in this text. Accordingly, each section discusses the most advanced concepts regarding **wide-field retinal angiography and imaging** of retinal disorders. In essence, a large amount of new information on **wide-field retinal angiography and imaging** has been compiled in this text in an authoritative and comprehensive format.

The topics discussed in this book include wide-field fluorescein angiography, wide-field ICG angiography, and wide-field autofluorescence on a variety of retinal conditions, including intraocular tumors and posterior uveitis. While there have been several publications which describe specific uses of **wide-field retinal angiography and imaging**, this textbook attempts to engage a select group of experts to elegantly describe and amply illustrate the variety of ocular abnormalities described in this *Atlas of Wide-Field Retinal Angiography and Imaging*. In short, Igor Kozak and Fernando Arevalo have achieved success in fulfilling a challenging goal in this concise, salient, and superbly illustrated and descriptive atlas. The editors and their expert contributors are to be congratulated for compiling an educational addition to **wide-field retinal angiography and imaging**. Essentially, this new text represents a wonderful labor by an elite group of expert clinical and scientific contributors. Their monumental efforts should be rewarded by the gratitude of clinicians and perhaps even some patients who will receive incalculable pleasure as a reader of their work.

Neil M. Bressler, MD
The James P. Gills Professor of Ophthalmology
Chief, Retina Division – Wilmer Eye Institute
Johns Hopkins University School of Medicine and Hospital
Baltimore, MD, USA

Preface

We were privileged to work together at King Khaled Eye Specialist Hospital (KKESH) in Riyadh, Saudi Arabia, and introduce several advancements in retinal imaging to the Middle East. The popularity of retinal imaging is based on the necessity to document and aid in the early detection and management of diseases that can affect both the retina and overall health. We as ophthalmologists need to be aware of recent advances in retinal imaging. The desire to view larger areas of the retina and the retinal periphery has been ongoing since the original fundus cameras were developed, and over the past two decades fundus cameras capable of obtaining wide field images, angiograms, and autofluorescence have emerged to help us better diagnose, understand, and treat disease.

Our experience at a very florid, high-volume Retina and Uveitis clinic at KKESH triggered a comprehensive presentation of the current clinical aspects of the *Atlas of Wide-Field Retinal Angiography and Imaging*. This book includes contributions from an internationally renowned group of experts from the United States, Spain, and Saudi Arabia. The topics discussed in this book do not pretend to be all-inclusive but include history and principles of wide-field retinal imaging, wide-field fluorescein angiography, wide-field indocyanine angiography, wide-field autofluorescence, wide-field retinal imaging of diabetic retinopathy, wide-field retinal imaging of branch retinal vein occlusions, wide-field retinal imaging of central retinal vein occlusions, wide-field retinal imaging of other retinal vascular diseases, wide-field retinal imaging of retinal dystrophies, wide-field retinal imaging of peripheral retinal degenerations, wide-field retinal imaging of pediatric retina, wide-field retinal imaging of retinal and choroidal tumors, wide-field retinal imaging of retinal and choroidal inflammatory diseases, wide-field retinal imaging of retinal and choroidal infectious diseases, and wide-field retinal imaging of other miscellaneous retinal diseases.

The impetus to edit this book has come from our students and colleagues in all fields of ophthalmology and internal medicine at KKESH and internationally. This book is intended for retina and vitreous specialists, uveitis and ocular oncology specialists, retina and vitreous fellows, uveitis and ocular oncology fellows, ophthalmology residents, comprehensive ophthalmologists, and physicians in general.

The principal objective of this atlas is to present the current information on wide-field retinal angiography and imaging from leading experts in the field. We hope their knowledge and experience will assist ophthalmologists, retina specialists, uveitis and ocular oncology specialists, and physicians in general approach a level of knowledge about wide-field retinal angiography and imaging to benefit their patients in everyday clinical practice.

Riyadh, Saudi Arabia — Igor Kozak, MD, PhD

Baltimore, MD, USA — J. Fernando Arevalo, MD, FACS

Acknowledgments

We would like to acknowledge the hard work and contribution of the members of the Photography Department at the King Khaled Eye Specialist Hospital in Riyadh, Saudi Arabia, namely Mizher Al Ghamdi, Abdulrahman Al Oraini, Saleh Al Dhafiri, Ayshah Al Twijeri, and Sami Al Ghamdi, and Nikhil Edward for image processing. We wish to extend this acknowledgment to other photographers and ophthalmic technicians from all participating centers.

Contents

List of Contributors

Editors

Igor Kozak, MD, PhD Senior Academic Consultant, Vitreoretinal Division, King Khaled Eye Specialist Hospital, Riyadh, Saudi Arabia

J. Fernando Arevalo, MD, FACS Edmund F. and Virginia B. Ball Professor of Ophthalmology, Chairman, Department of Ophthalmology, Johns Hopkins Bayview Medical Center, Retina Division, Wilmer Eye Institute, The Johns Hopkins University School of Medicine, Baltimore, MD, USA

Associate Editor

Szilárd Kiss, MD Division Chief, Retina Service, Director of Clinical Research, Associate Professor of Ophthalmology, Weill Cornell Medical College, Associate Attending Physician, NewYork-Presbyterian Hospital, NY, USA

Steven D. Schwartz, MD Ahmanson Professor in Ophthalmology, Chief, Retina Division, Jules Stein Eye Institute, Department of Ophthalmology, David Geffen School of Medicine, UCLA, Los Angeles, CA, USA

Contributors

Alfredo Adán Ocular Inflammation Section, Clínic Institute of Ophthalmology(ICOF), Clínic Hospital of Barcelona, University of Barcelona, Barcelona, Spain

David S. Boyer, MD Retina-Vitreous Associated Medical Group, Los Angeles, CA, USA

R.V. Paul Chan, MD Department of Ophthalmology, Weill Cornell Medical College, New York, NY, USA

Thomas G. Chu, MD, PhD Retina-Vitreous Associated Medical Group, Los Angeles, CA, USA

Netan Choudhry, MD Vitreoretinal Surgery Division, Herzig Eye Institute Toronto, Toronto, ON, Canada

Peter Coombs, MD Department of Ophthalmology, Weill Cornell Medical College, New York, NY, USA

Michael J. DaSilva, MD Department of Ophthalmology and Visual Science, Stanley M. Truhlsen Eye Institute, University of Nebraska Medical Center, Omaha, NE, USA

Diana V. Do, MD Department of Ophthalmology and Visual Science, Stanley M. Truhlsen Eye Institute, University of Nebraska Medical Center, Omaha, NE, USA

Mrinali Patel Gupta, MD Department of Ophthalmology, Weill Cornell Medical College, New York–Presbyterian Hospital, New York, NY, USA

Keegan A. Harkins, MD Department of Ophthalmology and Visual Science, Stanley M. Truhlsen Eye Institute, University of Nebraska Medical Center, Omaha, NE, USA

Florian M. Heussen, MD St. Paul's Eye Unit, Royal Liverpool University Hospital, Liverpool, UK

Karyn E. Jonas, BSN, RN Department of Ophthalmology and Visual Sciences, Illinois Eye and Ear Infirmary, University of Illinois at Chicago, Chicago, IL, USA

Szilárd Kiss, MD Department of Ophthalmology, Weill Cornell Medical College, New York–Presbyterian Hospital, New York, NY, USA

Byung Ro Lee, MD, PhD Department of Ophthalmology, Hanyang University, Seoul, South Korea

Ella H. Leung, MD Department of Ophthalmology, Bascom Palmer Eye Institute, University of Miami, Miami, FL, USA

Victor Llorenç, MD, PhD Ocular Inflammation Section, Clínic Institute of Ophthalmology (ICOF), Clínic Hospital of Barcelona, University of Barcelona, Barcelona, Spain

Marina Mesquida, MD, PhD Ocular Inflammation Section, Clínic Institute of Ophthalmology(ICOF), Clínic Hospital of Barcelona, University of Barcelona, Barcelona, Spain

Quan Dong Nguyen, MD, MSc Department of Ophthalmology and Visual Science, Stanley M. Truhlsen Eye Institute, University of Nebraska Medical Center, Omaha, NE, USA

Anton Orlin, MD Department of Ophthalmology, Weill Cornell Medical College, New York, NY, USA

Pradeep S. Prasad, MD Retina Division, Jules Stein Eye Institute, University of California, Los Angeles, Los Angeles, CA, USA

Carmen A. Puliafito, MD, MBA Keck School of Medicine, University of Southern California, Los Angeles, CA, USA

Richard Rosen, MD Retinal Services, New York Eye and Ear Infirmary of Mount Sinai, New York, NY, USA

Irene Rusu, MD Department of Ophthalmology, Weill Cornell Medical College, New York–Presbyterian Hospital, New York, NY, USA

SriniVas R. Sadda Medical Retina Service, Doheny Eye Institute, Keck School of Medicine, University of Southern California, Los Angeles, CA, USA

David Sarraf, MD Ophthalmology Division, Jules Stein Eye Institute, David Geffen School of Medicine, University of California, Los Angeles, Los Angeles, CA, USA

Carol L. Shields, MD Ocular Oncology Service, Wills Eye Hospital, Philadelphia, PA, USA

Jerry A. Shields, MD Ocular Oncology Service, Wills Eye Hospital, Philadelphia, PA, USA

Irena Tsui, MD Retina Division, Department of Ophthalmology, Jules Stein Eye Institute, University of California, Los Angeles, Los Angeles, CA, USA

Yoshihiro Yonekawa, MD Vitreoretinal Fellow, Associated Retinal Consultants, Royal Oak, MI, USA

1 Fundus Imaging in Wide-Field: A Brief Historical Journey

Ella H. Leung and Richard Rosen

Our ability to visualize has often limited our ability to conceptualize, in medicine as well as technology, science, and mathematics. Before we were able to see the retina, our perspective of ocular disease was largely confined to disorders of the anterior segment, such as strabismus, corneal disease, conjunctivitis, and cataracts. Our understanding of blindness and amaurosis was hidden behind the seemingly impenetrable pupillary curtain.

In 1704, Jean Méry (Fig. 1) first described to the French Royal Academy of Sciences in Paris the retinal vessels in a living cat by immersing the animal in water [1]. In 1709, physicist Philippe de la Hire (Fig. 2) elucidated the optics of water's neutralization of the corneal curvature (Fig. 3) [1].

E.H. Leung, MD
Department of Ophthalmology, Bascom Palmer Eye Institute, University of Miami, Miami, FL, USA
e-mail: leungehs@gmail.com

R. Rosen, MD (✉)
Retinal Services, New York Eye and Ear Infirmary of Mount Sinai, New York, NY, USA
e-mail: RRosen@nyee.edu

I. Kozak, J.F. Arevalo (eds.), *Atlas of Wide-Field Retinal Angiography and Imaging*, DOI 10.1007/978-3-319-17864-6_1

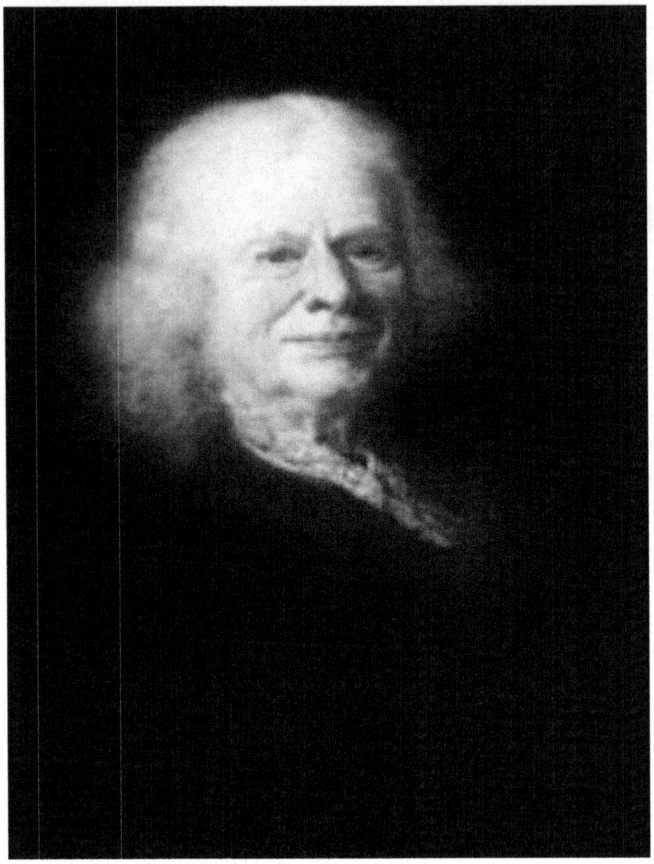

Fig. 1 Jean Méry (Reproduced from Heitz [1]; with permission)

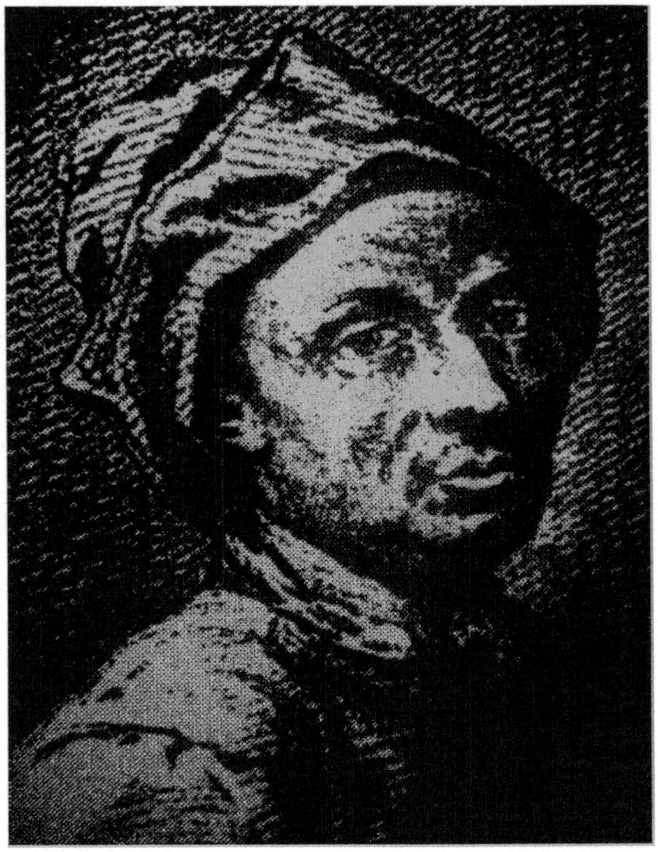

Fig. 2 Philippe de la Hire (Reproduced from Heitz [1]; with permission)

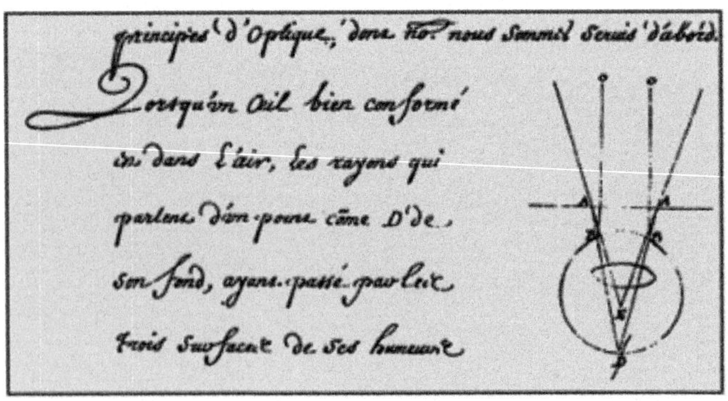

Fig. 3 The optics of water's neutralization of the corneal curvature (Reproduced from Heitz [1]; with permission)

However, it was Jan Evangista Purkinje (Fig. 4) who first described the principles of an ophthalmoscope in 1823 using the red reflex from a dog's eye (Figs. 5 and 6) [2, 3]. He had difficulty convincing clinicians to use the technique and his descriptions were lost for many years [2].

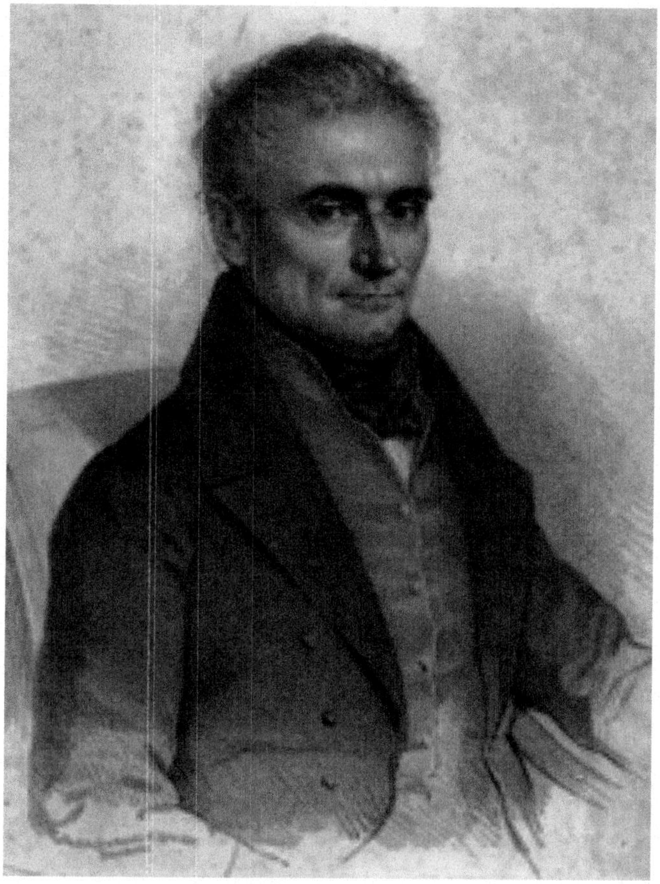

Fig. 4 Jan Evangiste Purkinje (Reproduced from Albert and Miller [2]; with permission)

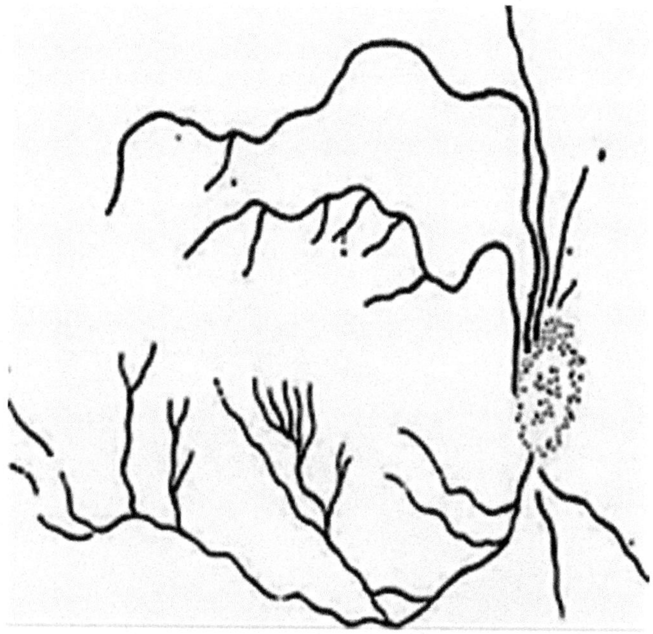

Fig. 5 Jan Evangiste Purkinje's drawing of the "tree of the eye" (Reproduced from Albert and Miller [2]; with permission)

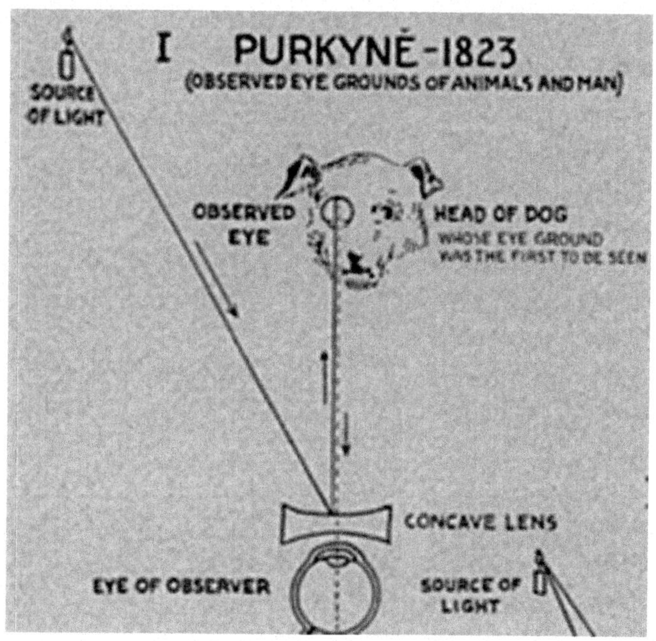

Fig. 6 Jan Evangiste Purkinje's optical description (Reproduced from Thau [3]; with permission)

Adolf Kussmaul, in 1845, recognizing the value of his predecessors' work, reproduced Méry's experiment and attempted to build his own ophthalmoscope but failed to produce a usable image [4]. In 1846, William Cumming used the light from a window to study the luminous internal reflecting membrane of the eye and made some intraocular diagnoses [5]. A year later, Charles Babbage (Fig. 7), the inventor of the computer, used a small silvered-glass to examine the retina (Fig. 8). Unfortunately, the ophthalmologist he consulted was unable to see a clear image and dismissed its potential value [6].

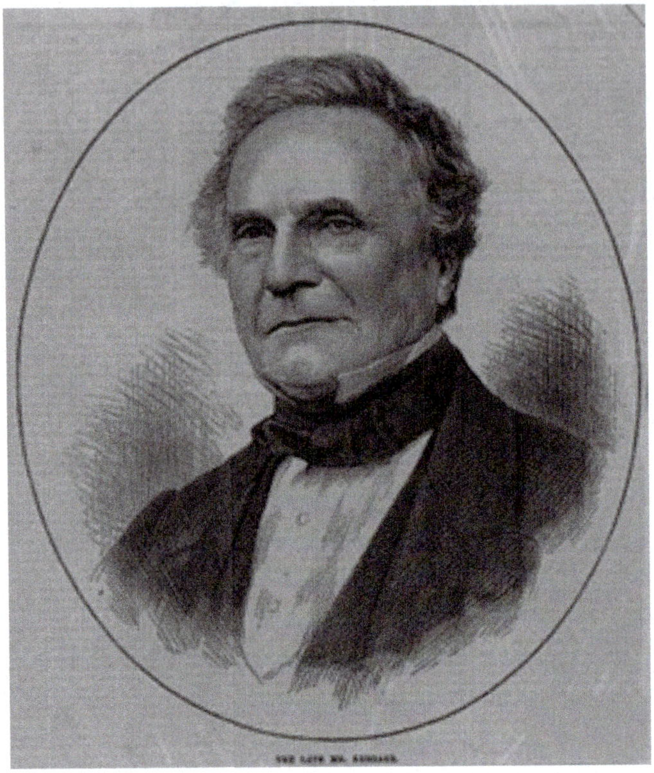

Fig. 7 Charles Babbage

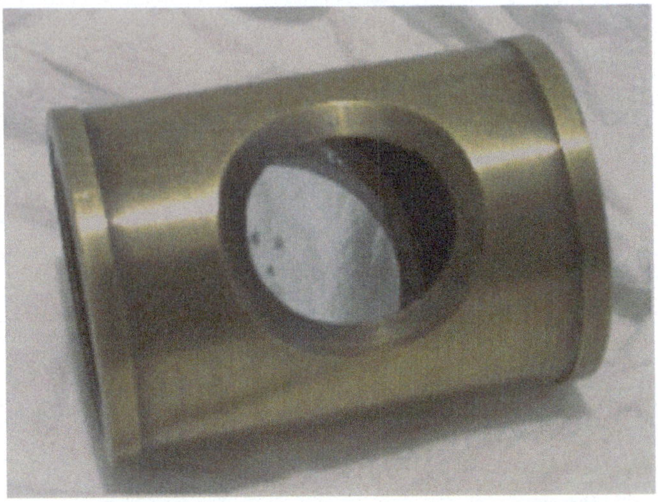

Fig. 8 Babbage's ophthalmoscope (Courtesy of The College of Optometrists, London)

It was Hermann von Helmholtz (Fig. 9) in 1951 who was thus credited with producing the first direct ophthalmoscope (Figs. 10 and 11) [7]. Semi-reflecting mirrors illuminated the patient's fundus, and the reflected parallel light rays were focused on to the retina of the observer. A flurry of fundus discoveries quickly followed, including the presence of retinal tears and detachments in 1853 by Coccius, drusen and pigmentary retinopathy in 1854 by Donders, venous occlusions in 1855 by Leibreich, diabetic retinopathy in 1856 by Jaeger, arterial occlusions in 1859 by von Graeffe, and macular degenerations in 1874 by Hutchinson [8].

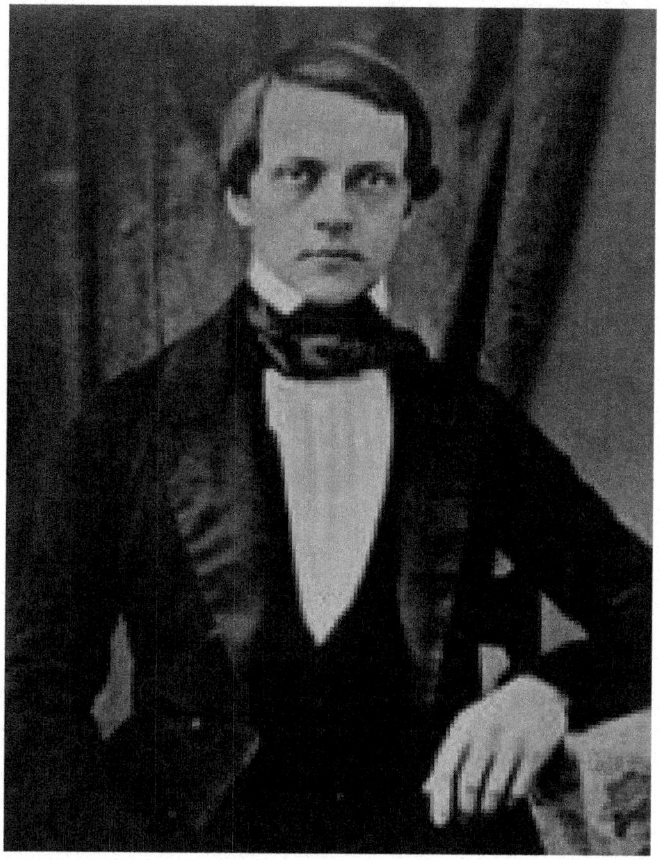

Fig. 9 Hermann von Helmholtz

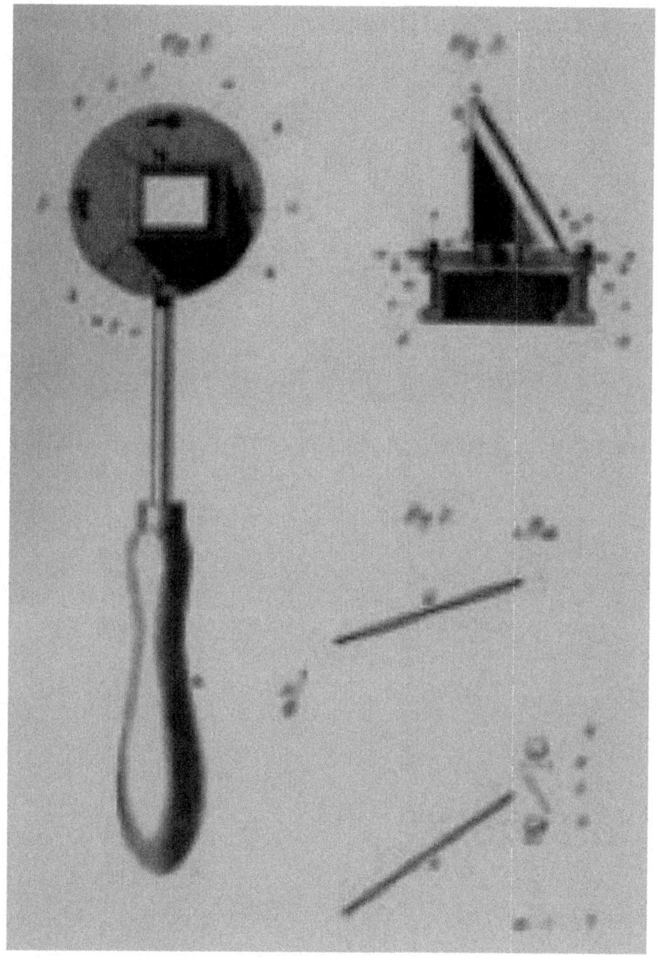

Fig. 10 Helmholtz's ophthalmoscope

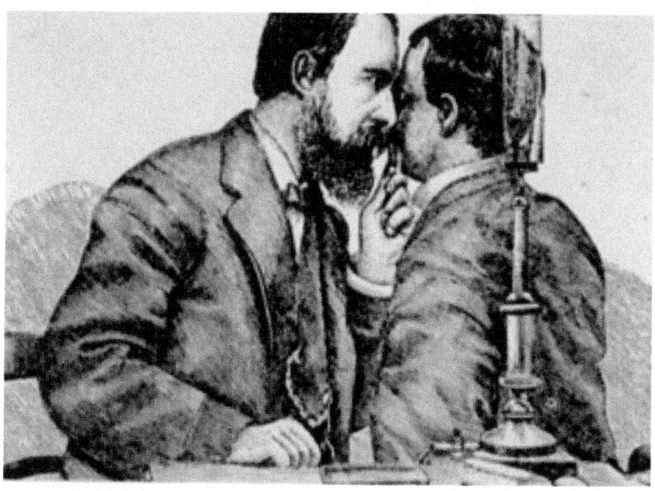

Fig. 11 Helmholtz's ophthalmoscope (Web archive historical)

Theodor Ruete introduced the indirect ophthalmoscope (Fig. 12) in 1852, which gave him a much wider field of view [9]. Nearly a century later, Charles Schepens (Fig. 13) in 1945 fastened the light source to a head band, leaving the user's hands free to hold a condensing lens and a scleral depressor, making complete evaluation of the peripheral retina possible [10]. Surgical outcomes from retinal detachment repairs rapidly improved as the techniques of the binocular indirect ophthalmoscopic exams and fundus drawings gained popularity [4, 11].

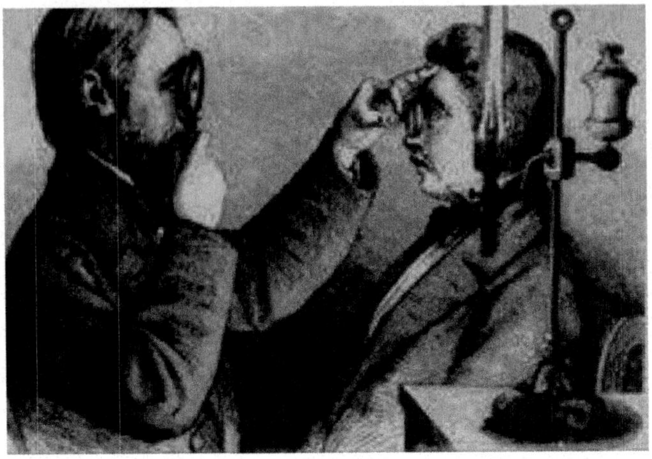

Fig. 12 Ruete indirect ophthalmoscope (Web archive historical)

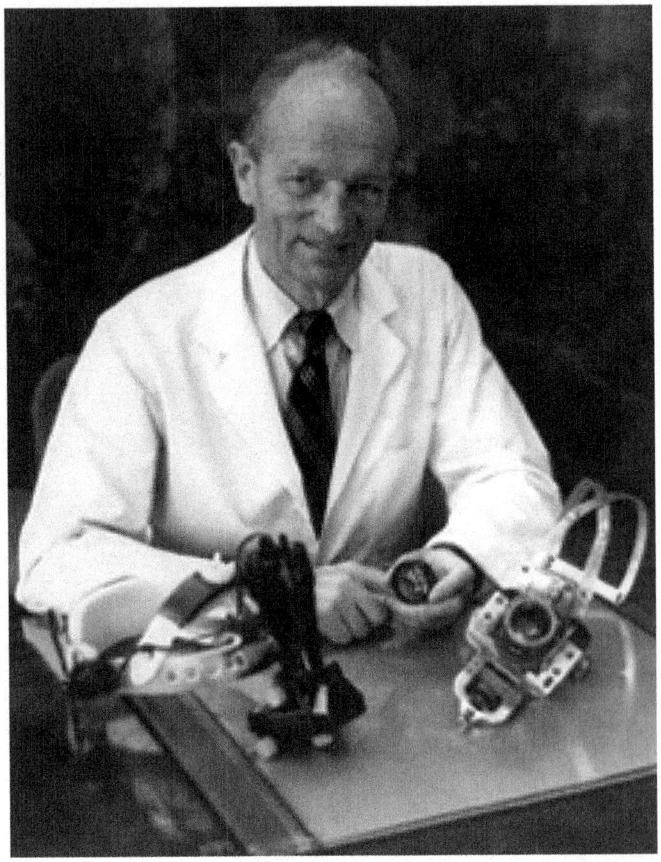

Fig. 13 Charles Scheppens with head-mounted binocular indirect ophthalmoscope (Courtesy of Schepens Eye Research Institute)

Photography was invented by Nicephore Niepce in 1823, and Louis Jacques Mande-Daguerre advanced the field with the introduction of the daguerreotype in 1839; however, the technology was still not sufficiently fast or portable enough to allow fundus photographs [12]. In 1851, Frederic Scott Archer improved the quality of images by coating glass plates with light-sensitive emulsions. While these plates had to be used wet, they were sensitive enough for Dr. Henry Noyes (Fig. 14) to photograph the first fundus of a living creature, a rabbit, in 1862. Later that year, Dr. Rosenbrugh obtained a retinal photograph of a cat. No pictorial records of these experiments remain, however, and it took another 20 years before Dr. Lucien Howe (Fig. 15) in 1885 produced the first photographic image of a human retina.

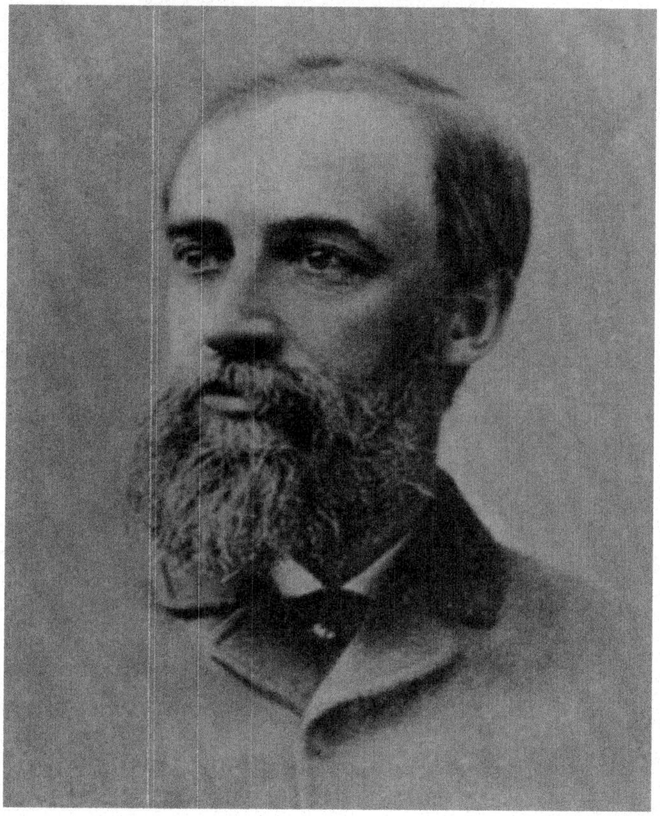

Fig. 14 Dr. Henry Noyes (From the American Ophthalmological Society; with permission)

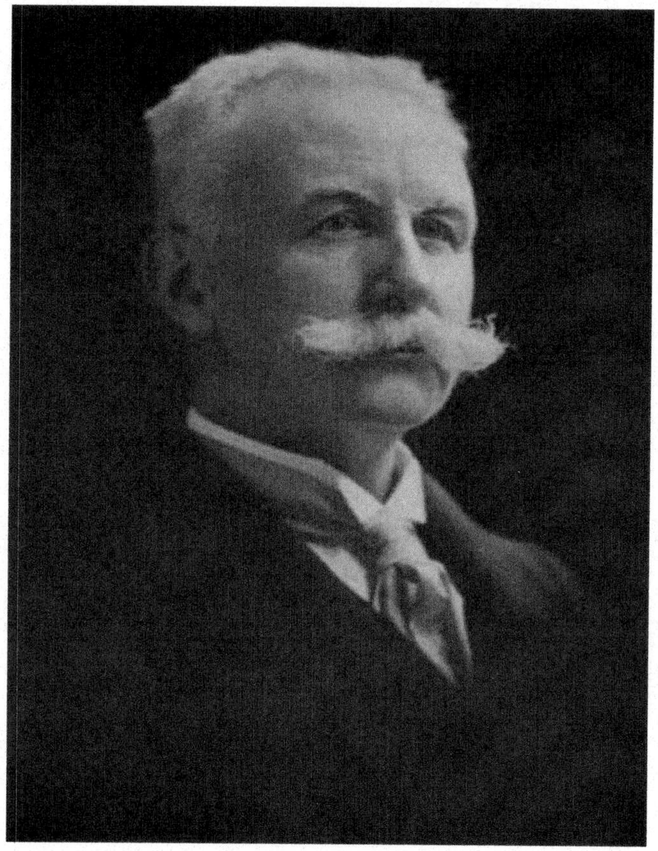

Fig. 15 Dr. Lucien Howe (Courtesy of the Museum of Vision and The American Academy of Ophthalmology)

Drs. Jackman and Webster were the first to publish an image in 1886 (Fig. 16). Although the 2.5-min exposure time and large central reflection artifact limited the detail that could be seen, the optic disc and some of the larger blood vessels could be appreciated (Fig. 17).

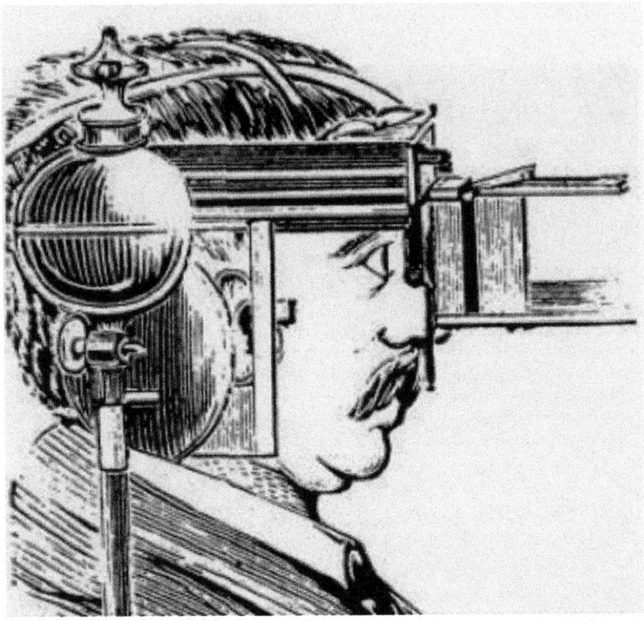

Fig. 16 Apparatus used to create the first published human fundus photograph. The light source was an albocarbon burner, and a 2.5-min exposure was required (Reproduced from Mark [13]; with permission)

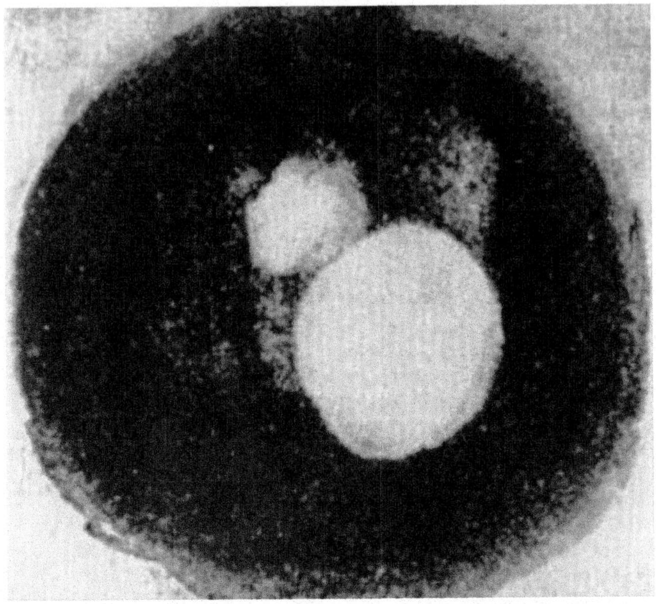

Fig. 17 First published fundus photo features a large light reflection artifact which all but obscures the blood vessels and optic nerve details (Reproduced from Mark [13]; with permission)

In 1891, Gerloff published a low-magnification retinal photograph (Fig. 18), which was much clearer than previous efforts [13, 14].

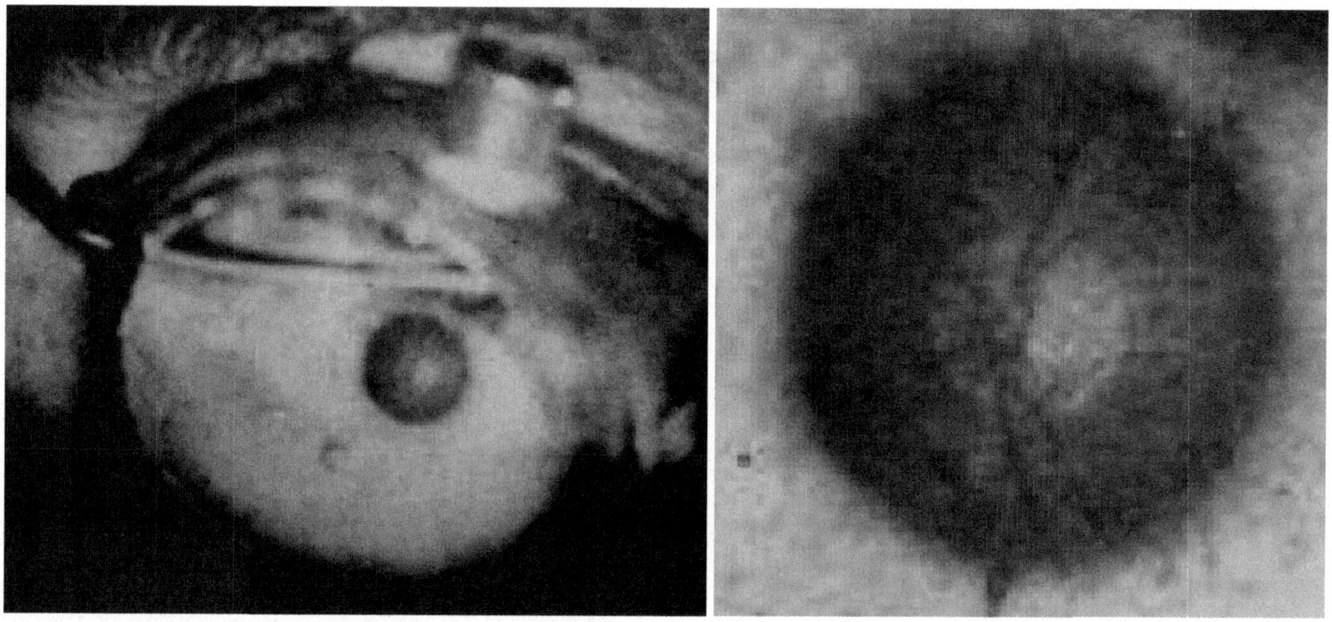

Fig. 18 Gerloff's fundus photograph (Reproduced from Gerloff [14]. Public domain)

Dr. Walter Thorner in 1899 developed an ophthalmoscope in conjunction with manufacturers F. Schmidt and Haensch in Berlin, which partially solved the reflex problem [15]. Thorner's ophthalmoscope later was attached to a camera, producing photographs with the artifact decentered inferiorly (Fig. 19).

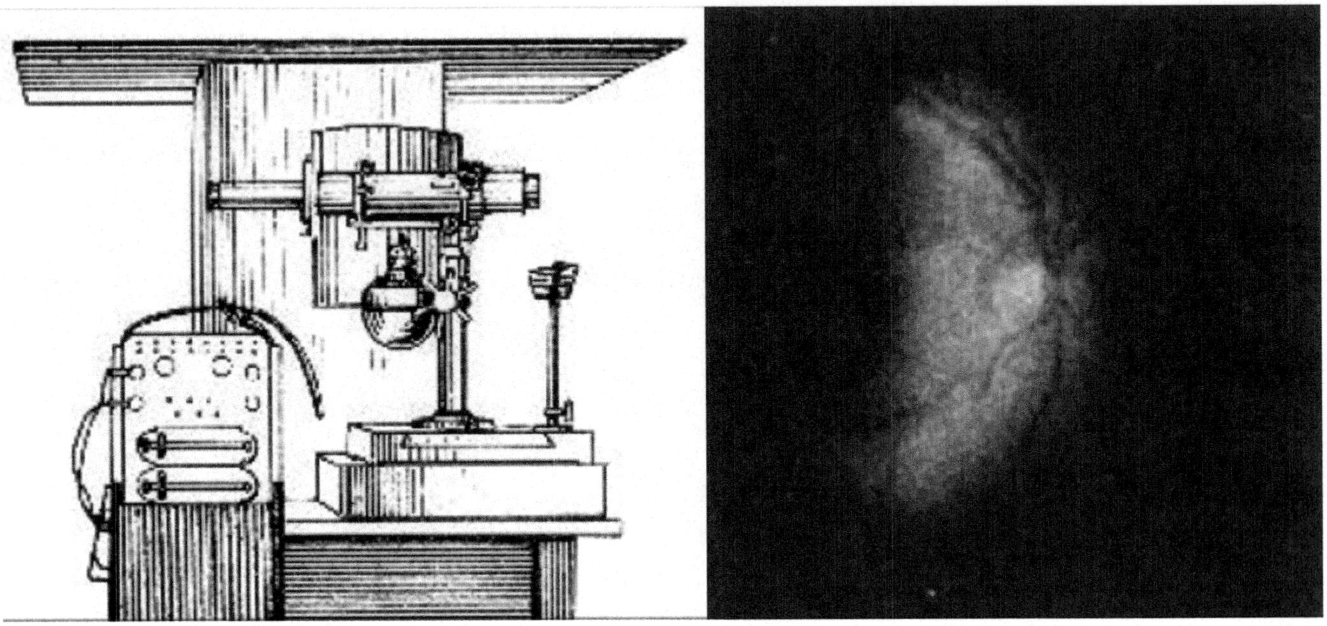

Fig. 19 Thorner's camera (*left*); Thorner's fundus images with good detail but uneven illumination (*right*) (Reproduced from Thorner [15]. Public domain)

In 1905, Dr. Dimmer collaborated with the Zeiss company in Jena to produce a large retinal camera that captured reflex-free photographs of the retina (Fig. 20 and 21) [16]. Dr. Dimmer's camera occupied an entire tabletop. Although only one such camera was ever produced, Dr. Dimmer's associate, Dr. Pillate, used it to create an atlas of the fundus in 1927, 2 years after Dr. Dimmer's death.

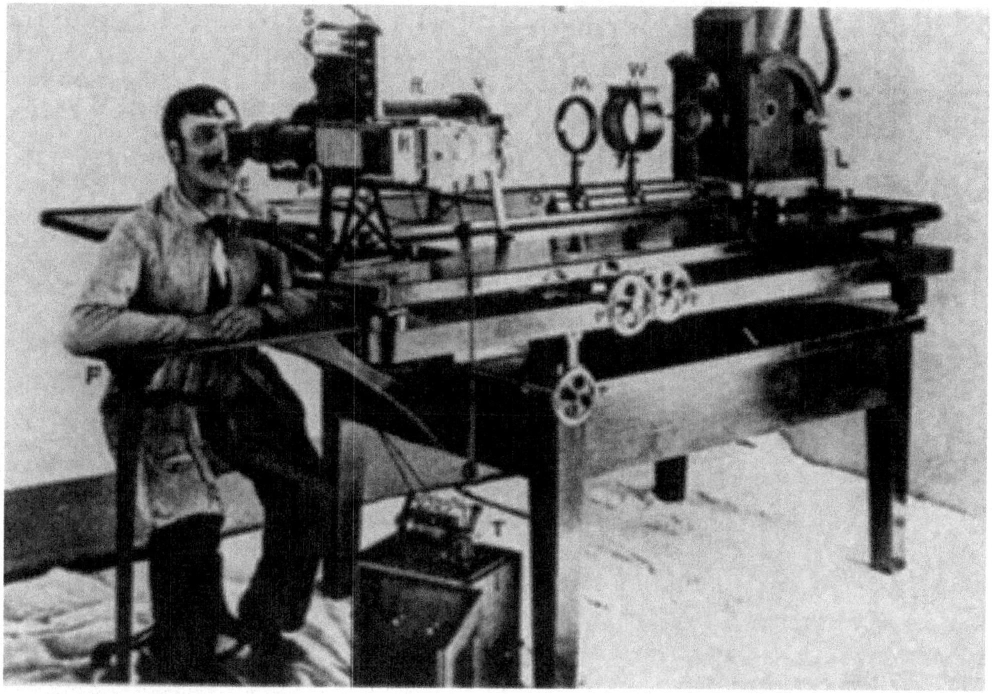

Fig. 20 Dimmer's camera (Reproduced from Dimmer [16]. Public domain)

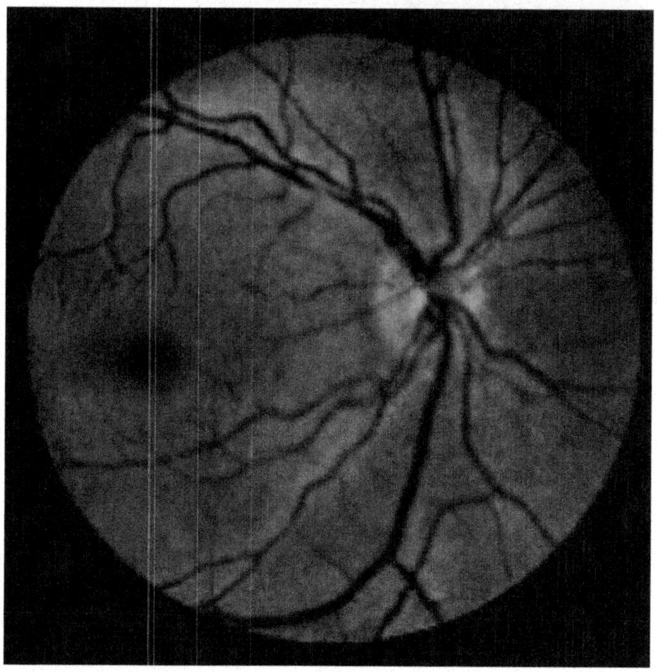

Fig. 21 Dimmer's fundus image (Reproduced from Dimmer [16]. Public domain)

In 1925, Dr. J. W. Nordenson in Stockholm working with the Zeiss Company used the Gullstrand principle of illumination to produce the Zeiss-Nordenson fundus camera [17]. It was widely used for many years with various light sources until 1953 when Hansell and Beeson added the first electronic flash (Figs. 22, 23, and 24) [18].

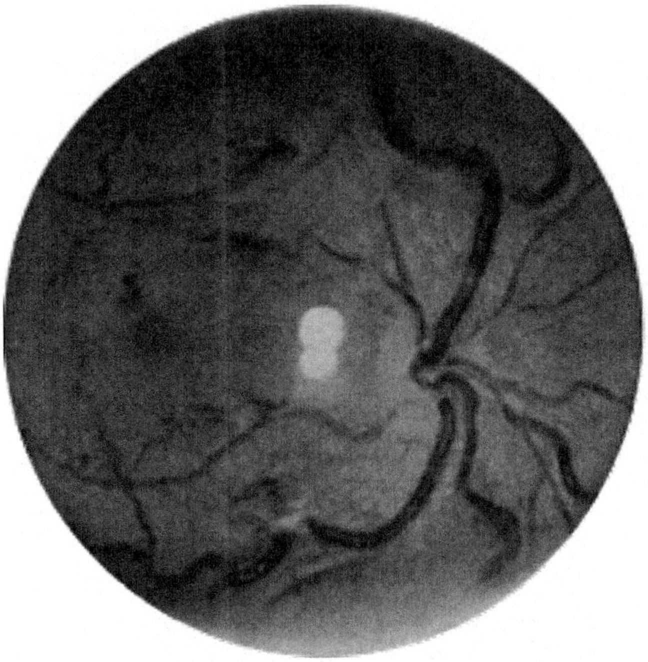

Fig. 22 Zeiss-Nordenson fundus camera image (Web archive historical)

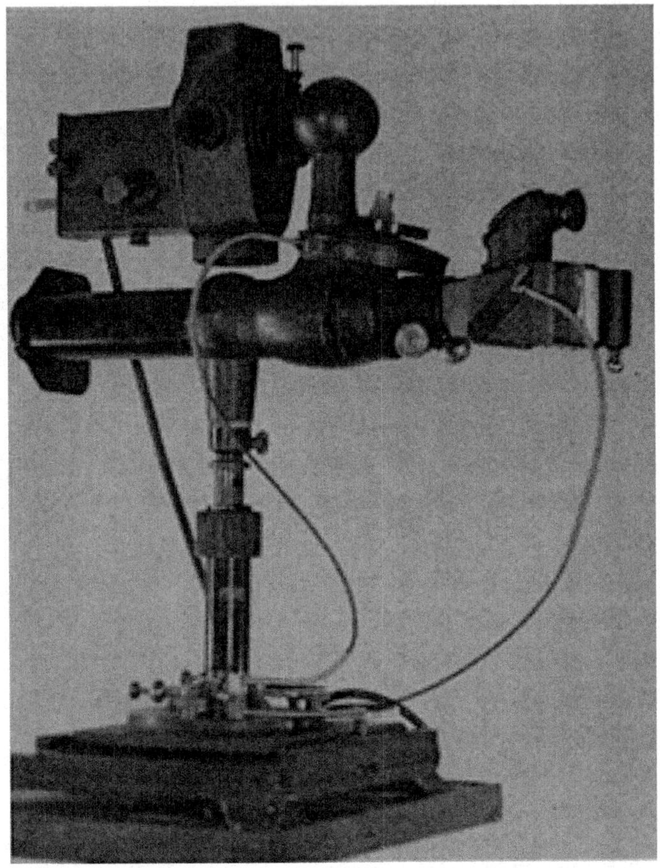

Fig. 23 Zeiss-Nordenson fundus camera (Reproduced from Saine [13]; with permission)

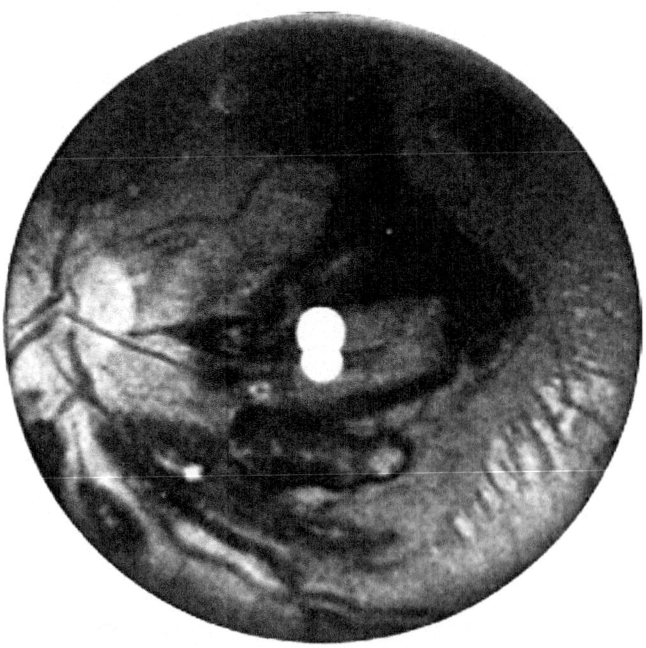

Fig. 24 Zeiss-Nordenson fundus camera image (Web archive historical)

Introduced in 1955 by Hans Littman (Fig. 25) at Zeiss, the modern fundus camera (Fig. 26) offered for the first time exact measurement on an object on the retina through the use a telecentric beam path (Fig. 27).

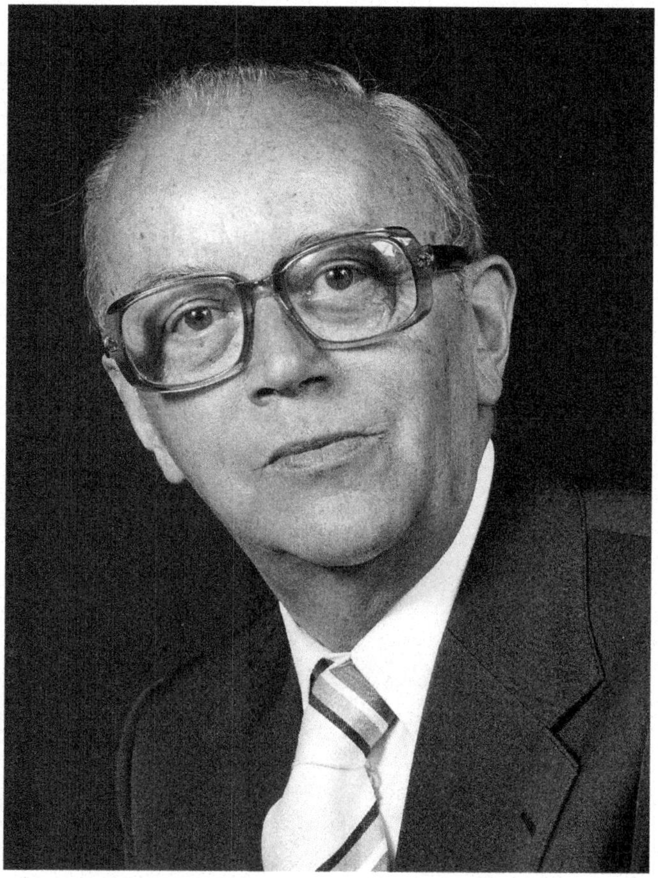

Fig. 25 Hans Littman (Courtesy of Carl Zeiss Archives)

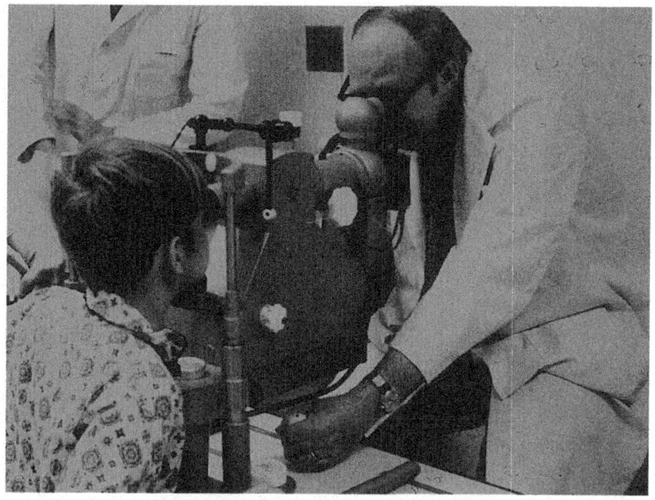

Fig. 26 Modern Zeiss fundus camera (Courtesy of New York Eye and Ear Infirmary Retina Service)

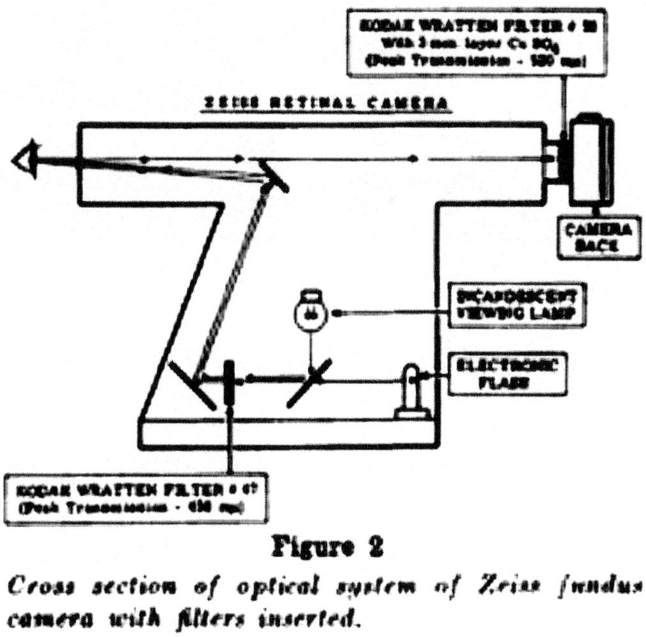

Fig. 27 Modern fundus camera optics (Web archive historical)

The addition of fluorescein angiography in 1961 brought another dimension to retinal imaging and increased the need to image the peripheral retina. Experiments in oral and intravenous dyes were performed as early as 1881, with the first fluorescein angiograms of the retinal vasculature being performed in 1958 by Milton Flocks and Peter Chao. Three years later, Harold Novotny (Fig. 28) and David Alvis (Fig. 29) improved the illumination and light filters and are credited with being the inventors of modern fluorescein angiography (Fig. 30) [17, 19].

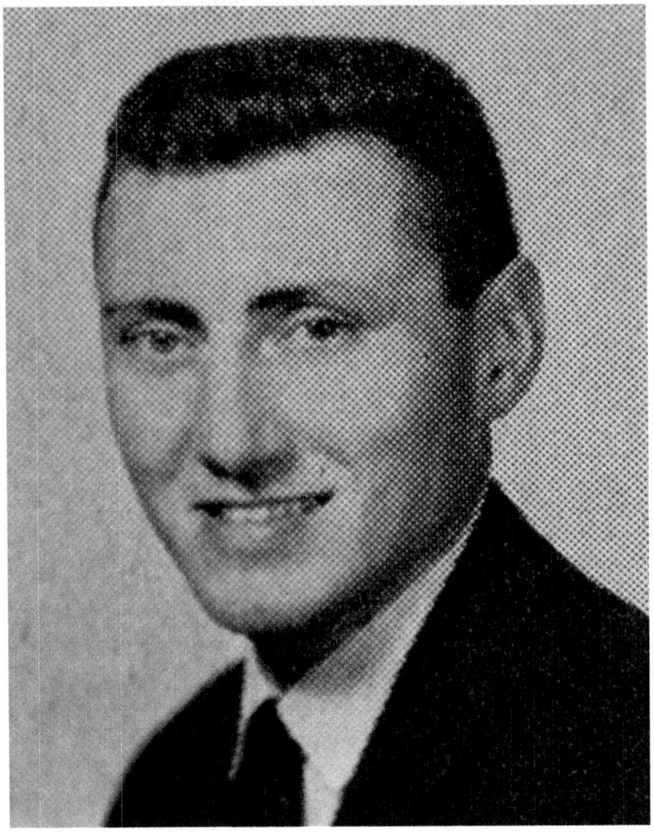

Fig. 28 Harold Novotny (Web archive historical)

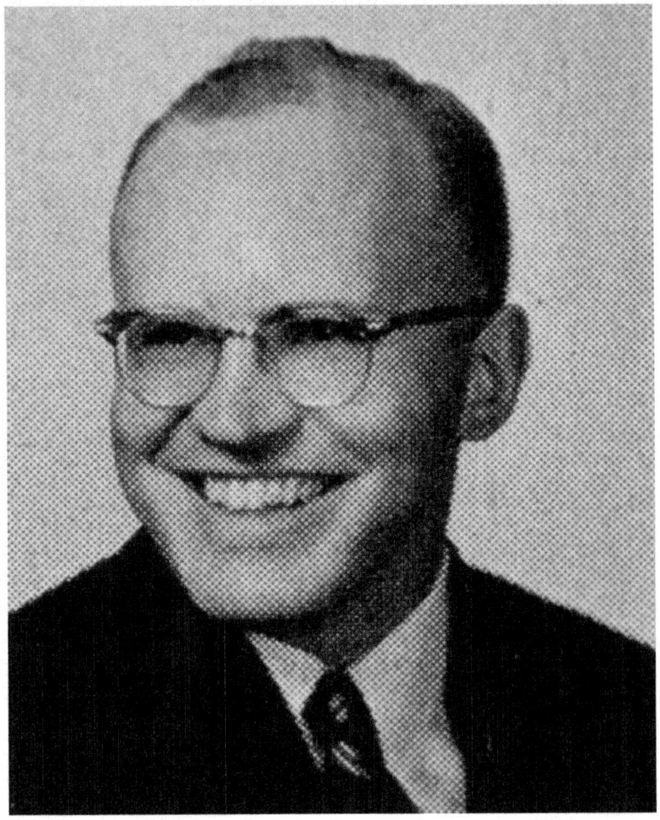

Fig. 29 David Alvis (Web archive historical) [19]

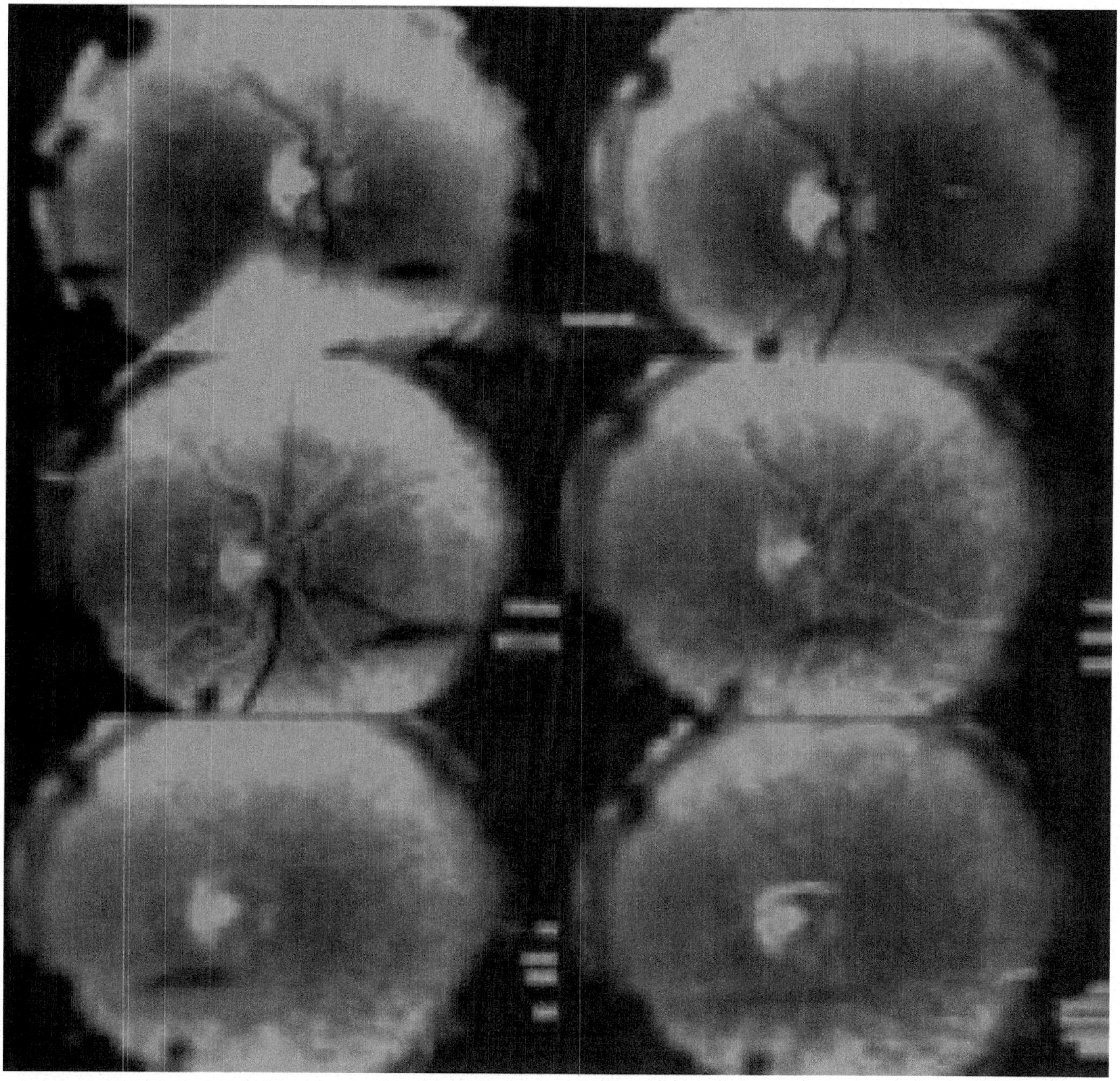

Fig. 30 First published fluorescein angiogram (Reproduced from Novotny [19]; with permission)

In 1977, Oleg Pomerantzeff (Fig. 31) created the first camera to image beyond the equator (Fig. 32), capturing up to 148° of the retina (Figs. 33 and 34) [20]. It featured a spring-loaded contact lens and transscleral illumination.

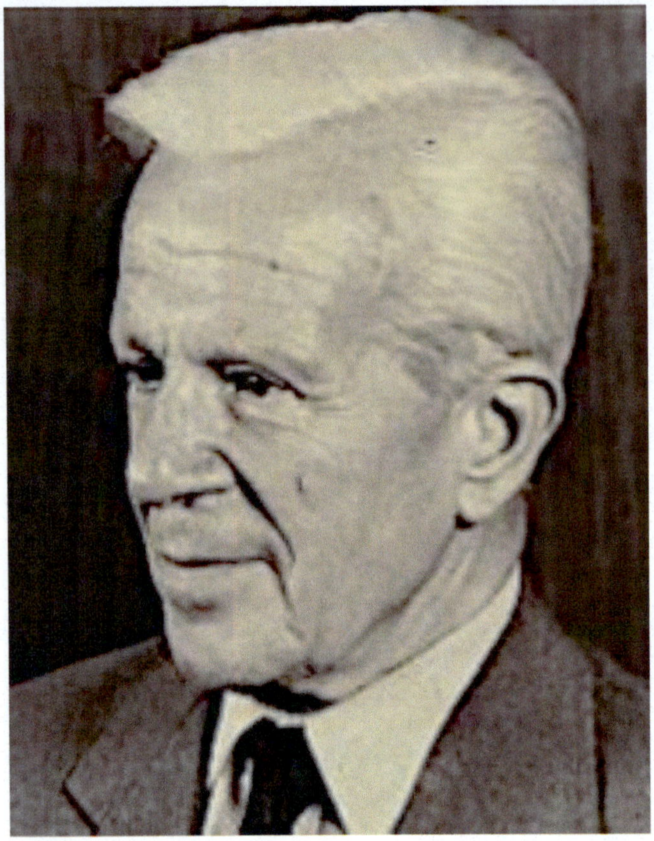

Fig. 31 Oleg Pomeranzeff (Courtesy of Schepens Eye Research Institute)

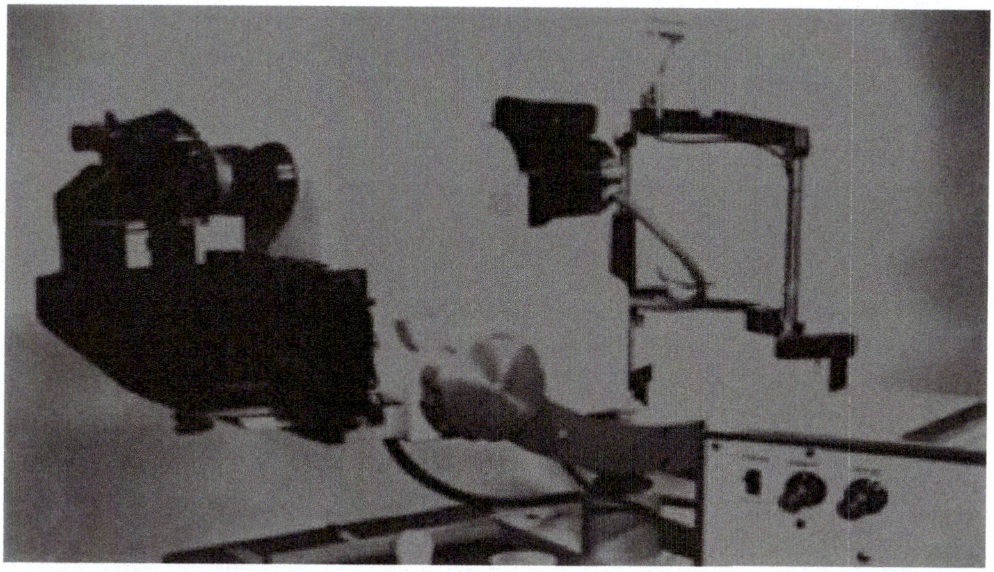

Fig. 32 Pomerantzeff's equator plus camera (Reproduced from Pomerantzeff [20]; with permission from the Association for Research in Vision and Ophthalmology)

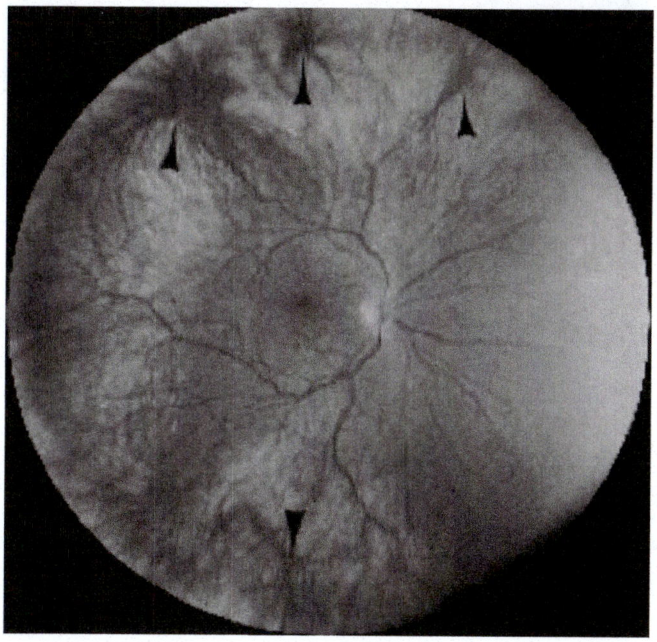

Fig. 33 Equator plus red-free image (Reproduced from Pomerantzeff [20]; with permission)

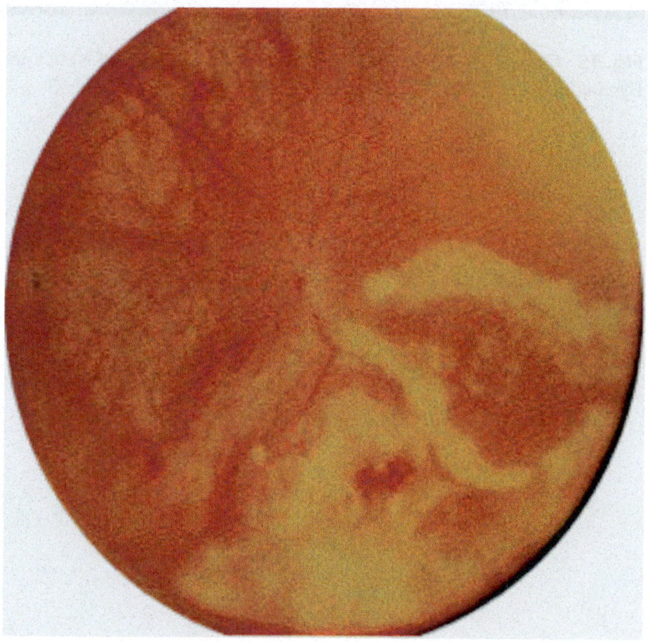

Fig. 34 Equator plus wide-field color fundus (Reproduced from Pomerantzeff [20]; with permission)

The most popular method to record the peripheral retina for some time was the montage of multiple overlapping images, such as the 75° views assembled for the Early Treatment Diabetic Retinopathy Study seven Standard Fields (Figs. 35 and 36) [21].

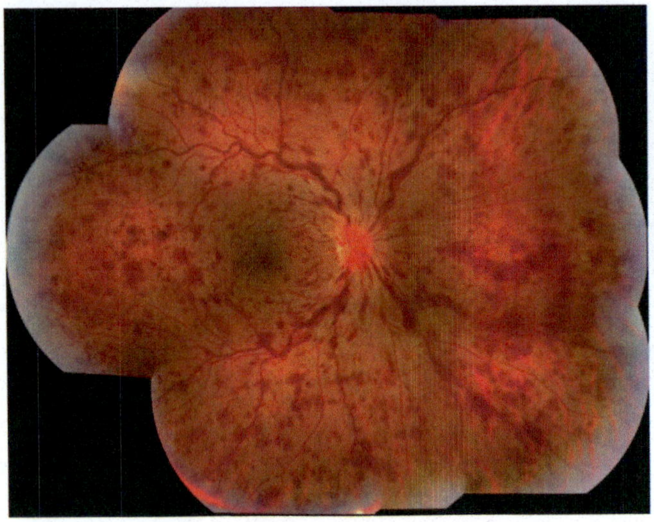

Fig. 35 Central retinal vein occlusion montage (Courtesy of New York Eye and Ear Infirmary Retina Service)

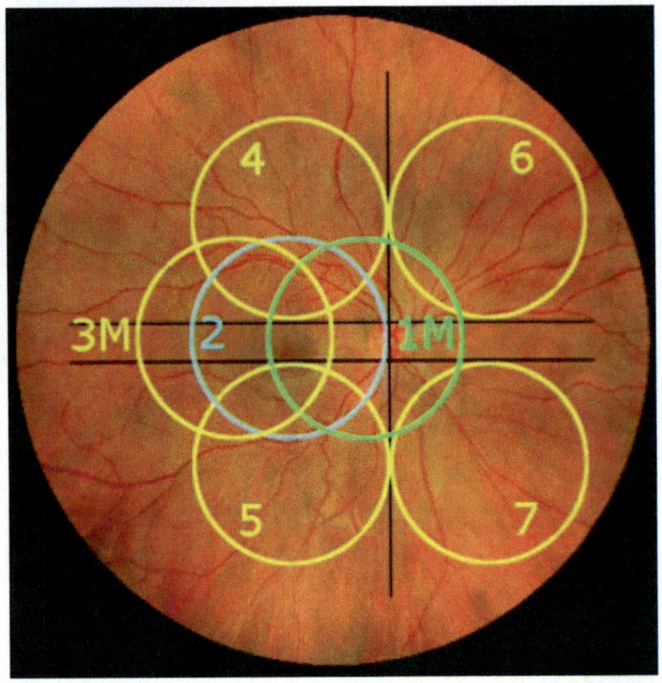

Fig. 36 ETDRS seven standard fields (Optos Brochure; Courtesy of Szilard Kiss)

In 1997, Bert Massie introduced the Retcam (Fig. 37), a portable wide-field imaging system employing a fiberoptic cable light source, interchangeable contact lenses, and the ability to capture up to 130°. It quickly gained popularity for imaging pediatric retinal disease and peripheral tumors, such as retinopathy of prematurity and retinoblastoma (Fig. 38). The main limitation of the device is its optical method of illumination, which demands a clear media, making it difficult to image adults with cataracts (Figs. 39, 40, and 41).

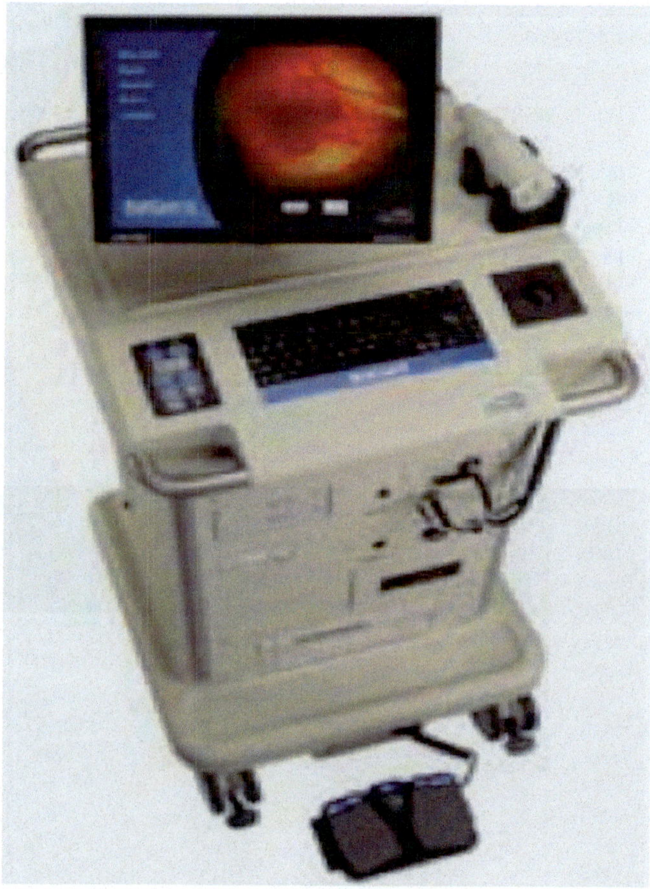

Fig. 37 RetCam II (Courtesy of Bert Massey)

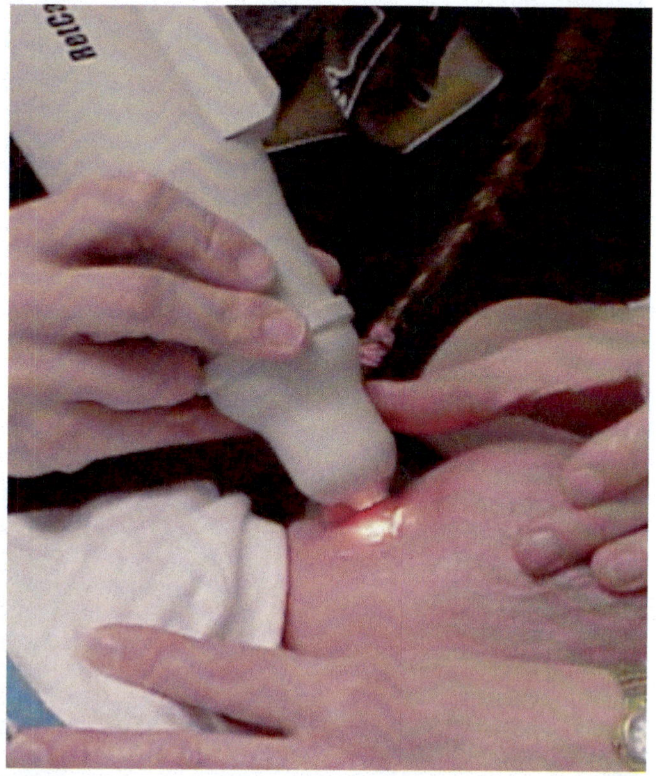

Fig. 38 Infant examination with the RetCam II (Courtesy of Bert Massey)

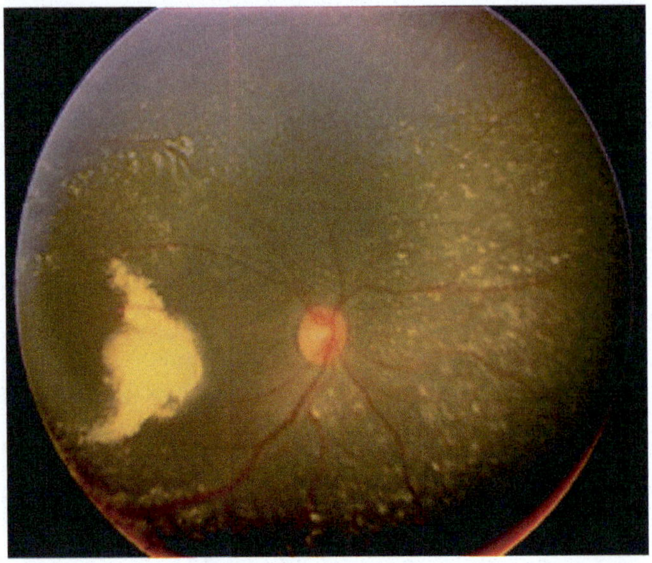

Fig. 39 Coats' disease (color fundus) showing exudate (Courtesy of New York Eye and Ear Infirmary Retina Service)

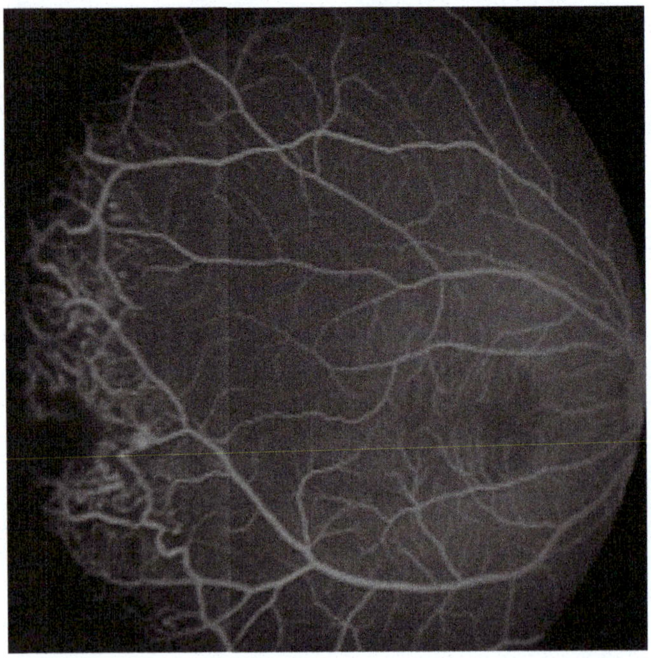

Fig. 40 Early fluorescein image showing nonperfusion (Courtesy of New York Eye and Ear Infirmary Retina Service)

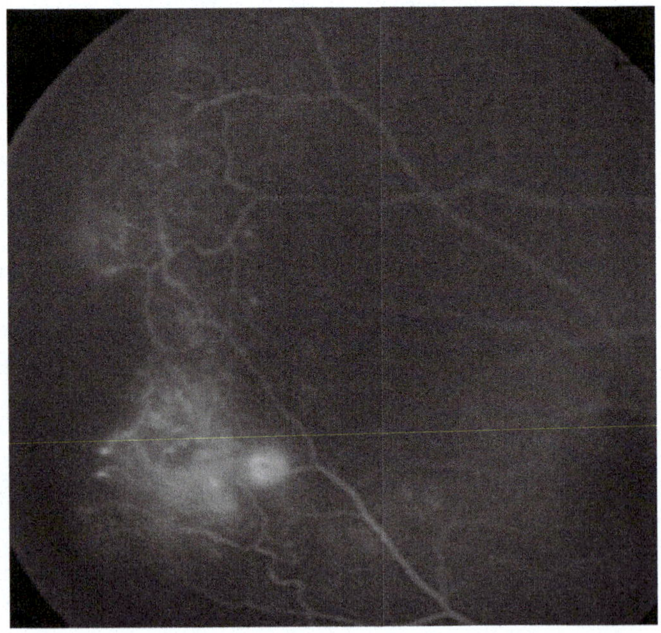

Fig. 41 Late fluorescein image showing leakage (Courtesy of New York Eye and Ear Infirmary Retina Service)

In 2003, Medibell introduced the Panoret-1000, which did not require pupillary dilation, could image up to 100° of the fundus, and was suitable for imaging adults [22]. Although its pictures had excellent quality, it was unwieldy and required two operators. Its high-resolution grayscale camera with a rotating color filter wheel produced high-resolution images, but its reliance on transscleral Illumination limited its ability to image darkly pigmented fundus (Figs. 42, 43, and 44).

In 1992, Douglas Anderson developed the Optos camera after his then 5-year-old son went blind in one eye when a retinal detachment was detected too late [21]. It uses an ellipsoidal mirror with one focal point located vir-

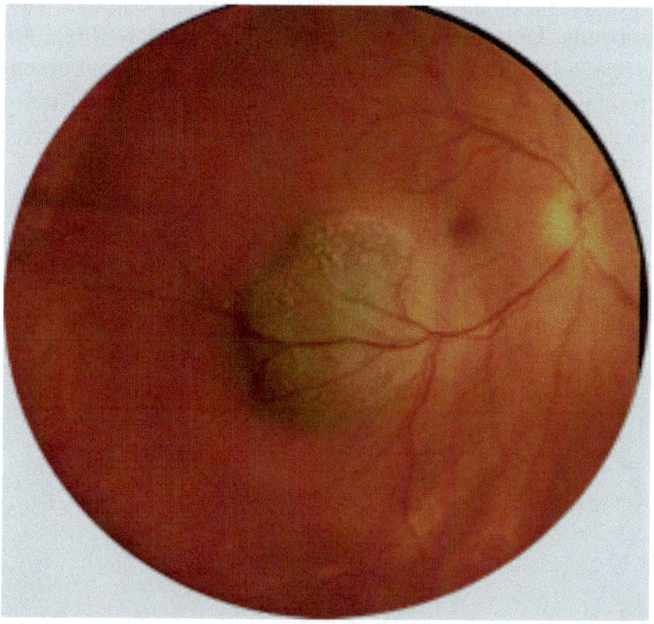

Fig. 42 Medibell transscleral illuminated image (Courtesy of New York Eye and Ear Infirmary Retina Service)

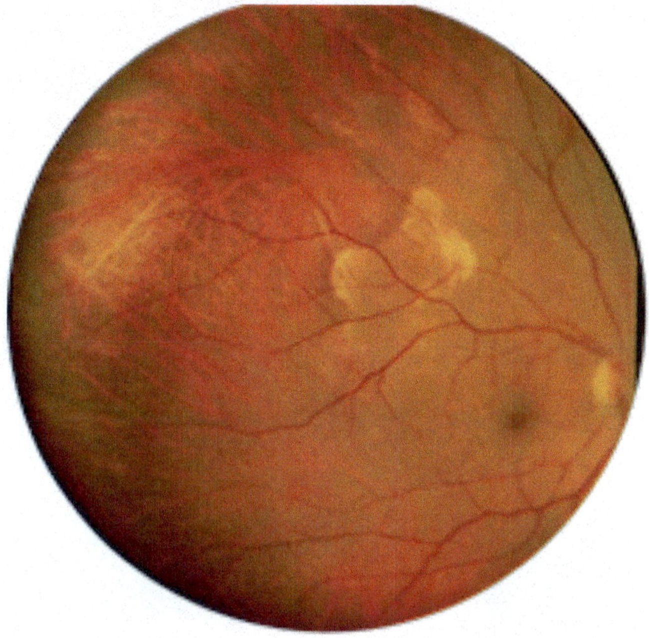

Fig. 43 Medibell imaging arrangement (Courtesy of New York Eye and Ear Infirmary Retina Service)

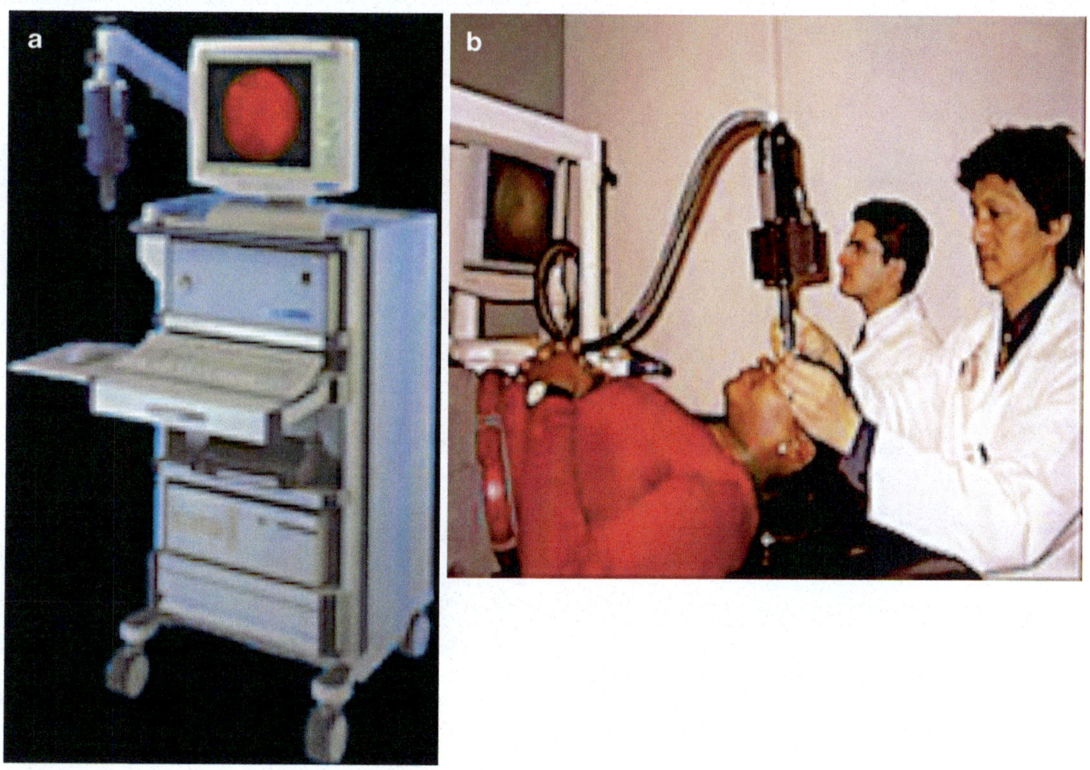

Fig. 44 (**a**) Optos 200 wide-field fundus Imager (Courtesy of New York Eye and Ear Infirmary Retina Service); (**b**) Medibell wide-field fundus camera (Courtesy of New York Eye and Ear Infirmary Retina Service)

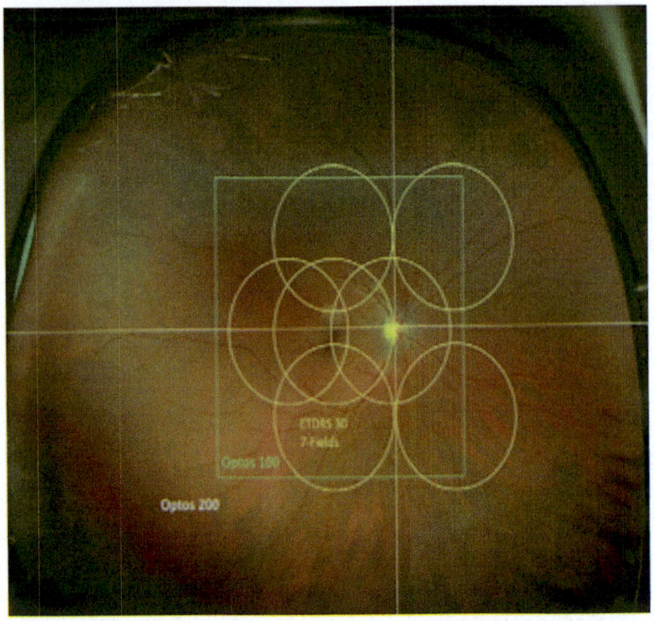

Fig. 45 Optos 200 wide-field imager (Optos brochure; Courtesy of Szilard Kiss)

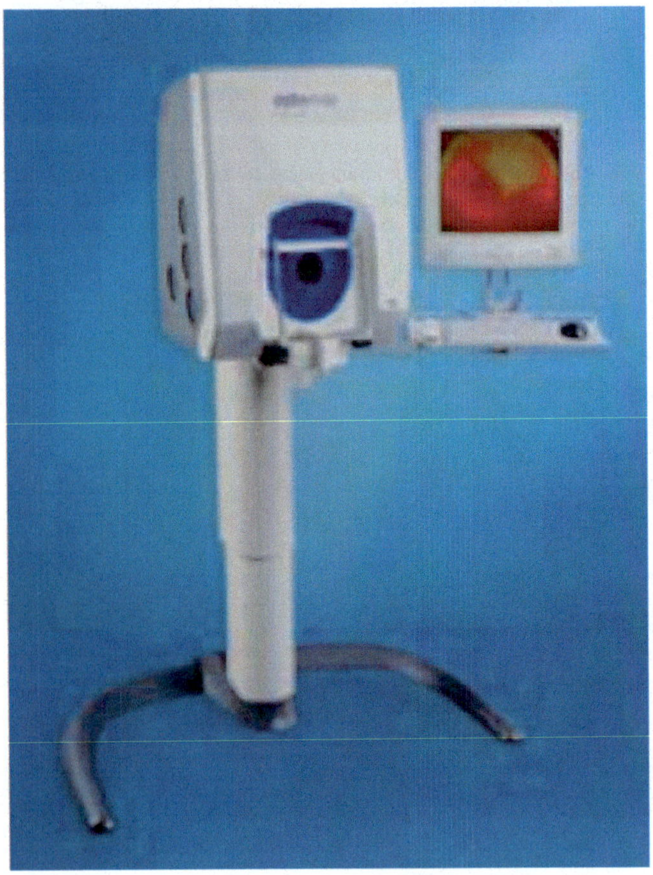

Fig. 46 Optos 200 wide-field imager (Optos brochure; Courtesy of Szilard Kiss)

tually behind the iris plane to capture up to 200° of the internal viewing angle of the retina. The addition of the ultra wide-field fluorescein angiography (UWFA) option expanded the clinician's ability to detect peripheral capillary nonperfusion, growth of masses, and pediatric diseases. An indocyanine green (ICG) mode was also recently introduced [23]. Limitations of the Optos, however, include laser speckling, abnormal colors, peripheral distortions, lack of stereopsis, and eyelid artifacts (Figs. 45, 46, 47, 48, and 49) most color images are the actual green-red laser while others (e.g. page 113) have the 'false' color overlay provided by the software in the Optos device.

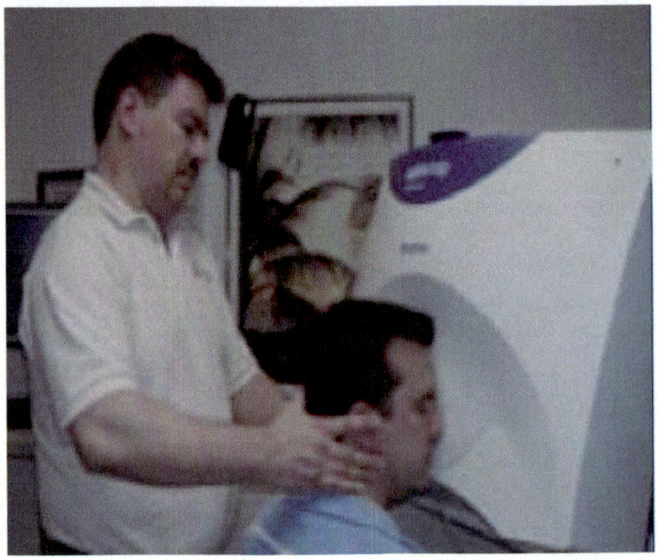

Fig. 47 Optos patient interface (Optos brochure; Courtesy of Szilard Kiss)

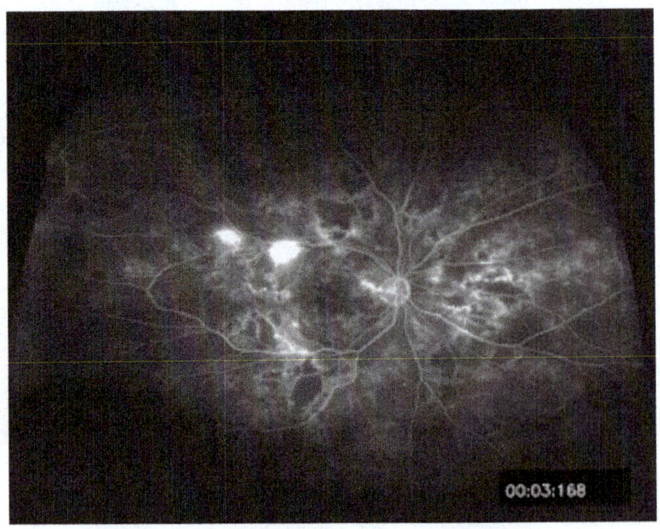

Fig. 48 Optos wide-field fluorescein (Courtesy of Szilard Kiss)

In 2005, Giovan ni Staurenghi introduced the handheld Staurenghi 230 SLO Retina Lens [24], which uses a contact lens for expanding the view of a confocal scanning laser ophthalmoscope to 150° of the retina for both color fundus photography and fluorescein angiography (Figs. 50, 51, and 52)

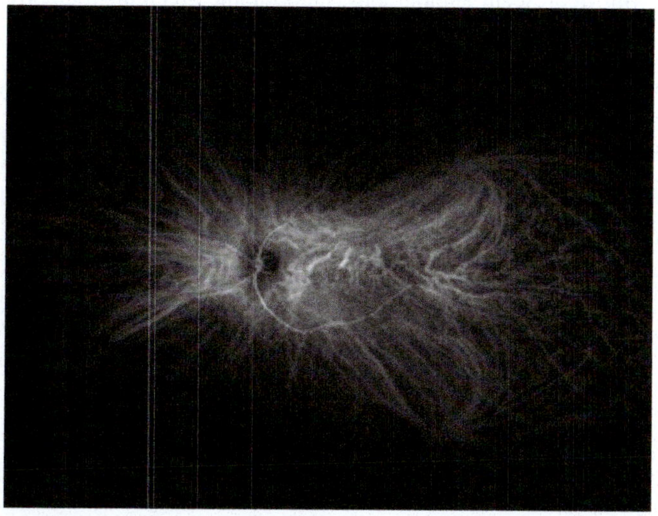

Fig. 49 Optos wide-field ICGA and not a fluorescein as labeled

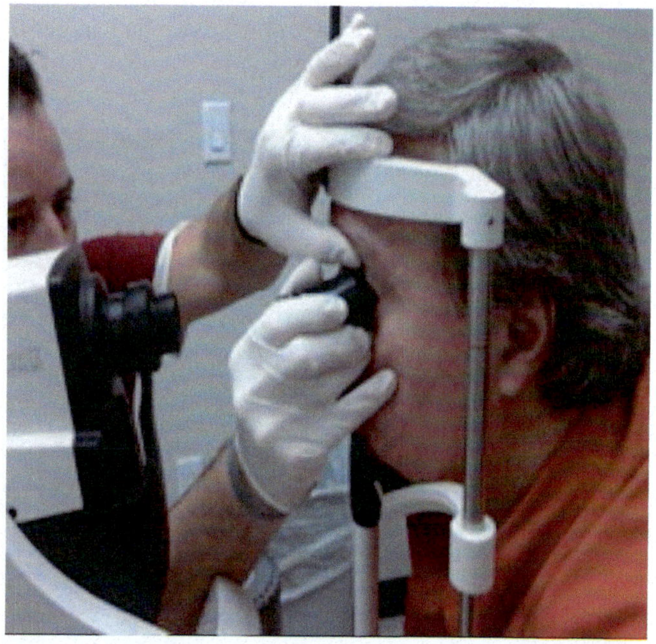

Fig. 51 Staurenghi lens placement (Courtesy of Eric Kegley)

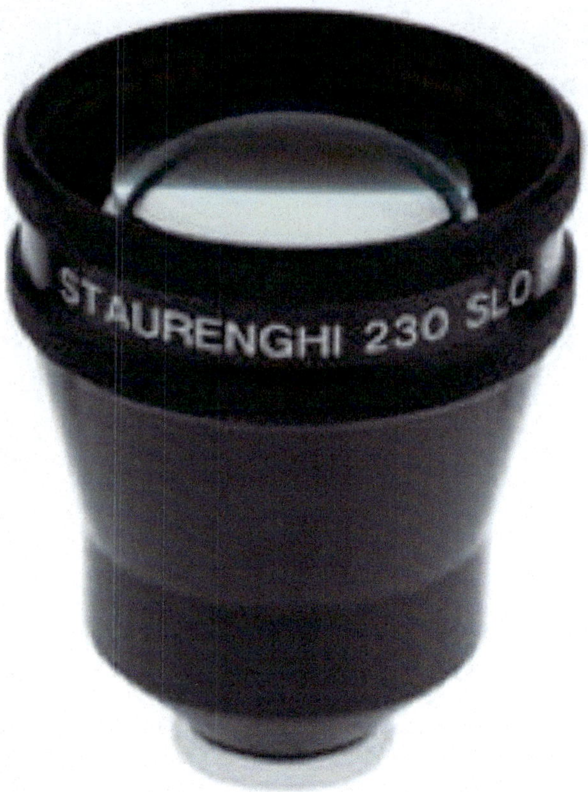

Fig. 50 Staurenghi wide-field lens (Courtesy of Eric Kegley)

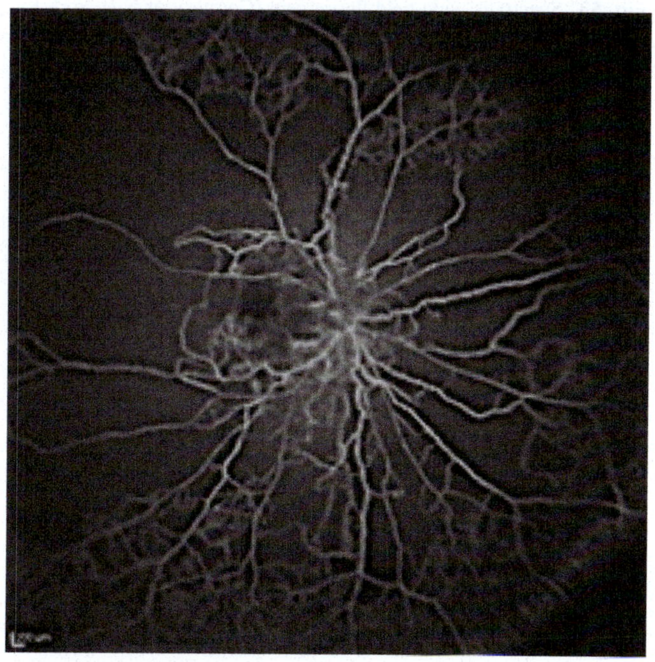

Fig. 52 Staurenghi lens view of ischemic fundus (Courtesy of Eric Kegley)

Spectalis introduced its wide-field imaging solution most recently using a noncontact version of the Staurenghi lens incorporated into their Spectralis HRA. Although its field of view is only about 100°, instructing the patient to look in extreme fields of gaze provides extended viewing of the periphery while taking advantage of the dynamic features of Spectralis system (Figs. 53 and 54).

The field of ocular photography continues to expand. The ultimate goal will be to image the entire retina, from ora to ora. Future photography platforms will likely be multifunctional, capable of combining ocular coherence tomography (OCT) with fluorescein angiography, indocyanine green angiography, adaptive optics, and perhaps laser photocoagulation to allow for a more comprehensive evaluation and treatment of the eye [25].

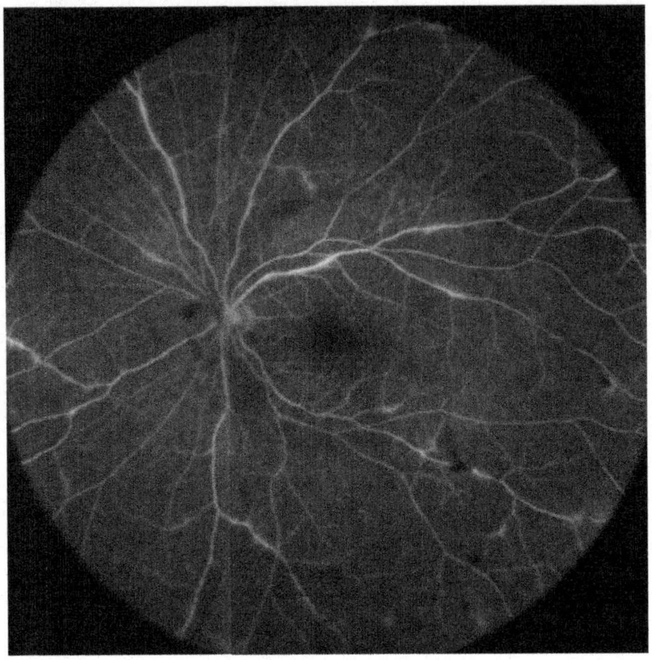

Fig. 53 Spectralis wide-field fluorescein (Courtesy of New York Eye and Ear Infirmary Retina Service)

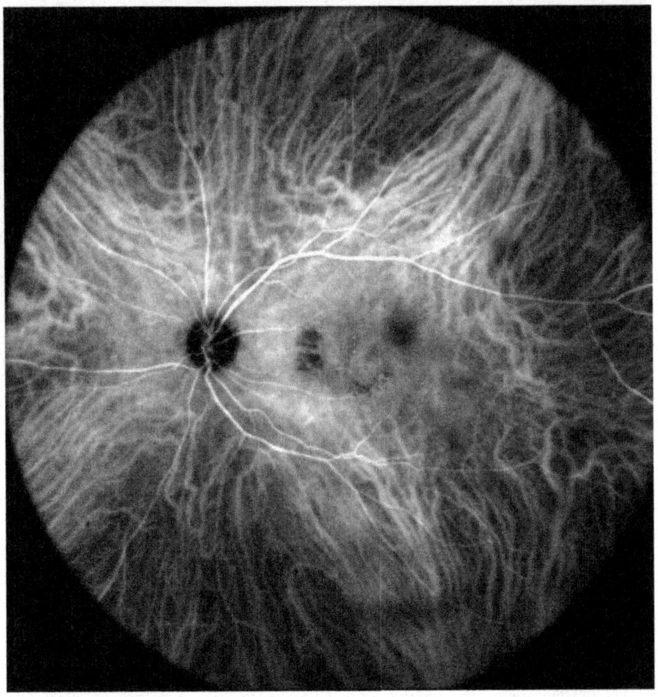

Fig. 54 Spectralis wide-field ICG (Courtesy of New York Eye and Ear Infirmary Retina Service)

References

1. Heitz RF. The earliest visualizations of the living eye's fundus by immersion in water. Archiwum Historii I Filozofii Medycyny. 2012;75:11–5.
2. Albert DM, Miller WH. Jan Purkinje and the ophthalmoscope. Am J Ophhalmol. 1973;76:494–9.
3. Thau W. Purkyně: a pioneer in ophthalmoscopy. Arch Ophthalmol. 1942;27:299–316.
4. Mark HH. The first ophthalmoscope. Arch Ophthalmol. 1970;84: 520–1.
5. Cumming W. On a luminous appearance of the human eye, and its application to the detection of disease of the retina and posterior part of the eye. Med Chir Trans. 1846;29:283–96.
6. Lyons HG. Charles Babbage and the ophthalmoscope. Rec R Soc London. 1940;3:146–8. doi:10.1098/rsnr.1940.0019.
7. Mark HH. On the evolution of binocular ophthalmoscopy. Arch Ophthalmol. 2007;125:830–3.
8. Miller D. Ophthalmic technology for the clinician: direct ophthalmoscopy revisited. Ann Ophthalmol. 1982;14:1107–10.
9. Jacklin HN. 125 years of indirect ophthalmoscopy. Ann Ophthalmol. 1979;11:643–6, 649–50.
10. Snead MP, Rubinstein MP, Jacobs PM. The optics of fundus examination. Surv Ophthalmol. 1992;36:439–45.
11. Colenbrander A. Principles of ophthalmoscopy. Duane's Ophthalmology, Lippencott Williams Wilkens, Philadelphia 2006; 1.
12. Van Cader TC. History of ophthalmic photography. J Ophthalmic Photogr. 1978;1:7–9.
13. Saine PJ. Landmarks in the historical development of fluorescein angiography. J Ophthalmic Photogr. 1993;15:17–23.
14. Gerloff O. Ueber die fotografie des augenhintergrundes. Klin Monat Augenheil. 1891;29:397.
15. Thorner W. A new stationary ophthalmoscope without reflexes. Am J Ophtholmol. 1899;16:376–91.
16. Dimmer F. Ueber Die Photographic Des Augenhintergrundes. Wiesbaden: Bergmann; 1907. p. 1.
17. Rosen E. Fundus cameras. Trans Ophthalmol Soc U K. 1981; 101:146–8.
18. Hansell P, Beeson EJG. Retinal photography in colour. Br J Ophtholmol. 1953;37:65–9.
19. Novotny HR, Alvis DL. A method of photographing fluorescence in circulating blood in the human retina. Circulation. 1961;24:82–6.
20. Pomerantzeff O. Wide-angle noncontact and small-angle contact cameras. Invest Ophthalmol Vis Sci. 1980;19:973–9.
21. Witmer MT, Kiss S. Wide-field imaging of the retina. Surv Ophthalmol. 2013;58:143–54.
22. Shields C, Materna M, Shields J. Panoramic imaging of the ocular fundus. Arch Ophtholmol. 2003;121:1603–7.
23. Patel M, Kiss S. Ultra-wide-field fluorescein angiography in retinal disease. Curr Opin Ophthalmol. 2014;25:213–20.
24. Staurenghi G, Viola F, Mainster MA, Graham RD, Harrington PG. Scanning laserophthalmoscopy and angiography with a wide-field contact lens system. Arch Ophthalmol. 2005;123:244–52.
25. Min Sagong, Jano van Hemert, Lisa C. Olmos de Koo, Cullen Barnett, SriniVas R. Sadda. Assessment of Accuracy and Precision of Quantification of Ultra-Widefield Images. Ophthalmology 2015 Apr;122(4):864–6.

Wide-Field Fluorescein Angiography

2

Thomas G. Chu and David S. Boyer

Historical

In 1886, the first ophthalmic photographs were taken by Jackman and Webster with an improvement in technique by Dr. Frederick Dimmer, who, in 1921, published an ophthalmic textbook on his images. The first commercially available fundus camera was produced by Carl Zeiss and had a 20° field of vision.

Fluorescein dye was first synthesized in 1871 by Adolf von Baeye. The dye was first used in humans by MacClean and Maumenee in 1955 [1]. It was not, however, widely accepted or utilized until Novotny and Alvis developed a system to photographically document the transit of fluorescein dye through the ocular fundus [2]. Their findings allowed for the widespread use of this technique to document, understand, and treat a variety of retinal and choroidal diseases.

Sodium fluorescein is a water-soluble and relatively inert organic plant resin that exhibits its maximum fluorescence at a near-normal blood pH of 7.4. Excitation of fluorescein occurs when it is exposed to blue wavelengths between 465 and 490 nm, resulting in emission of yellow-green frequencies (520–530 nm). The molecular size of fluorescein prevents its passage through the tight endothelial junctions of retinal blood vessels and zonula occludens in retinal pigment epithelium while allowing for rapid diffusion of the dye into potential spaces.

Administration

After a consent to perform surgery is obtained and the patient's eyes are dilated, the photographer should determine which eye is the primary eye and the location of pathology. The lens of the camera and the machine should be cleaned. The patient's chin is placed in the chin rest and the patient is placed in a comfortable position.

The usual dose of fluorescein dye is 5 mL of 10 % sodium fluorescein solution or 2 mL of 25 % fluorescein dye administered intravenously. A small butterfly needle is attached to the syringe containing the dye. The needle is placed in a vein and blood is refluxed into the tubing before injection to ensure entry into the vein. Administration is carefully observed to avoid extravasation of dye, which may cause severe localized pain and even skin necrosis. Blood precautions should be observed and gloves are recommended for those placing the intravenous line and administering the dye. The butterfly needle is left in until the procedure is over to allow drugs to be administered, if necessary.

Side Effects

Fluorescein dye is a relatively safe diagnostic compound. Nausea and emesis are the most commonly reported reactions, occurring with a frequency of 5 % or less, and may be reduced by administering the dye slowly and in lesser amounts. The nausea appears to be related to the difference in the pH of sodium fluorescein to the pH of the body pH 8–9.8. Syncope, thrombophlebitis, temperature elevation, nerve palsy, and local tissue necrosis are classified as moderate adverse reactions occurring in less than 1 %. Severe adverse reactions include laryngeal edema, bronchospasm, and anaphylaxis [3–5]. An emergency tray and oxygen should be available whenever fluorescein is administered. Leaving the butterfly needle in until the procedure is done and no untoward reactions have occurred will allow venous access in case of a severe medical complication [6–19]. Although there have been no reports of human fetal complications secondary to fluorescein injection during pregnancy, most physicians avoid administration, if possible, in pregnant patients. The dye does pass into the breast milk in nursing mothers [20, 21], and it is recommended that breastfeeding mothers store their milk and refrain from breastfeeding for 48 h after the fluorescein injection. The dye is metabolized by the kidneys and is eliminated through the urine within 24–36 h.

T.G. Chu, MD, PhD • D.S. Boyer, MD (✉)
Retina-Vitreous Associated Medical Group,
Los Angeles, CA, USA
e-mail: thomaschu@laretina.com; VITDOC@aol.com

I. Kozak, J.F. Arevalo (eds.), *Atlas of Wide-Field Retinal Angiography and Imaging*, DOI 10.1007/978-3-319-17864-6_2

Wide-Field Imaging Systems

The desire to view larger areas of the retina and the retinal periphery has been ongoing since the original fundus cameras were developed. Over 80 years, the field of view has increased from 20° to 50°. Recently, the blending of several digital images enables a composite montage image to afford a larger angle of view of the retina (~75°) (Figs. 1 and 2).

In 1975, Pomerantzeff et al. reported on a camera system involving the use of a dilated pupil, a contact lens, and an external illumination device that was applied to the sclera that allowed visualization of up to about 150° of the retina [22–24].

In 1997, the Retcam (Clarity Medical Systems, Inc., Pleasanton, CA), which utilizes a digital format, was introduced. This system is in wide use in the neonatal intensive care unit to screen for retinopathy of prematurity [25]. The illumination system passes through the pupil and lens and can be used with a variety of contact lenses to obtain a 130° view of the retina. This system allows for patients to be lying on their back to obtain images. It needs clear media to get good overall images. Intravenous fluorescein angiography can be done with this system (Fig. 3) [26].

The Panoret-1000 developed by Medibell Medical Vision Technologies, Inc. (Haifa, Israel), is a hand-held system that uses a contact lens and an external light source to capture digital fundus images. This device does not require pupil dilation [27].

In 2000, the Optos camera (Optos PLC, Dunfermline, UK) was introduced. This camera uses the principles of a scanning laser ophthalmoscope (SLO) to capture ultra-wide-angle digital fundus images. The system employs an ellipsoid mirror that allows the laser light to pass through it; the patient's eye is positioned to be in line with the mirror's focal point. The system does not require a dilated pupil and easily passes through lens opacities that would preclude visualization by other cameras (Fig. 4).

A 200° field of view of the retina is possible. Both fluorescein angiography and fundus autofluorescence are available. New steering qualities allow an even larger area of the retina to be viewed. Nasal and temporal areas of the retina are usually well seen, with superior and inferior areas not as well visualized.

Staurenghi et al. introduced a contact lens system (OcularStaurenghi 230 SLO Retina Lens; Ocular Instrument Inc., Bellevue, WA.) compatible with existing SLO cameras. This is a contact lens that requires the photographer to hold the lens. With this system, approximately 150° of the retina can be viewed (Figs. 5, 6, and 7) [26].

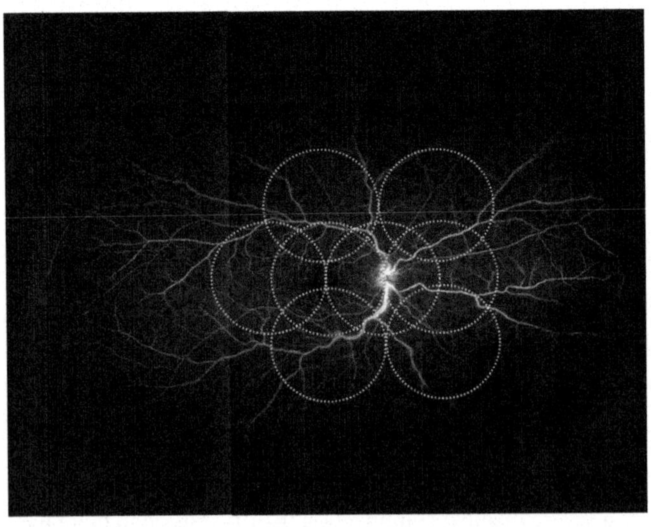

Fig. 1 Seven field photographs compared with the wide-field image

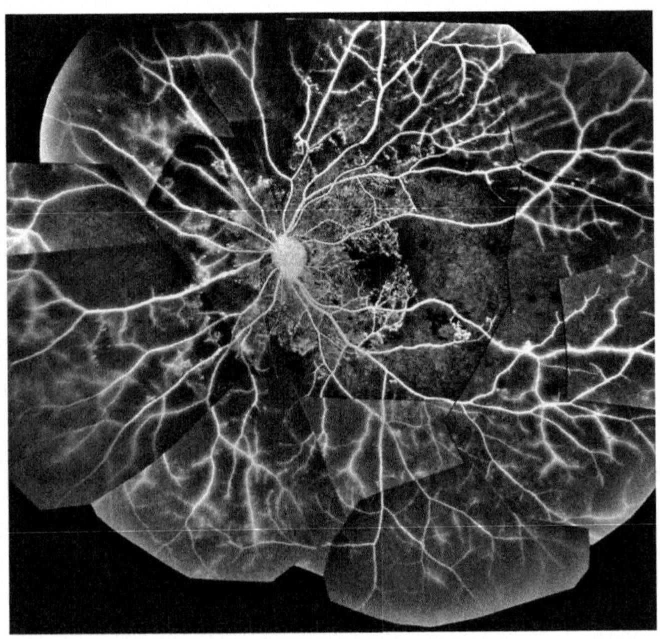

Fig. 2 Dr. Shimazu popularized montage photographs to create a larger field of view

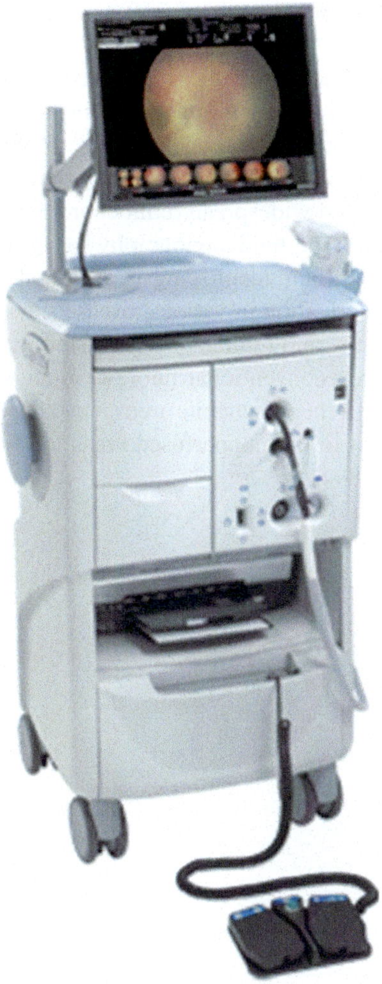

Fig. 3 Retcam instrument and photo obtained

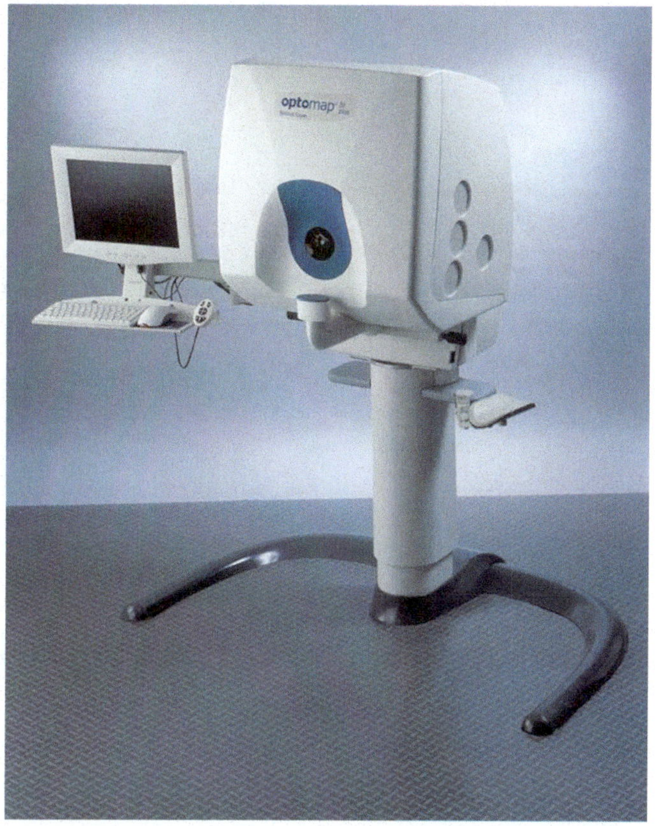

Fig. 4 Optos machine. Note that the image comes up on the monitor adjacent to the machine

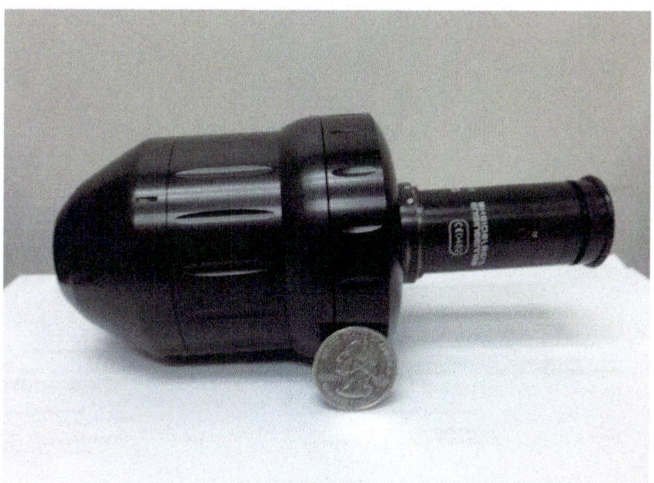

Fig. 5 Staurenghi lens

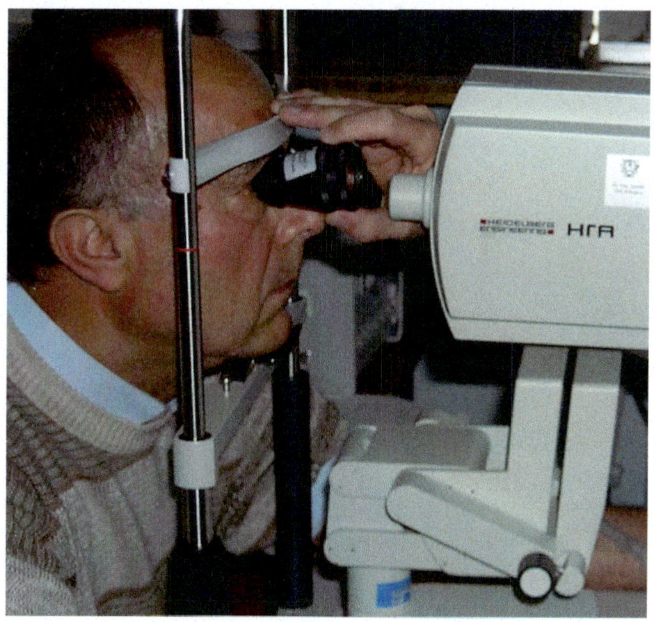

Fig. 6 Staurenghi lens

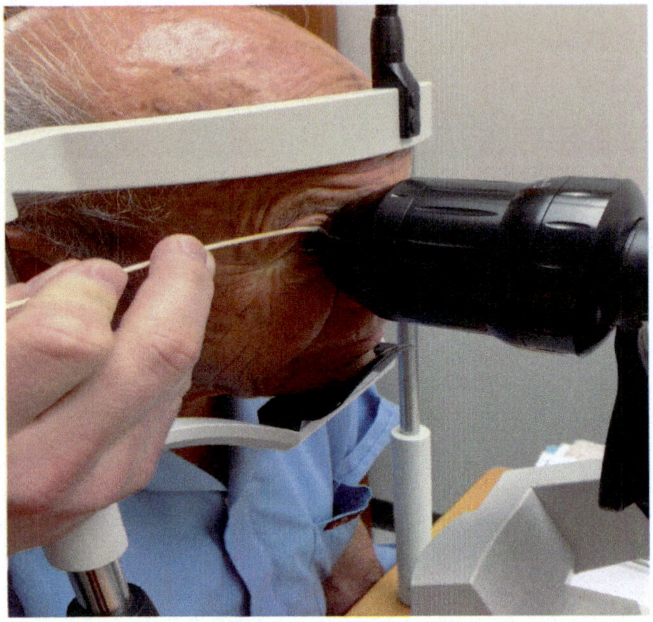

Fig. 7 Staurenghi lens being placed and cotton applicators used to help open the eye

Disease States

The utility of wide-field angiography has been demonstrated in a number of ocular conditions Including diabetic retinopathy, uveitis, retinal vascular occlusions, choroidal and retinal masses, sickle cell retinopathy, pediatric retinal disease, retinal vasculitis, and widespread retinochoroidal dystrophies.

In diabetes, wide-field angiography has been shown to be particularly helpful in identifying areas of both nonperfusion and neovascularization in various disease states such as diabetic retinopathy and retinal vein occlusion that are not easily identified on conventional fluorescein angiography. The identification of these ischemic areas may allow for selective laser treatment to the nonperfused areas to minimize tissue destruction [28–41].

Artifacts

The major cause of artifacts in fundus photography arises from the reflection of light from interfaces in the ocular media. The SLO and the Optos imaging system reduce this problem.

For all wide-angle cameras, positioning of the patients eye is critical. For the Optos, this is extremely important to avoid unusual artifacts. All hair must be cleared away from the face and forehead before imaging. Patients should be positioned so they are leaning forward into the camera, leading with the chin, not the forehead. To image the right eye, the chin cup will be moved to the left position with the face of the patient also turned left (reverse to image right eye). Anything near the center of the face mask will be imaged by the Optos (*e.g.*, hair, lashes, nose, photographer's fingers, cotton tip applicators). Removing the forehead strap on the camera allows for increased space to hold the eyelids open and allows for increased room for patient positioning (Fig. 8).

To remove eyelash, finger, and nose artifacts, have the patient blink several times, maintain a clear view, and ask her or him to open the eyes as wide as possible. If the eyelids or eyelashes are still present, the photographer can artificially widen the palpebral fissure by placing his or her finger or a cotton-tip applicator on the lateral canthus and elevating slightly (Figs. 9, 10, 11, 12, 13, 14, 15, and 16).

Cataracts may result in soft focus. In patients with nuclear sclerotic cataracts, camera fixation at the margin of the pupil, rather than the center, may improve the clarity. In patients with cortical cataracts, the camera should be focused through the least involved area. It may require the photographer to take several images before a clear image is obtained.

Green light artifacts occur when a patient's face is pressed too far into the face mask. To counteract this, the photographer can press on the (–) on the hand control or have the patient pull slightly back from the mask. Only a slight adjustment may be needed. If the patient's head is too far away from the face mask, the field of view will be decreased. If the patient is too far away from the face mask, the pupillary margin or even the sclera may be visible.

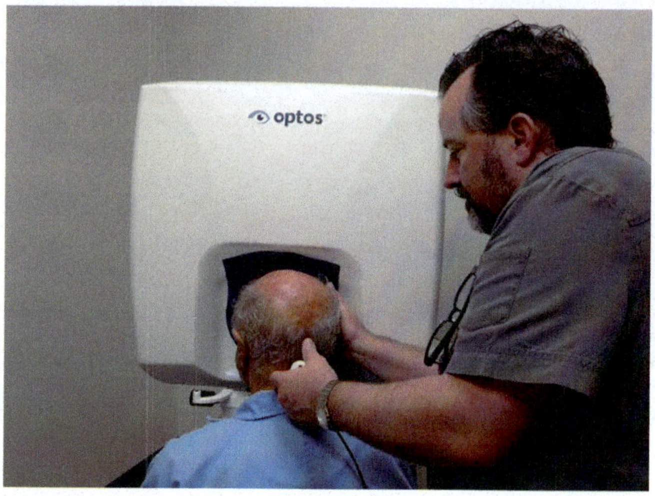

Fig. 8 Proper positioning for Optos photographs is critical

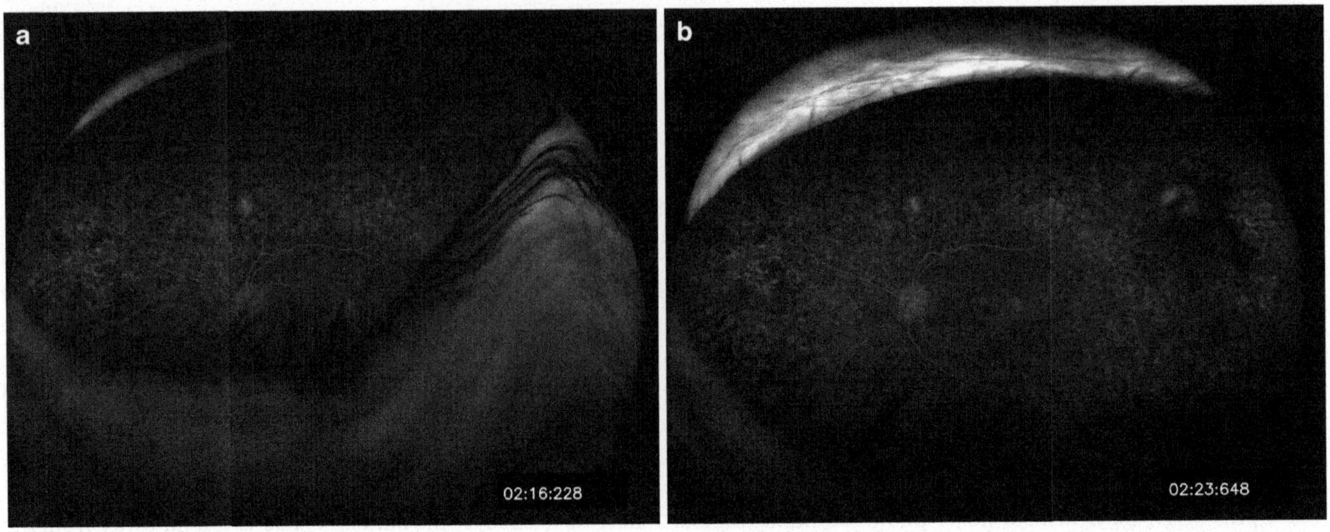

Fig. 9 (**a**) The artifact observed on the Optos camera when the patient blinks while the fluorescein angiogram is being taken. (**b**) Corrected view

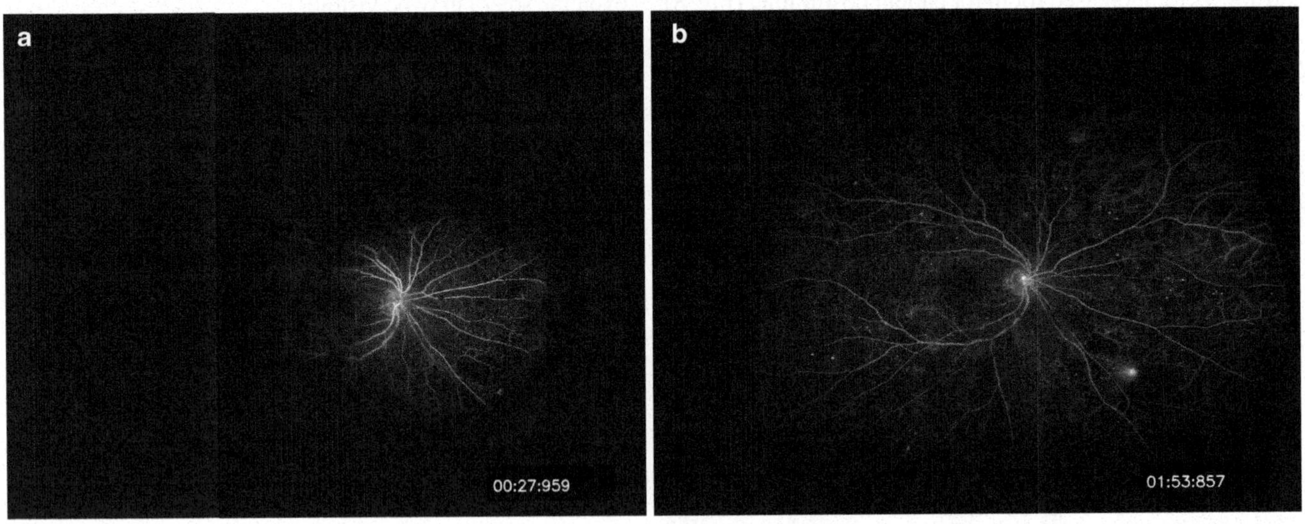

Fig. 10 (**a**) The focus on the eye is too far out, giving a very small field of view. (**b**) Corrected view

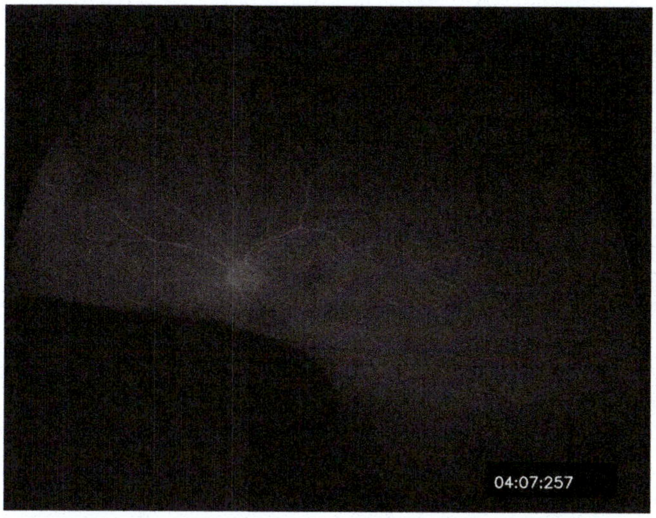

Fig. 11 The photographer's finger, which is trying to open the eyelid, is visualized in the photograph

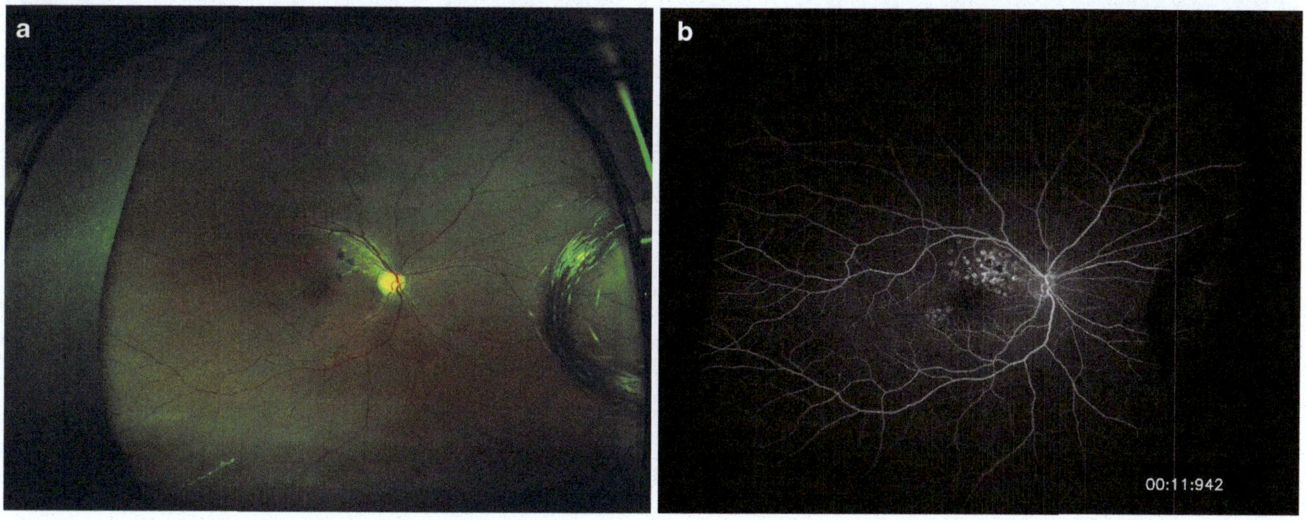

Fig. 12 The patient's hair is visualized in both the color photograph (**a**) and the fluorescein angiogram (**b**)

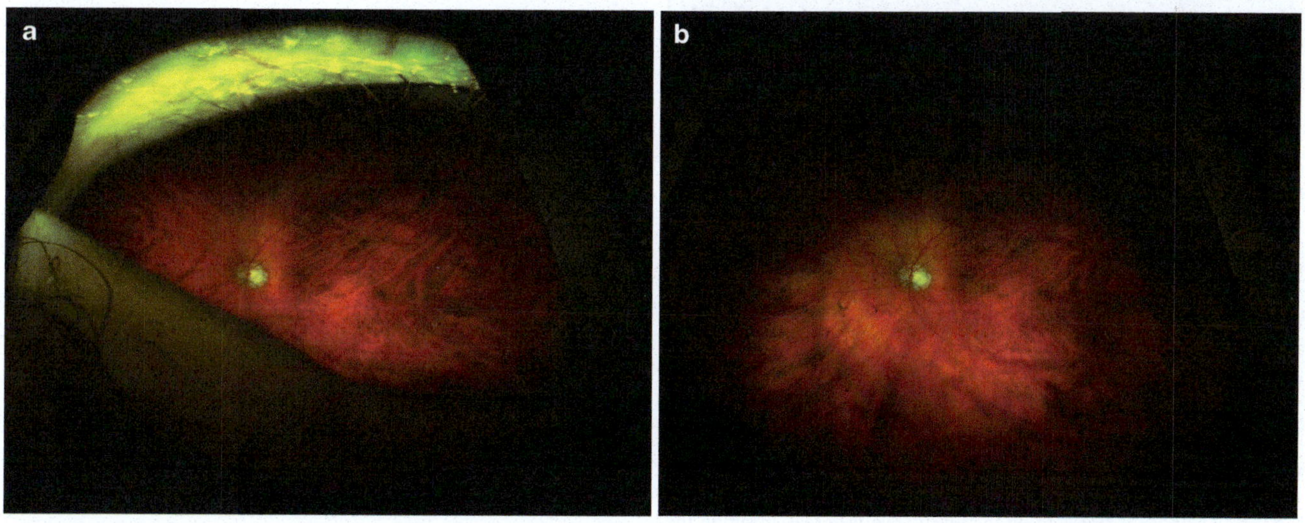

Fig. 13 (**a**) The focus of the camera is in too close. (**b**) Corrected view

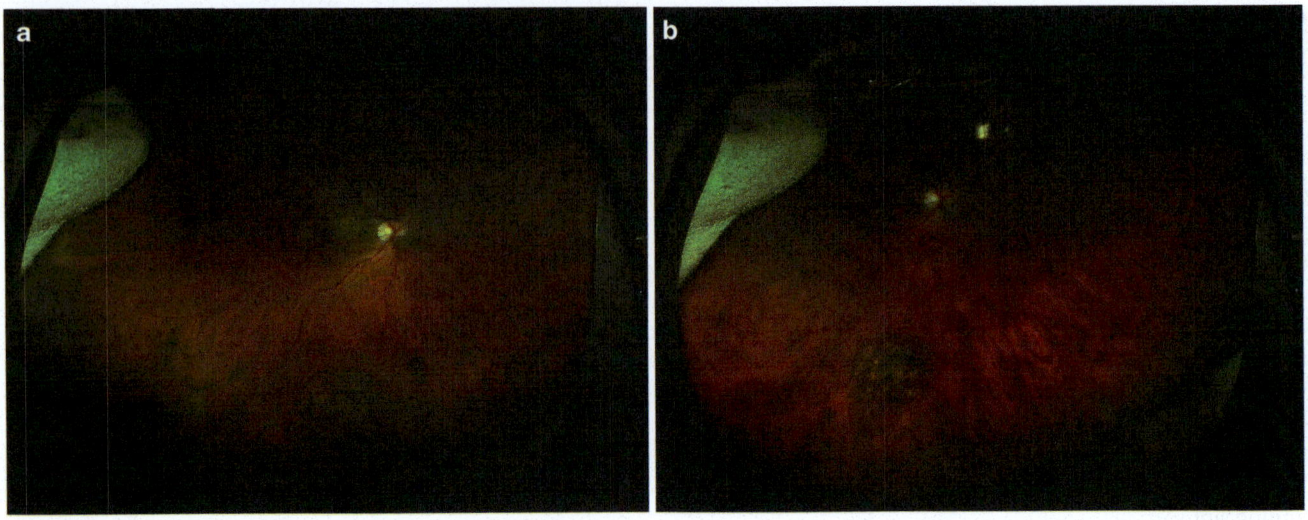

Fig. 14 (**a**) The nose of the patient is in view. (**b**) Corrected view

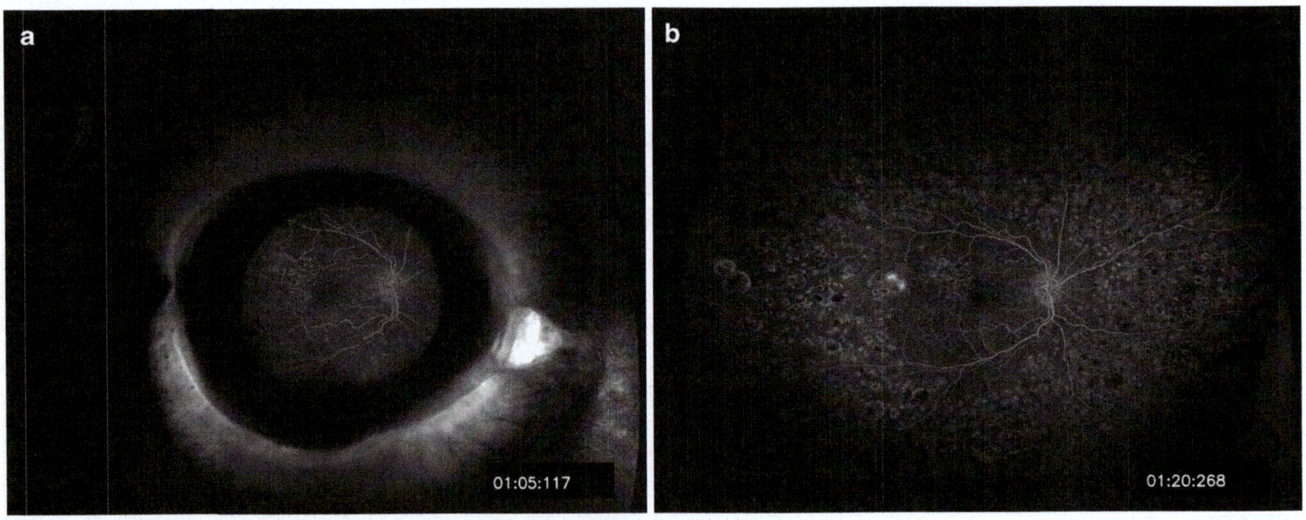

Fig. 15 (**a**) The focus of the camera is out too far. The eye itself is visualized and the view is very small. (**b**) Corrected view

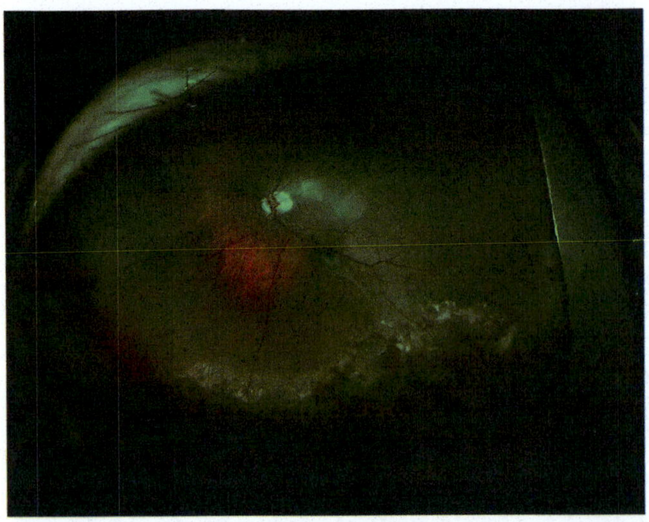

Fig. 16 The nose is pressing on the plastic eye/face rest, bringing the plastic edge into view

Comparisons

The Optos provides a substantially larger view of the retina than that of the Heidelberg SLO. Optos captures a retinal area averaging 151.362 pixels versus the Heidelberg Spectralis, averaging 101.786. Heidelberg has a new non-contact lens that makes it much easier to obtain images because it does not require the photographer to hold the lens.

Wide-field angiography was compared in a study at the Wilmer Eye Institute. They compared the percentage of patients that the wide-field Optos fluorescein changed management of the patients. Seventy-one patient visits from 23 patients were analyzed. Examination plus wide-field photography and fluorescein detected disease activity in 68 % of visits compared with examination and standard fluorescein angiography, in which only 45 % of patients were identified. The addition of ultra-wide-field angiography caused a change in management 51 % of the time [42].

Conclusion

Wide-field angiography offers additional information that may change the treatment of many retinal vascular diseases. The ability to penetrate through small pupils or media opacities offer additional benefits to wide-angle angiography. The administration of the fluorescein dye and the precautions and side effects of the injection are unchanged from conventional fluorescein angiography.

References

1. Jackman WT, Webster JD. On photographing the retina of the living eye. Philadelphia Photographer. 1886;23:340–1.
2. Ciardella A, Brown D. Wide field imaging. In: Agarwal A, editor. Fundus fluorescein and indocyanine green angiography: a textbook and atlas. New York: Slack Incorporated; 2007. p. 79–83.
3. Novotny HR, Alvis DL. A method of photographing fluorescence in circulating blood in the human retina. Circulation. 1961;24:82–6.
4. Hitosugi M, Omura K, Yokoyama T, Kawato H, Motozawa Y, Nagai T, et al. An autopsy case of fatal anaphylactic shock following fluorescein angiography: a case report. Med Sci Law. 2004;44(3):264–5.
5. Kinsella FP, Mooney DJ. Anaphylaxis following oral fluorescein angiography. Am J Ophthalmol. 1988;106(6):756–6.
6. Gomez-Ulla F, Gutierrez C, Seoane I. Severe anaphylactic reaction to orally administered fluorescein. Am J Ophthalmol. 1991; 112(1):94.
7. Kwan AS, Barry C, McAllister IL, Constable I. Fluorescein angiography and adverse drug reactions revisited: the Lions eye experience. Clin Experiment Ophthalmol. 2006;4(1):33–8.
8. Jennings BJ, Mathews DE. Adverse reactions during retinal fluorescein angiography. J Am Optom Assoc. 1994;65(7):465–71.
9. Kwiterovich KA, Maguire MG, Murphy RP, Schachat AP, Bressler NM, Bressler SB, et al. Frequency of adverse systemic reactions after fluorescein angiography. Results of a prospective study. Ophthalmology. 1991;98(7):1139–42.
10. Chazan BI, Balodimos MC, Koncz L. Untoward effects of fluorescein angiography in diabetic patients. Ann Ophthalmol. 1971;3(1):42.
11. Pacurariu RI. Low incidence of side effects following intravenous fluorescein angiography. Ann Ophthalmol. 1982;14(1):32–6.
12. Butner RW, McPherson AR. Adverse reactions in intravenous fluorescein angiography. Ann Ophthalmol. 1983;15(11):1084–6.
13. Marcus DF, Bovino JA, Williams D. Adverse reactions during intravenous fluorescein angiography. Arch Ophthalmol. 1984; 102(6):825.
14. Kwiterovitch KA, Maguire MG, Murphy RP, Schachat AP, Bresssler NM, Bressler SB, et al. Frequency of adverse systemic reactions occurring after fluorescein angiography—results of a prospective study. Ophthalmology. 1991;98(7):1139–42.
15. Buchanan RT, Levine NS. Blood pressure drop as a result of fluorescein injection. Plast Reconstr Surg. 1982;70(3):363–8.
16. Gombos GM, Lieberman RM. Seizures associated with fluorescein angiography. Ann Ophthalmol. 1989;21(3):89–90.
17. Kelly SP, MacDermott NJ, Saunders DC, Leach FN. Convulsion following fluorescein angiography. Br J Ophthalmol. 1989;73(8): 655–6.
18. Hess JB, Pacurariu RI. Acute pulmonary edema following intravenous fluorescein angiography. Am J Ophthalmol. 1976;82(4): 567–70.
19. Ascaso FJ, Tiestos MT, Navales J, Iturbe F, Paloma A, Ayala JI. Fatal acute myocardial infarction after intravenous fluorescein angiography. Retina. 1993;13(3):238–9.
20. Schatz H. Sloughing of skin following fluorescein extravasation. Ann Ophthalmol. 1978;10(5):625.
21. Halperin LS, Olk RJ, Soubrane G, Coscas G. Safety of fluorescein angiography during pregnancy. Am J Ophthalmol. 1980;109(5):563–6.
22. Greenberg F, Lewis RA. Safety of fluorescein angiography during pregnancy [letter]. Am J Ophthalmol. 1991;110(3):323–5.
23. Pomerantzeff O. Equator-plus camera. Invest Ophthalmol. 1975;14(5):401–6.
24. Pomerantzeff O. Wide-angle noncontact and small-angle contact cameras. Invest Ophthalmol Vis Sci. 1980;19(8):973–9.
25. Ducrey N, Pomerantzeff O, Schepens CL, Delori FC, Schneider J. Clinical trials with the equator-plus camera. Am J Ophthalmol. 1977;84(6):840–6.
26. Wu C, Petersen RA, VanderVeen DK. RetCam imaging for retinopathy of prematurity screening. J AAPOS. 2006;10(2):107–11.
27. Staurenghi G, Viola F, Mainster MA, Graham RD, Harrington PG. Scanning laser ophthalmoscopy and angiography with a wide-field contact lens system. Arch Ophthalmol. 2005;123(2):244–52.
28. Shields CL, Materin M, Shields JA. Panoramic imaging of the ocular fundus. Arch Ophthalmol. 2003;121(11):1603–7.
29. Prasad PS, Oliver SC, Coffee RE, Hubschman JP, Schwartz SD. Ultra wide-field angiographic characteristics of branch retinal and hemicentral retinal vein occlusion. Ophthalmology. 2010;117(4):780–4.
30. Heussen FM, Vasconcelos-Santos DV, Pappuru RR, Walsh AC, Rao NA, Sadda SR. Ultra-wide-field green-light (532-nm) autofluorescence imaging in chronic Vogt-Koyanagi-Harada disease. Ophthalmic Surg Lasers Imaging. 2011;42(4):272–7.
31. Kaines A, Oliver S, Reddy S, Schwartz SD. Ultrawide angle angiography for the detection and management of diabetic retinopathy. Int Ophthalmol Clin. 2009;49(2):53–9.
32. Kaines A, Tsui I, Sarraf D, Schwartz SD. The use of ultra wide field fluorescein angiography in evaluation and management of uveitis. Semin Ophthalmol. 2009;24(1):19–24.
33. Kernt M, Schaller UC, Stumpf C, Ulbiq NW, Kampik A, Neubauer AS. Choroidal pigmented lesions imaged by ultra-wide-field scanning laser ophthalmoscopy with two laser wavelengths (Optomap). Clin Ophthalmol. 2010;4:829–36.
34. Lorenz B, Spasovska K, Elflein H, Schneider N. Wide-field digital imaging based telemedicine for screening for acute retinopathy of prematurity (ROP). Six-year results of a multicentre field study. Graefes Arch Clin Exp Ophthalmol. 2009;247(9):1251–62.

35. Spaide RF. Peripheral areas of nonperfusion in treated central retinal vein occlusion as imaged by wide-field fluorescein angiography. Retina. 2011;31(1):829–37.
36. Wessel MM, Aaker GD, Parlitsis G, Cho M, D'Amico DJ, Kiss S. Ultra-wide-field angiography improves the detection and classification of diabetic retinopathy. Retina. 2012;32(4):785–91.
37. Win PH, Young TA. Optos Panoramic 200A fluorescein angiography for proliferative diabetic retinopathy with asteroid hyalosis. Semin Ophthalmol. 2007;22(2):67–9.
38. Witmer MT, Kozbial A, Daniel S, Kiss S. Peripheral autofluorescence findings in age related macular degeneration. Acta Ophthalmol. 2012;90(6):e428–33.
39. Schwartz SD, Harrison SA, Ferrone PJ, Trese MT. Telemedical evaluation and management of retinopathy of prematurity using a fiberoptic digital fundus camera. Ophthalmology. 2000; 107(1):25–8.
40. Scott KE, Kim DY, Wang L, Kane SA, Coki O, Starren J, et al. Telemedical diagnosis of retinopathy of prematurity intraphysician agreement between ophthalmoscopic examination and image-based interpretation. Ophthalmology. 2008;115(7):228.e3.
41. Seidensticker F, Neubauer AS, Wasfy T, Stumpf C, Thurau SR, Kampik A, et al. Wide-field fundus autofluorescence corresponds to visual fields in chorioretinitis patients. Clin Ophthalmol. 2011;5:1667–71.
42. Leder HA, Campbell JP, Sepah YJ, Gan T, Dunn JP, Hatef E, et al. Ultra-wide-field retinal imaging in the management of non-infectious retinal vasculitis. J Ophthalmic Inflamm Infect. 2013;3:30.

Wide-Field Indocyanine Green Angiography

3

Irene Rusu, Peter Coombs, and Szilárd Kiss

Indocyanine green angiography (ICGA) is an important diagnostic tool in many retinal diseases including central serous chorioretinopathy (CSCR), uveitis, age-related macular degeneration (AMD), and polypoidal choroidal vasculopathy. ICGA was first reported for retinal angiography in humans in 1971 [1, 2]. Indocyanine green (ICG) is a tricarbocyanine dye with a molecular weight of 751.4 Da [3]. The excitation wavelength of ICG is 750–800 nm and it fluoresces at over 800 nm wavelengths. These near-infrared wavelengths have better tissue penetrance than wavelengths used in fluorescein angiography, allowing a better view of deeper anatomical and pathological structures such as the choroid with minimal signal disruption from overlying retinal tissue, retinal pigment epithelium, or any fluid, exudate, or hemorrhage that may be present [4]. In addition, ICG is more than 98 % bound to blood lipoproteins, which keeps it almost completely confined to the intravascular space in the absence of pathology and makes it ideal for imaging disorders with choroidal neovascular membranes [5–7].

ICGA has an excellent patient safety profile. A typical dose given is 20–25 mg/mL in a 2-mL bolus injection into the arm. Relatively few patients (<1 %) will experience nausea, vomiting, syncope, fever, or hives. Very rarely, in 0.05 % of patients, an anaphylactic or bronchospastic reaction to ICG may occur [4]. Patients allergic to shellfish or iodide should not undergo ICGA testing because the administered mixture includes a 5 % iodine powder. ICG has a short half-life in circulation and is rapidly excreted via the liver into bile [8]. Liver disease, Metformin use, and kidney disease are relative contraindications to ICGA. Even though side effects are rare, patients should still be informed of the risks and provide written consent prior to testing.

Like fluorescein angiography, ICGA has distinct phases. The early phase precedes the filling of the retinal artery (Fig. 1), the mid phase occurs with the filling of the arteries and veins (Fig. 2) and the late phase occurs 10 min after injection (Fig. 3). The choroidal vasculature fills sequentially from posterior to anterior and from large vessels to smaller vessels, starting with Haller's layer, then Sattler's layer, then finally with the choriocapillaris. The first choroidal vessels seen on ICGA are those fed directly by the posterior ciliary arteries (PCAs). Initially, distinct zones of perfusion can often be seen emanating from the medial and lateral PCAs. The filling of the choriocapillaris is characterized by a diffuse "choroidal flush." In the late phases of ICGA, vortex veins can be identified [9, 10].

The strength of fluorescence of ICG is only 4 % that of fluorescein dye, so a digital imaging system or a scanning laser ophthalmoscope is required to produce reliable and interpretable images. Because of this greater dependence on equipment, ICGA was much less commonly used than fluorescein angiogram until the early 1990s when digital technology improvements made it more widely available [10]. An example of a popular camera-based platform for ICGA imaging is the TRC-50DX ICG by Topcon (Tokyo, Japan) and a popular scanning laser ophthalmoscopy system is the Spectralis HRA by Heidelberg Engineering (Heidelberg, Germany). These offer excellent resolution but fields of view only as wide as 50° by 55°. Wide-angle angiography including ICGA with up to 160° fields of view was described in 1995 using the contact lens system and a fundus camera [11, 12]. Since then, a number of contact-based and noncontact-based systems have been developed to image the peripheral retina. In 2005, a new noncontact ultra-wide-field (UWF) fluorescein angiography system (Optos 200 MA/200Tx) was developed that could image up to 200° of the ocular fundus [13]. This system was modified to perform UWF-ICGA with a module capable of emitting 805-nm laser light and a filter with a cutoff of 835 nm to collect the cyanescence [14]. In a

I. Rusu, MD • S. Kiss, MD (✉)
Department of Ophthalmology, Weill Cornell Medical College, New York–Presbyterian Hospital, New York, NY, USA
e-mail: irr7002@med.cornell.edu; szk7001@med.cornell.edu

P. Coombs, MD
Department of Ophthalmology, Weill Cornell Medical College, New York, NY, USA
e-mail: pgcoombs@gmail.com

I. Kozak, J.F. Arevalo (eds.), *Atlas of Wide-Field Retinal Angiography and Imaging*, DOI 10.1007/978-3-319-17864-6_3

series of 138 eyes, UWF-ICGA proved clinically valuable providing high-resolution images of both the central and the peripheral choroidal circulation sufficient for diagnosis, evaluation, and monitoring of a variety of vitreoretinal disorders. In 67.4 % of eyes imaged in this study, the presence of peripheral pathology was found outside the 50–60° field of view of standard ICGA imaging systems [15]. In clinical practice, the most common uses for ICGA are for the evaluation of polypoidal choroidal vasculopathy, neovascular AMD, CSCR, and posterior uveitis with choroiditis, including birdshot retinochoroidopathy, acute zonal occult outer retinopathy, and multifocal choroiditis [15, 16].

In CSCR, UWF-ICGA shows patchy areas of hyperfluorescence in early- and mid-phase frames that fades in later frames (Fig. 4). Prominent dilated vessels may also be seen that correspond to areas of leakage on fluorescein angiography as well as areas that appear normal on fundus photography and fluorescein angiography (Figs. 5 and 6). In one study of 65 eyes with CSCR, UWF-ICGA revealed dilated choroidal vessels and choroidal hyperpermeability in areas corresponding to altered autofluorescence on UWF autofluorescence [17, 18].

In neovascular AMD, UWF-ICGA shows excellent visualization of posterior pole choroidal hyperfluorescence (Fig. 7) consistent with classic choroidal neovascularization (CNV) (Figs. 8, 9, and 10) while also showing peripheral mid-phase hypofluorescent areas up to 1 disc diameter in size consistent with extramacular serous pigment epithelial detachment without CNV (Fig. 11). Peripheral UWF-ICGA findings in non-neovascular AMD are evident as areas of hypofluorescence consistent with blockage from peripheral drusen or retinal pigment epithelium atrophy (Fig. 12).

In polypoidal choroidal vasculopathy, early UWF-ICGA images show a dilated network of vessels corresponding to an abnormal inner choroidal vascular network (Fig. 13). On clinical examination and fundus photography, this choroidal abnormality may result in clinically visible reddish-orange polyps. Slow leakage from these dilated choroidal vessels leads to corresponding areas of hyperfluorescence in later frames (Fig. 14). Far peripheral networks of polyps may also be seen in the mid-phase ICGA that display a characteristic "washout" in later-phase ICGA images.

In ocular syphilis, UWF fluorescein angiography shows areas of peripheral nonperfusion and leakage. On UWF-ICGA, multiple mid-phase peripheral diffuse round areas of hypofluorescence are seen (Figs. 15, 16, 17, and 18). In the posterior pole, mid-phase hyperfluorescent lesions suggestive of vascular anastomosis versus retinal cystic changes are seen (Fig. 17). The late-phase frames show inferior hypofluorescence and a choroidal filling defect consistent with nonperfusion. In sarcoidosis, UWF-ICGA shows multiple areas of choroidal hypofluorescence suggestive of a choroidal vascular filling defect versus blockage from retinal granulomas (Figs. 19, 20, and 21). In birdshot chorioretinopathy, UWF-ICGA shows areas of choroidal hypofluorescence corresponding to white lesions on clinical examination (Figs. 22, 23, and 24). In uveitis, UWF-ICGA shows a wide variety of peripheral pathological choroidal vasculature changes in a number of different conditions (Figs. 25, 26, and 27). In CMV retinitis, UWF-ICGA shows areas of hyperfluorescence corresponding to areas of retinal necrosis on Optos WF fundus photography and areas of staining and leakage on UWF-fluorescence angiography (Figs. 28, 29, and 30).

UWF-ICG angiography is an important diagnostic tool that provides simultaneous imaging of the peripheral and posterior pole choroidal vasculature comparable with that seen on UWF fluorescein angiography (~200° in a single shot). Abnormalities in the peripheral retina that may otherwise be missed on conventional ICG imaging are increasingly reported in a variety of retinal disorders. The clinical significance of these peripheral findings is becoming progressively apparent.

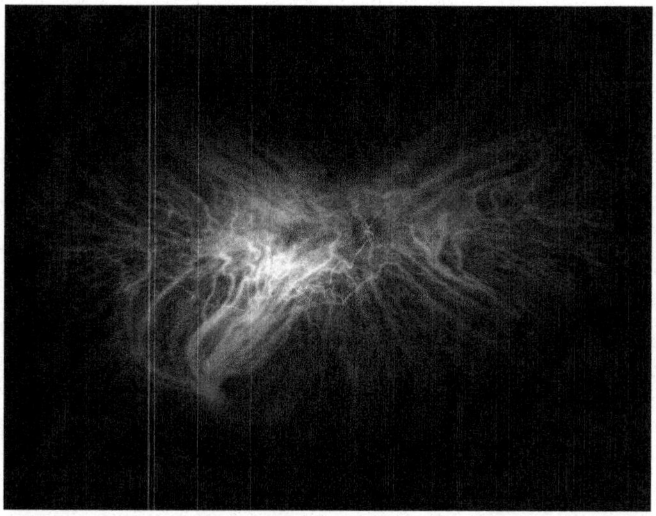

Fig. 1 Early-phase UWF-ICGA

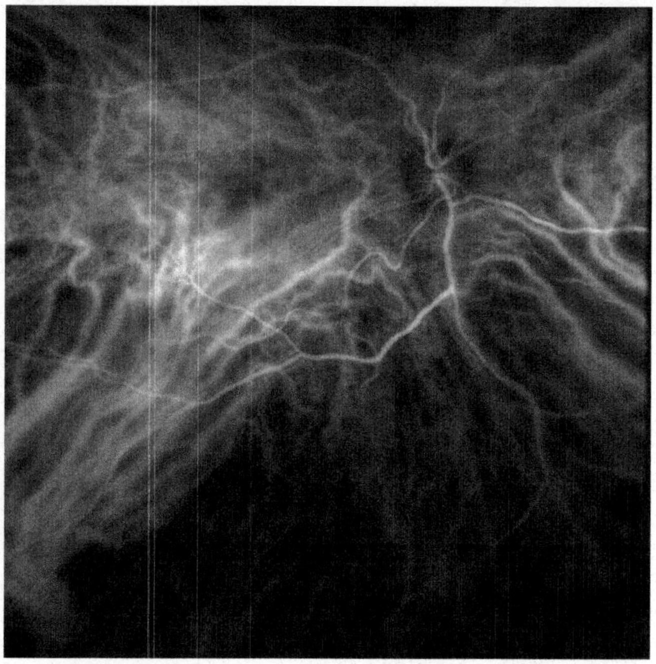

Fig. 2 Mid-phase Optos UWF-ICGA zoomed on the macula

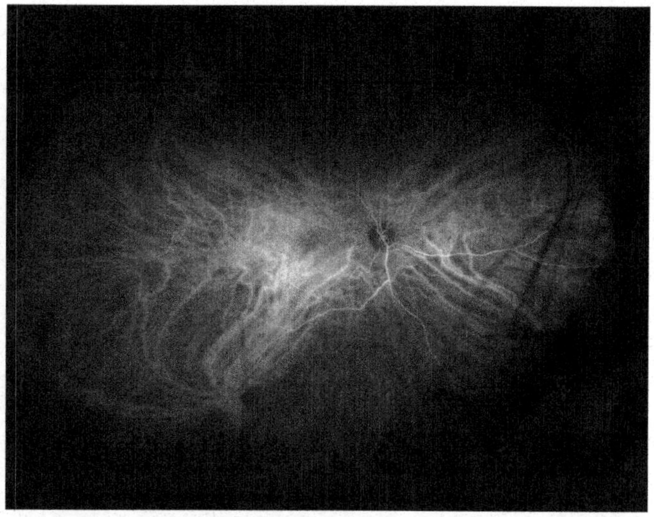

Fig. 3 Late-phase UWF-ICGA

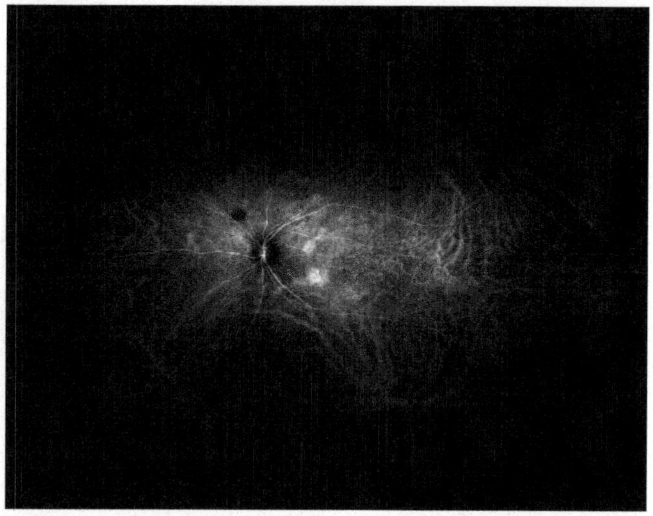

Fig. 4 CSCR. Heidelberg wide-field ICGA of the left eye shows patchy areas of hyperfluorescence and hypofluorescence

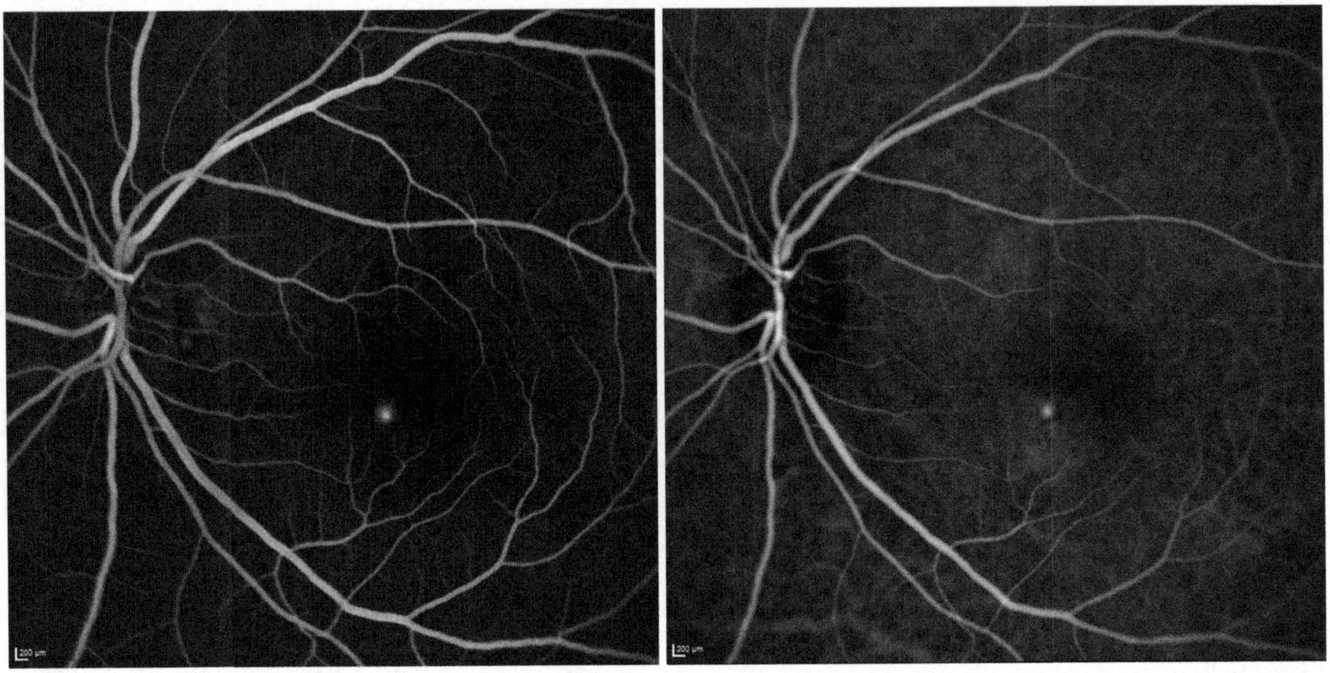

Fig. 5 CSCR. Heidelberg fluorescein angiography/ICGA of the left eye shows an area of hyperfluorescence consistent with expansile dot pattern of CSCR. Note the choroidal hyperfluorescence at the same location as the expansile dot pattern of leakage on fluorescein angiography suggesting active CSCR. Dilated vessels corresponding to areas of leakage on FA

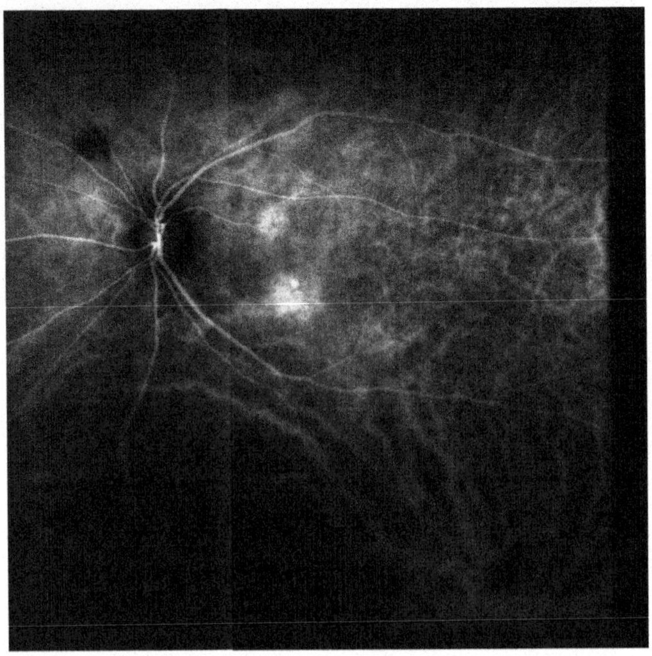

Fig. 6 CSCR. The macula resolution of the wide-field images is comparable with 50° Heidelberg ICGA imaging above

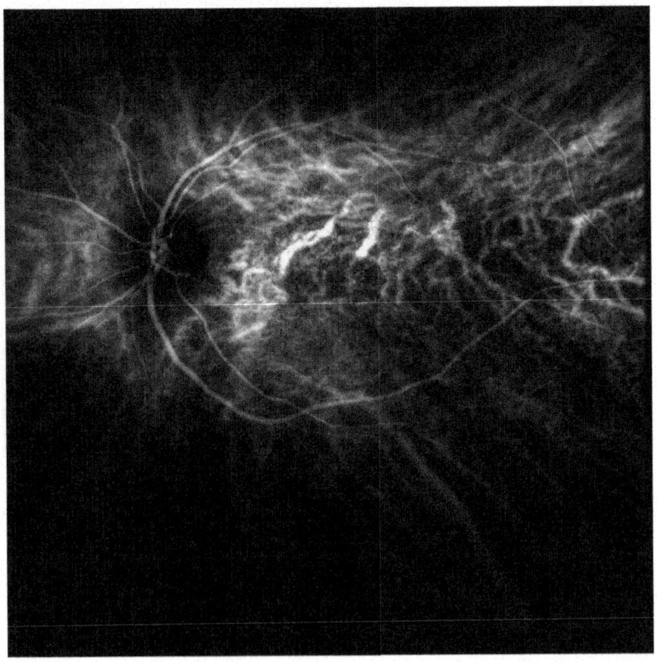

Fig. 7 Neovascular AMD. Optos UWF-ICGA, macular section, with choroidal hyperfluorescence

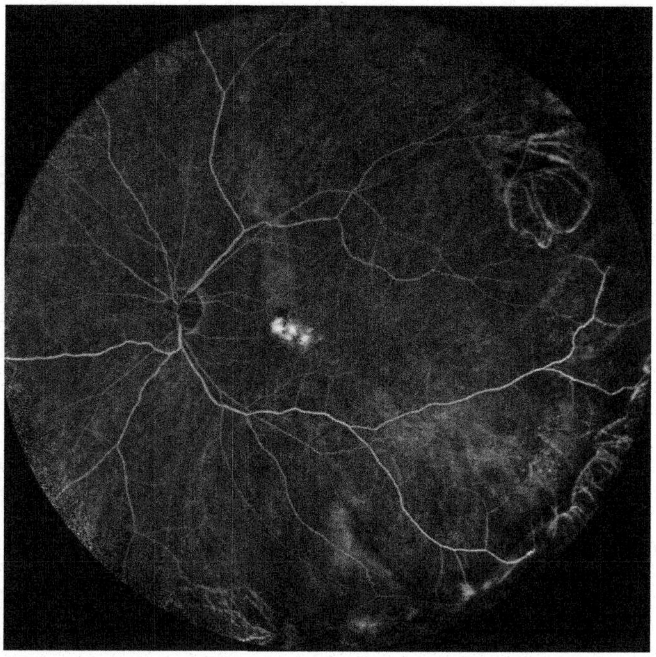

Fig. 8 An example of choroidal neovascularization as seen on Heidelberg wide-field ICGA

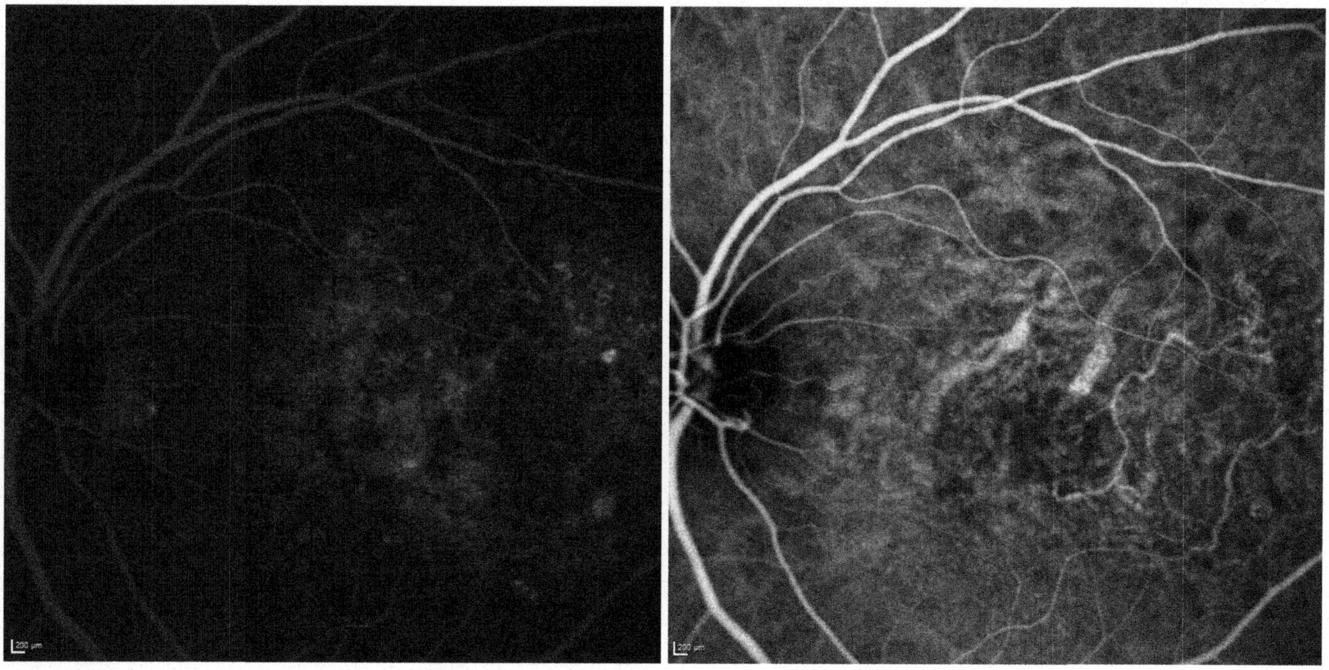

Fig. 9 Neovascular AMD. The resolution of the macular image of the Optos UWF-ICGA above is comparable with a Heidelberg 50° fluorescein angiography/ICG image below

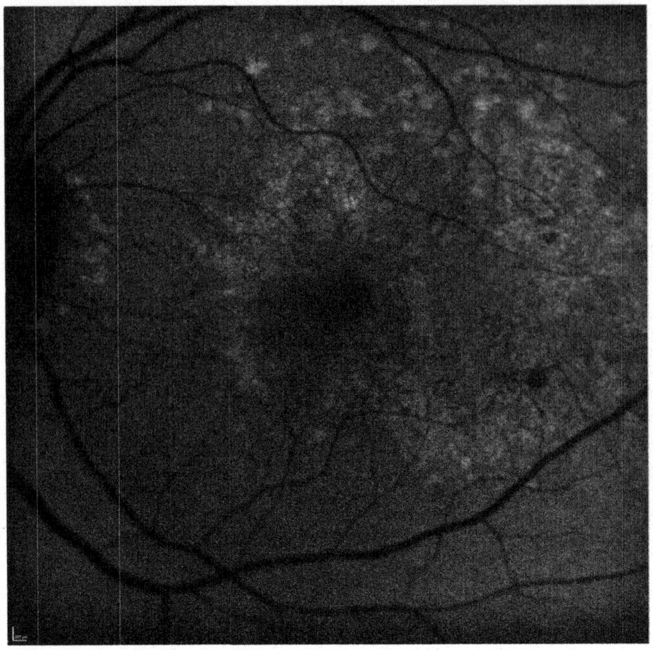

Fig. 10 Neovascular AMD. Heidelberg autofluorescence of the left eye shows mottled areas of hyperautofluorescence consistent with drusen and hypoautofluorescence consistent with retinal pigment epithelium atrophy

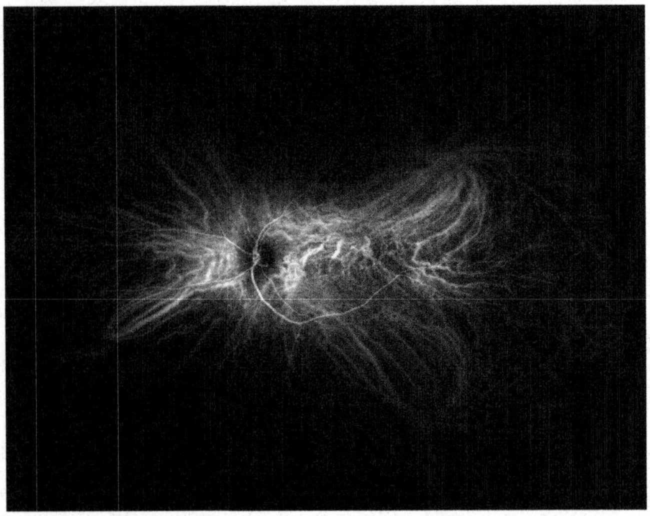

Fig. 11 Neovascular AMD. Optos UWF-ICGA shows excellent visualization of posterior pole, choroidal hyperfluorescence consistent with CNV, and hypofluorescent areas consistent with serous pigment epithelial detachment

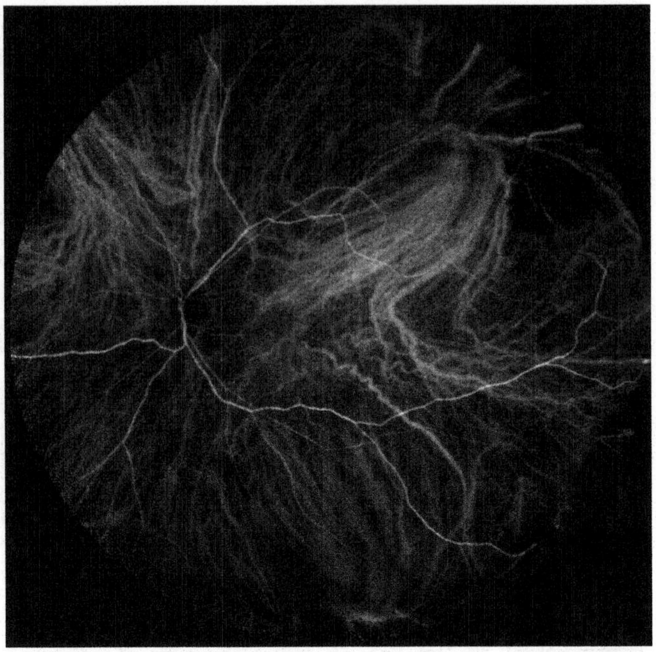

Fig. 12 Non-neovascular AMD. WF ICGA shows blockage from drusen or retinal pigment epithelium (*RPE*) atrophy

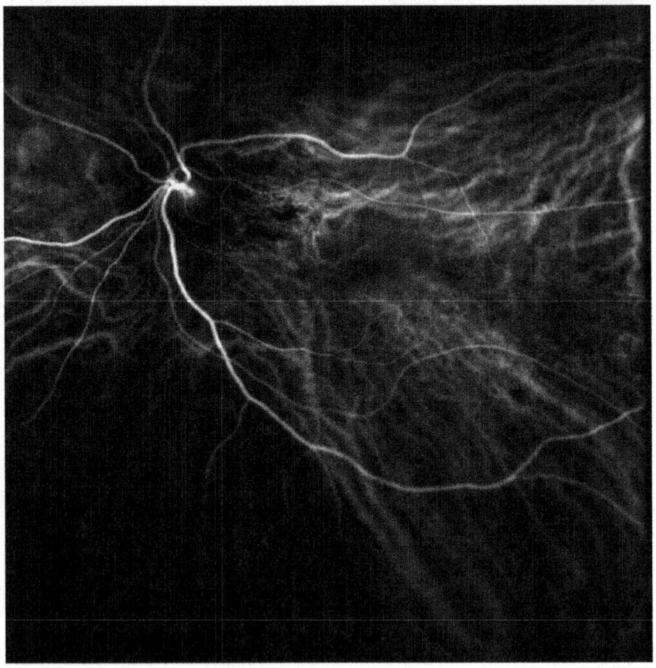

Fig. 13 Polypoidal choroidal vasculopathy. Early Optos UWF-ICGA shows polyps and dilated networks of vessels

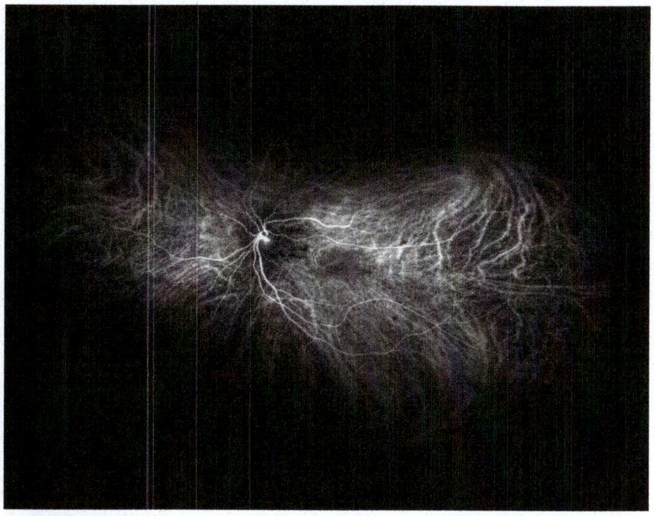

Fig. 14 Polypoidal choroidal vasculopathy. Optos UWF-ICGA shows hyperfluorescence corresponding to the areas of dilated vessels

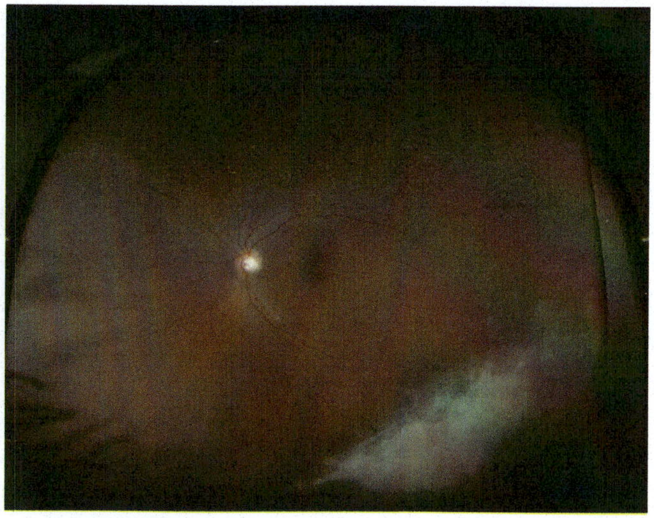

Fig. 16 Syphilis. Optos UWF photo

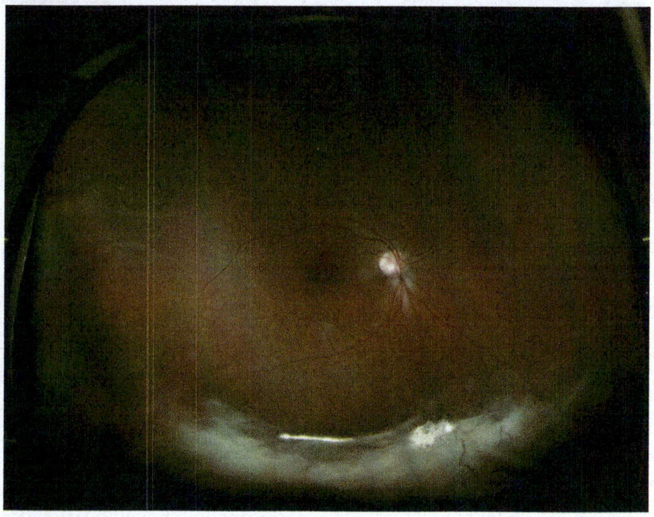

Fig. 15 Syphilis. Optos UWF photo

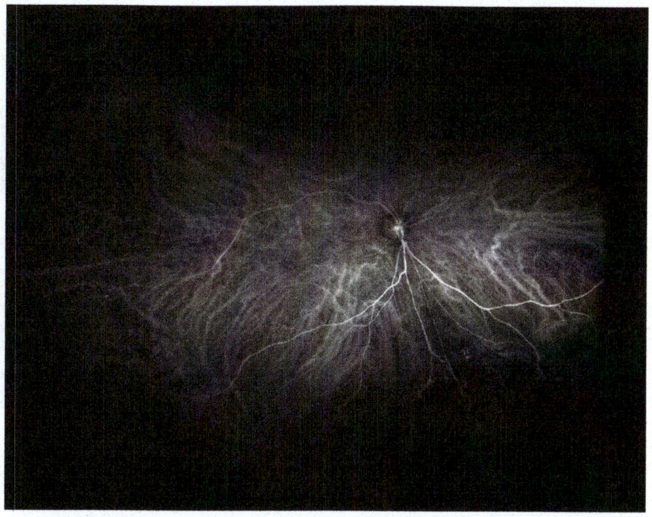

Fig. 17 Syphilis. Mid-phase UWF-ICG of the right eye shows diffuse round areas of hypofluorescence and vascular anastomosis

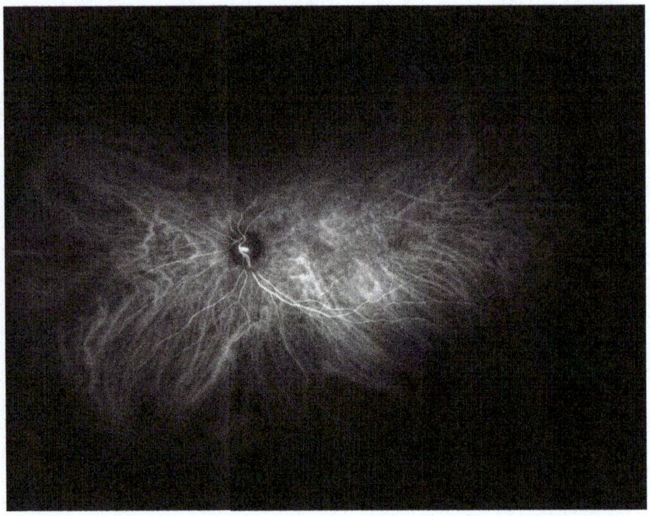

Fig. 18 Tertiary syphilis. Mid-phase UWF-ICG of the left eye shows mild hyperfluorescence consistent with chronic intraretinal cystic changes

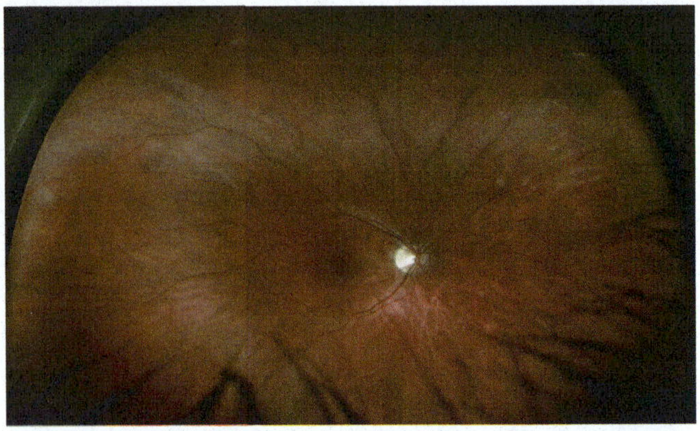

Fig. 19 Sarcoidosis. Optos fundus photograph of the right eye shows multiple chorioretinal lesions in the periphery outside the macula

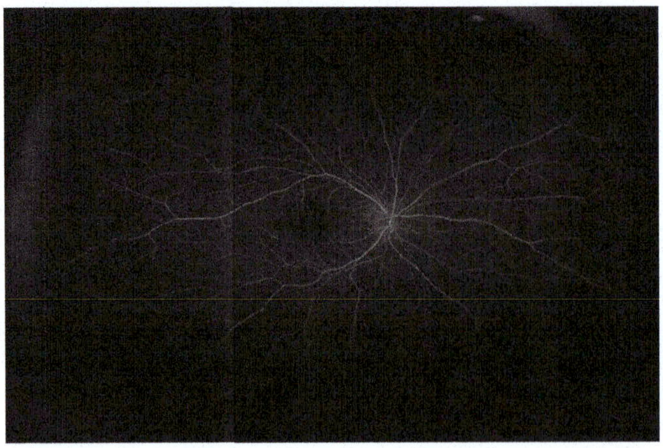

Fig. 20 Sarcoidosis. UWF fluorescein angiogram of the right eye shows blockage by chorioretinal lesions

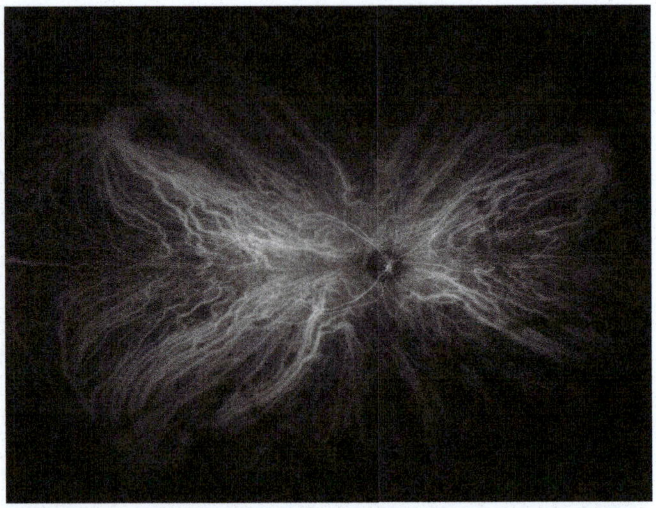

Fig. 21 Sarcoidosis. UWF-ICG of the right eye shows multiple round areas of choroidal hypofluorescence

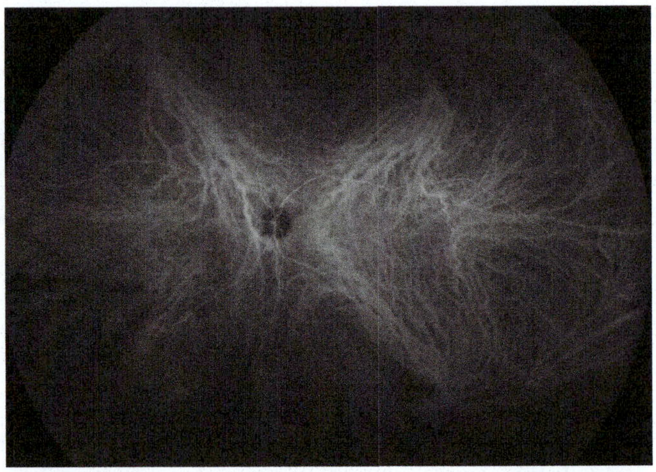

Fig. 22 Birdshot chorioretinopathy. UWF-ICGA of the left eye shows areas of choroidal hypofluorescence corresponding to white lesions on clinical examination

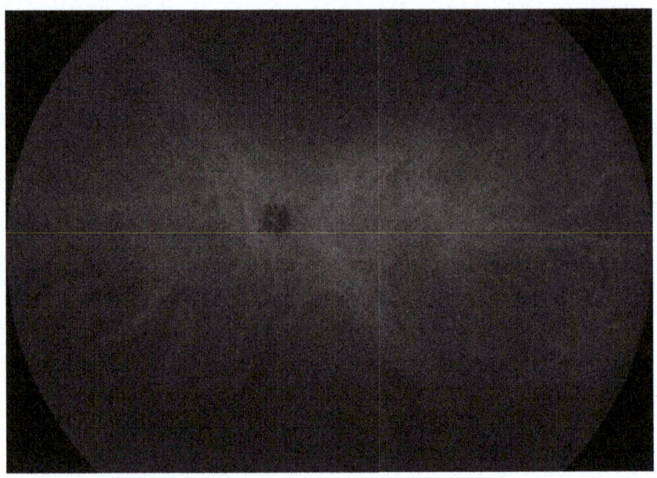

Fig. 23 Birdshot chorioretinopathy. Mid-phase UWF-ICG with choroidal hypofluorescence

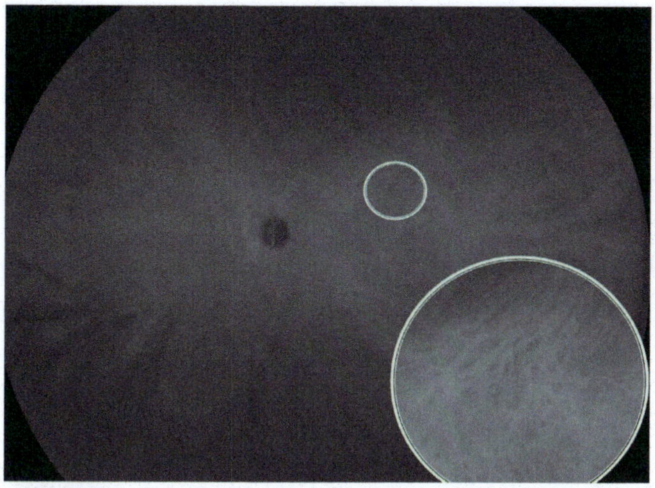

Fig. 24 Birdshot chorioretinopathy. UWF-ICGA of the left eye with close ups that show the areas of choroidal hypofluorescence

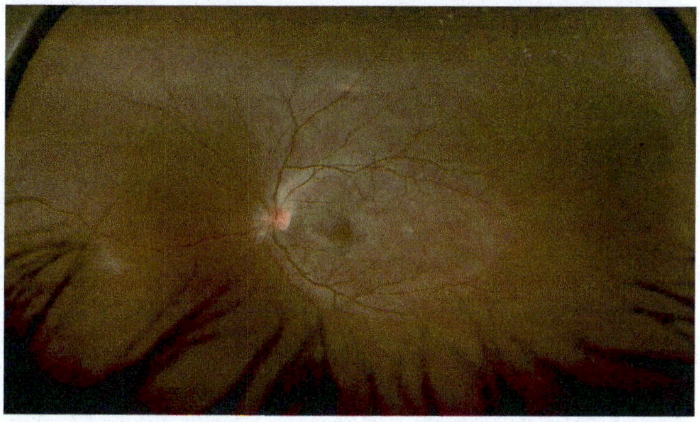

Fig. 25 Uveitis. Optos UWF image of the left eye

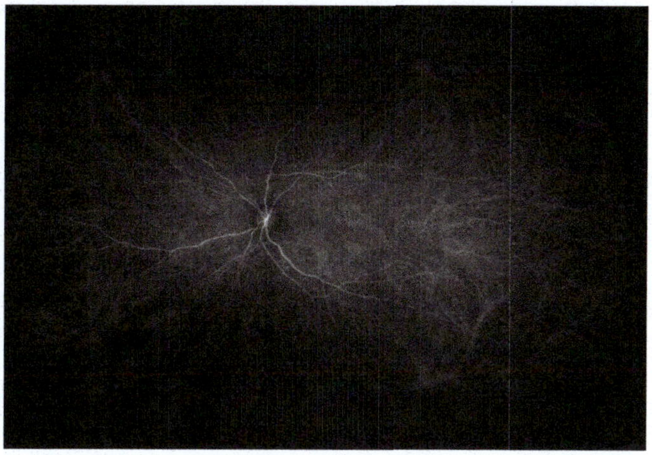

Fig. 26 Uveitis. UWF ICGA showing leakage

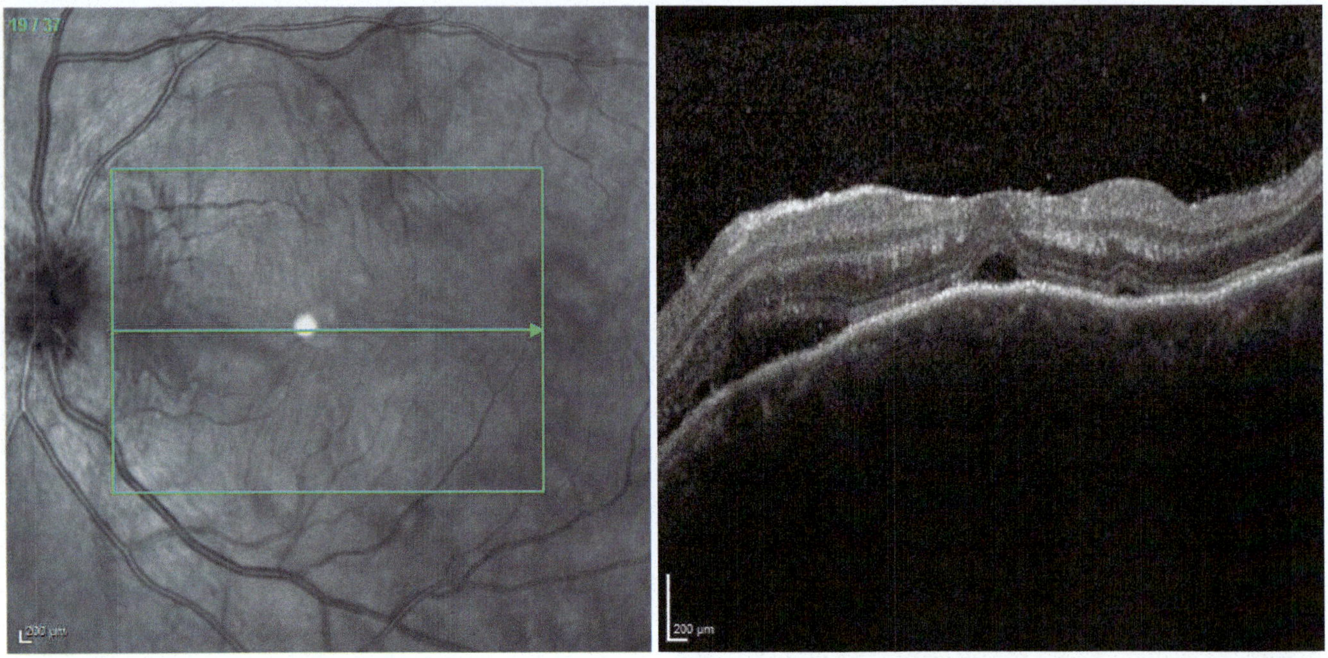

Fig. 27 Uveitis. OCT with subretinal fluid

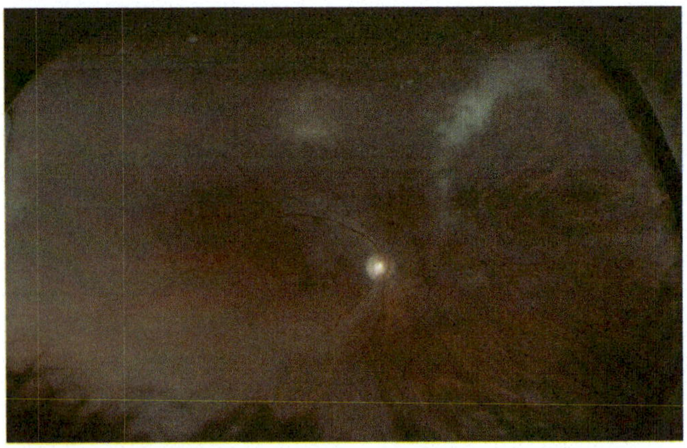

Fig. 28 Cytomegalovirus retinitis Optos wide-field photograph

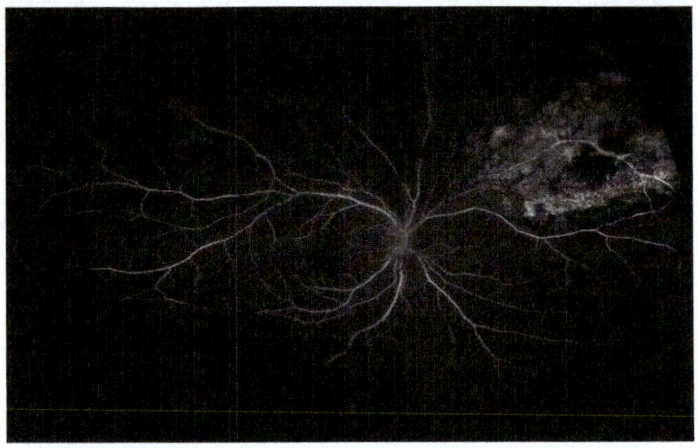

Fig. 30 Cytomegalovirus retinitis. UWF fluorescein angiography shows staining and leakage

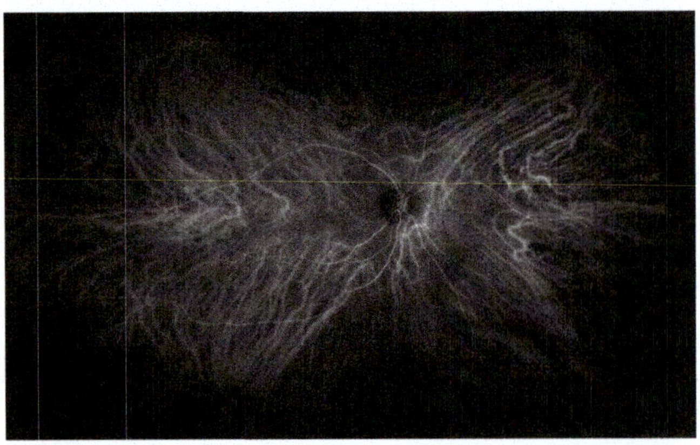

Fig. 29 Cytomegalovirus retinitis. UWF-ICGA shows hypofluorescence corresponding to areas of retinal necrosis in the photograph

References

1. Hochheimer BF. Angiography of the retina with indocyanine green. Arch Ophthalmol. 1971;86:564–5.
2. Flower RW. Injection technique for indocyanine green and sodium fluorescein dye angiography of the eye. Invest Ophthalmol. 1973;12:881–95.
3. Mishra A, Behera RK, Behera PK, Mishra BK, Behera GB. Cyanines during the 1990s: a review. Chem Rev. 2000;100:1973–2011.
4. Alander JT, Kaartinen I, Laakso A, Pätilä T, Spillmann T, Tuchin W, et al. A review of indocyanine green fluorescent imaging in surgery. Int J Biomed Imaging. 2012;2012:940585.
5. Slakter JS, Yannuzzi LA, Guyer DR, Sorenson JA, Orlock DA. Indocyanine-green angiography [review]. Curr Opin Ophthalmol. 1995;6:25–32.
6. Yannuzzi LA, Slakter JS, Sorenson JA, Guyer DR, Orlock DA. Digital indocyanine green videoangiography and choroidal neovascularization. Retina. 1992;12:191–223.
7. Guyer DR, Puliafito CA, Monés JM, Friedman E, Chang W, Verdooner SR. Digital indocyanine-green angiography in chorioretinal disorders. Ophthalmology. 1992;99:287–91.
8. Miwa M, Shikayama T. ICG fluorescence imaging and its medical applications. In: Ye S, Zhang G, Ni J, editors. Proceedings of the 2008 international conference on optical instruments and technology: optoelectronic measurement technology and applications, vol. SPIE-7160. Beijing: The International Society for Optical Engineering; 2009.
9. Hayreh SS. Physiological anatomy of the choroidal vascular bed. Int Ophthalmol. 1983;6:85–93.
10. Ryan SJ, Schachat AP, Wilkinson CP, Hinton DR, Sadda SR, Wiedemann P. Retina. 5th ed. Cambridge: Elsevier Health Sciences; 2012.
11. Guyer C, Yannuzzi LA, Slakter JS, Sorenson JA, Orlock S. The status of indocyanine-green videoangiography. Curr Opin Ophthalmol. 1993;4:3–6.
12. Takahashi K, Muraoka K, Kishi S, Shimizu K. Watershed zone in the human peripheral choroid. Ophthalmology. 1996;103:336–42.
13. Spaide RF, Orlock DA, Herrmann-Delemazure B, Ciardella AP, Yannuzzi LA, Freund KB, et al. Wide-angle indocyanine green angiography. Retina. 1998;18:44–9.
14. Manivannan A, Plskova J, Farrow A, Mckay S, Sharp PF, Forrester JV. Ultra-wide-field fluorescein angiography of the ocular fundus. Am J Ophthalmol. 2005;140:525–7.
15. Klufas MA, Yannuzzi NA, Pang CE, Srinivas S, Sadda SR, Freund KB, et al. Feasibility and clinical utility of ultra-widefield indocyanine green angiography. Retina. 2014;35:508–20.
16. Stanga PE, Lim JL, Hamilton P. Indocyanine green angiography in chorioretinal diseases: an evidence-based update. Ophthalmology. 2003;110:15–21.
17. Yannuzzi LA. Indocyanine green angiography: a perspective on use in the clinical setting. Am J Ophthalmol. 2011;151:745–51.
18. Pang CE, Shah VP, Sarraf D, Freund KB. Ultra-widefield imaging with autofluorescence and indocyanine green angiography in central serous chorioretinopathy. Am J Ophthalmol. 2014;158:362–71.e2.

4 Wide-Field Autofluorescence

Florian M. Heussen, Carmen A. Puliafito, and SriniVas R. Sadda

Fundus autofluorescence (FAF) has seen a remarkable rise in popularity in recent years. It provides high-contrast gray-scale images of the retinal fundus that carry a degree of cellular metabolic information. In principle, it is based on the excitation of fluorophores within the retinal fundus. The major contributing fluorophore is lipofuscin found in the retinal pigment epithelial (RPE) cells [1].

With increasing age, there is a build-up of lipofuscin inside the RPE, comparable with other post-mitotic cell lines. Lipofuscin itself is heterogeneous in nature and results from metabolic breakdown of various substrates like proteins and fatty acids. Its excessive accumulation over time can be regarded as indicator of oxidative cellular stress. One of the attributes of lipofuscin is its photo activity, which is leveraged through autofluorescence imaging.

Light of a certain wavelength, typically between 480 nm (blue light) and 560 nm (green light), is used to excite lipofuscin and induce autofluorescence. Cut-off filters limit the emitted autofluorescent light to a useful spectrum and minimize interference from other autofluorescent sources. This filtered autofluorescent light is captured by an acquisition module and a map of fundus autofluorescence is generated (Figs. 1, 2, and 3) [2].

Areas of altered fundus autofluorescence can be described as hyperfluorescent or hypofluorescent compared with background fluorescence. Because fundus autofluorescence is closely linked to the vitality of the RPE, hyperfluorescence indicates increased oxidative stress to RPE and possible impending cell death, where hypofluorescent areas mark RPE loss as sign of an advanced disease process.

For some diseases, autofluorescence presents in unique patterns and provides valuable information in the differential diagnosis. FAF images should always be considered when making the diagnosis of central serous chorioretinopathy or retinal dystrophies for their pathognomonic appearance in this respect (Figs. 4, 5, 6, and 7). Other diseases, like chloroquine maculopathy and age-related macular degeneration (AMD), benefit greatly from follow-up performed via FAF [3, 4]. Imaging of advanced dry AMD in particular has sparked new discussions on the usefulness of FAF because specific patterns of autofluorescence were identified in the marginal zone of geographic atrophy. Aside from being descriptive of phenotype, these patterns correlate with the rate of disease progression and allow a clinically meaningful characterization of the disease based on FAF [5]. It is imperative though not to isolate fundus autofluorescence from clinical fundus appearance when interpreting areas of hyper- and hypofluorescence (Figs. 14 and 15).

F.M. Heussen, MD
St. Paul's Eye Unit, Royal Liverpool University Hospital, Liverpool, UK
e-mail: florian.heussen@gmail.com

C.A. Puliafito, MD, MBA
Dean of the Keck School of Medicine, Keck School of Medicine, University of Southern California, Los Angeles, CA, USA
e-mail: cpuliafito@usc.edu

S.R. Sadda (✉)
Medical Retina Service, Doheny Eye Institute, Keck School of Medicine, University of Southern California, Los Angeles, CA, USA
e-mail: ssadda@doheny.org

I. Kozak, J.F. Arevalo (eds.), *Atlas of Wide-Field Retinal Angiography and Imaging*, DOI 10.1007/978-3-319-17864-6_4

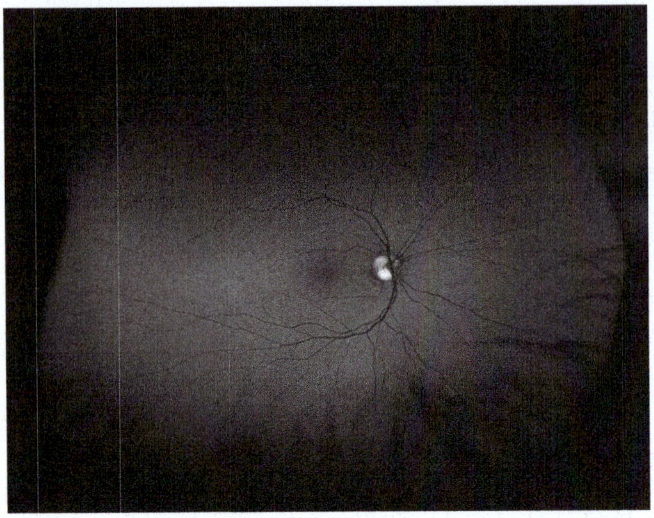

Fig. 1 Almost-normal-looking wide-field FAF image of a right eye. At second look, the optic nerve head appears hyperfluorescent. Clinically, a diagnosis of optic nerve drusen was made

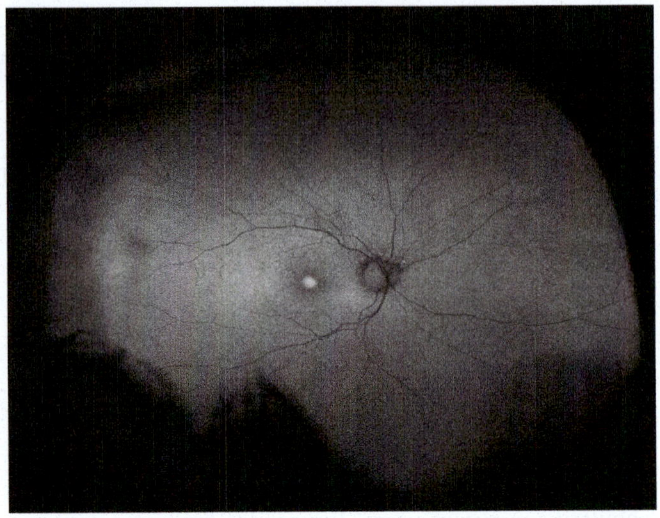

Fig. 2 FAF image of a patient who had been diagnosed with AMD. In conjunction with optical coherence tomography (OCT) images, the hyperfluorescent spot in the center was indicative of pseudovitelliform material, making a diagnosis of pattern dystrophy more likely

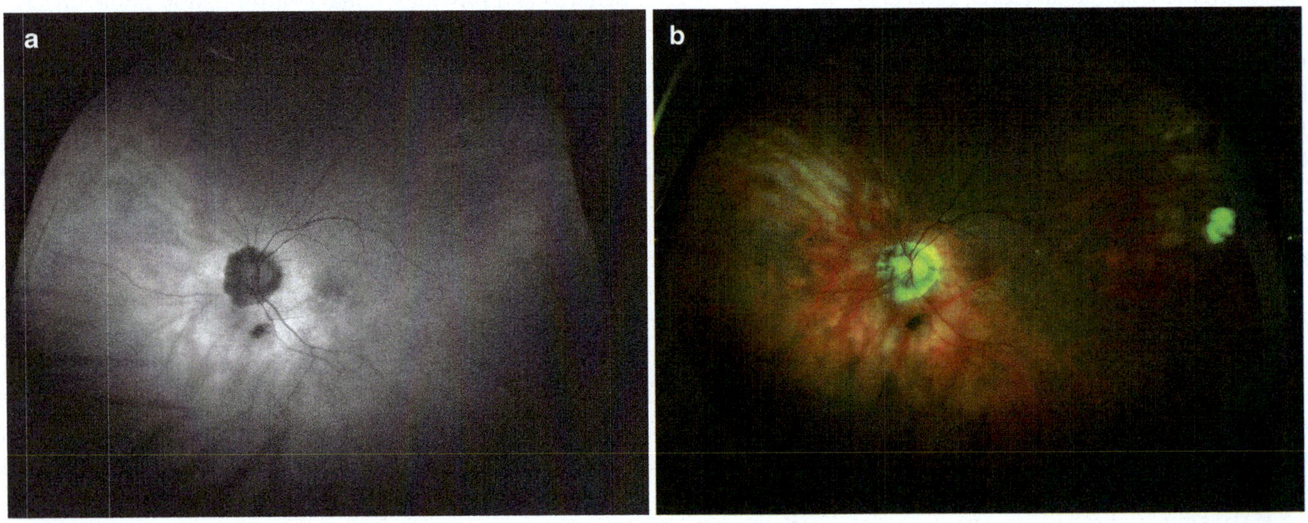

Fig. 3 A myopic fundus on FAF (**a**) and color fundus (**b**). The hypofluorescent ring around the optic nerve head represents peripapillary RPE atrophy. Overall, the background autofluorescence is slightly increased owing to the light pigmentation and increasing visibility of scleral autofluorescence

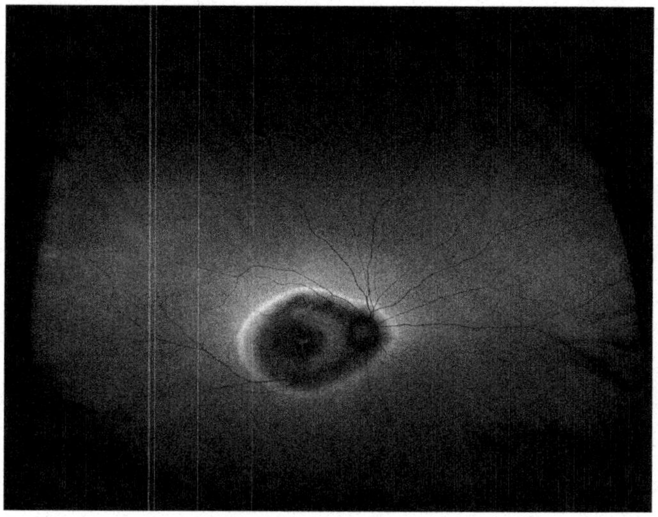

Fig. 4 A patient with cone dystophy. The FAF abnormalities are limited to the posterior pole. Patchy areas of hypofluorescence are indicative of retinal and RPE atrophy, whereas the hyperfluorescent ring around the central pathology most likely represents the area of current disease activity with future atrophy to follow

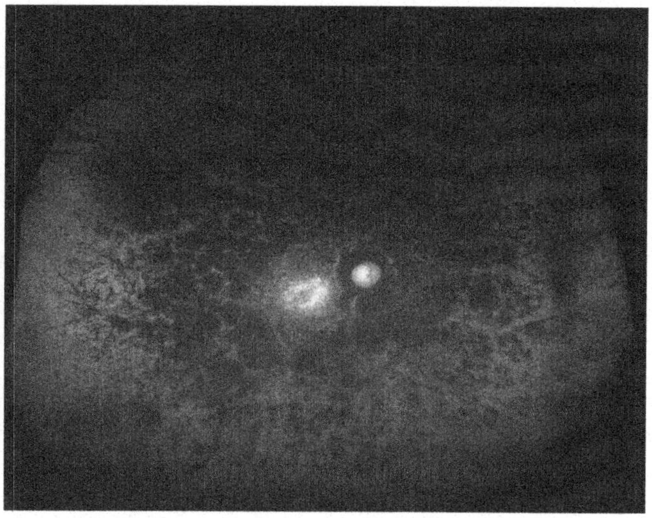

Fig. 6 Another case with severe rod/cone dystrophy. Extreme changes are visible on FAF with almost no healthy retina left

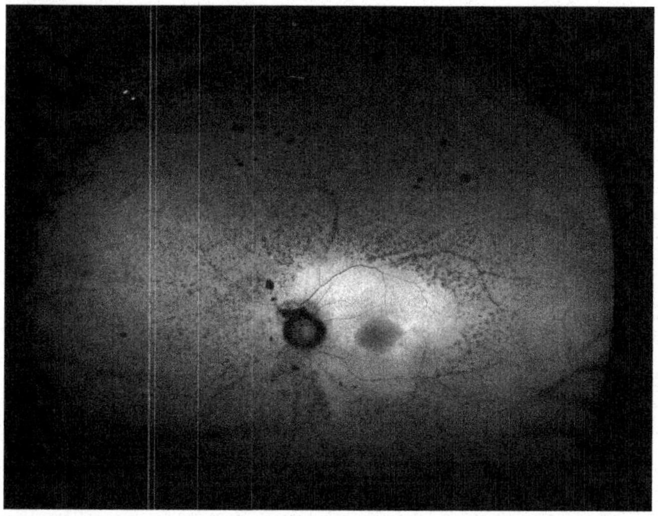

Fig. 5 This patient suffers from retinitis pigmentosa. The central FAF is not normal; however, the most striking changes can be seen peripherally with patchy, spotlike areas of RPE atrophy

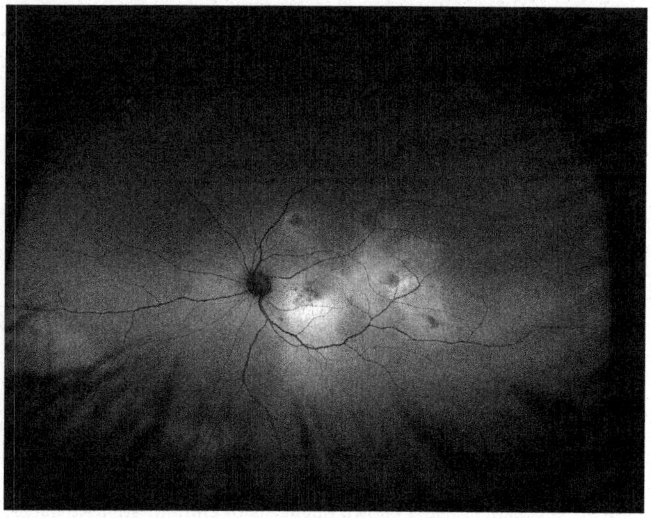

Fig. 7 Typical appearance of multifocal central serious chorioretinopathy. The hyperfluorescent "gutters" are a landmark for chronic subretinal fluid and secondary RPE changes

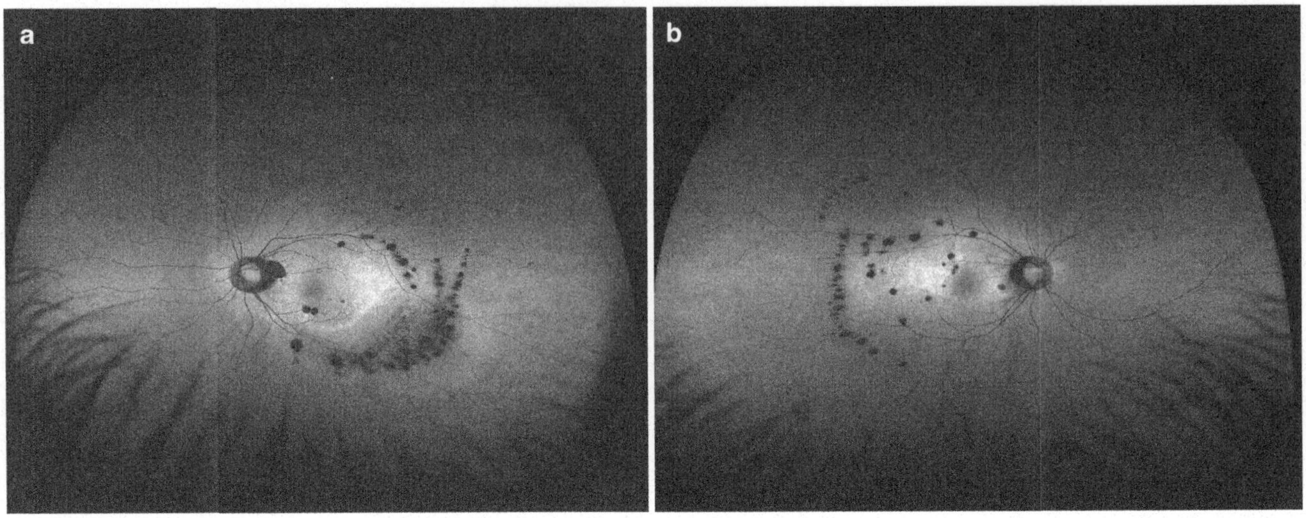

Fig. 8 FAF images of the left (**a**) and right (**b**) eyes show a unique symmetrical array of mid-peripheral scars. This patient was diagnosed with multifocal chorioretinitis

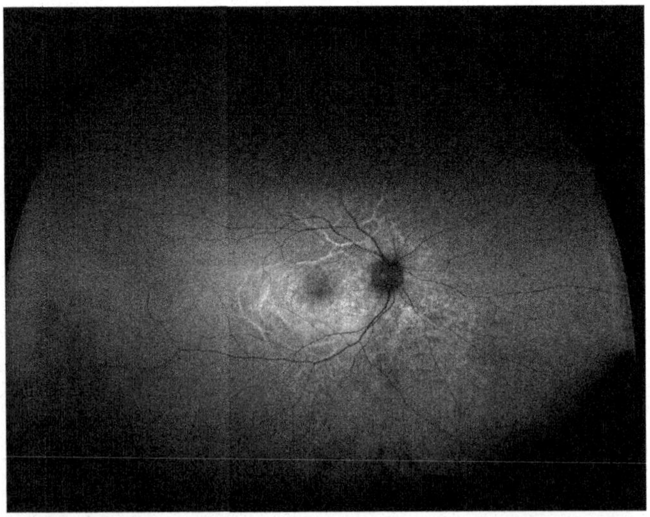

Fig. 9 This patient had a known diagnosis of chronic Vogt-Koyanagi-Harada disease. Striking are the banded hyperfluorescent changes centered around the posterior pole

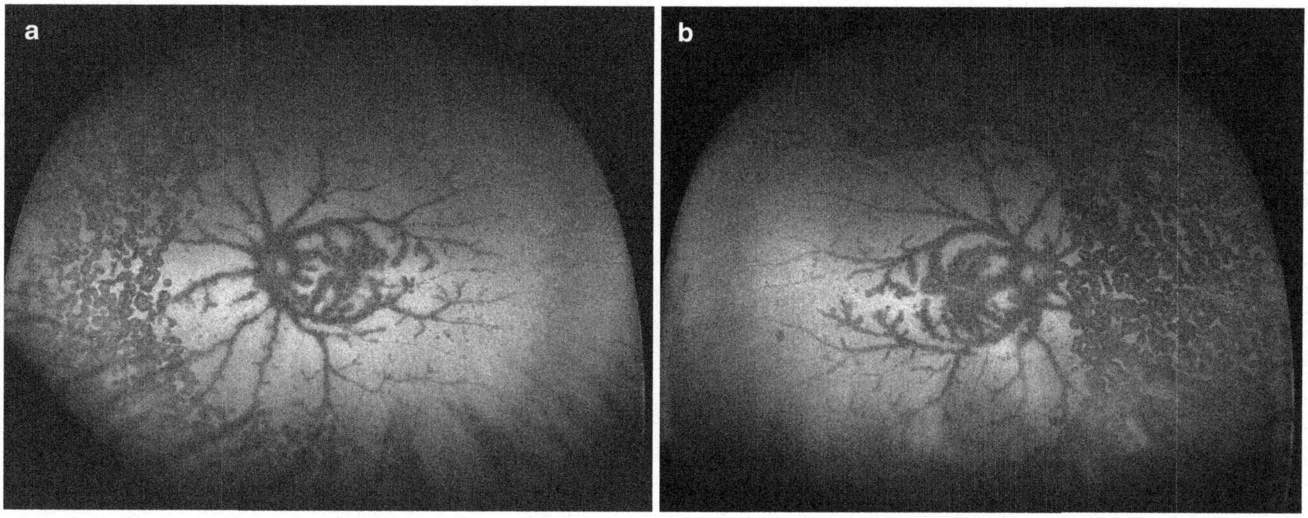

Fig. 10 Both eyes (**a**, *left*; **b**, *right*) of a patient who was diagnosed with idiopathic vasculitis after extensive workup. On top of the paravascular hypofluorescent changes, there are confluent scarlike changes in the nasal periphery as well. The patient had not received retinal laser treatment at any time

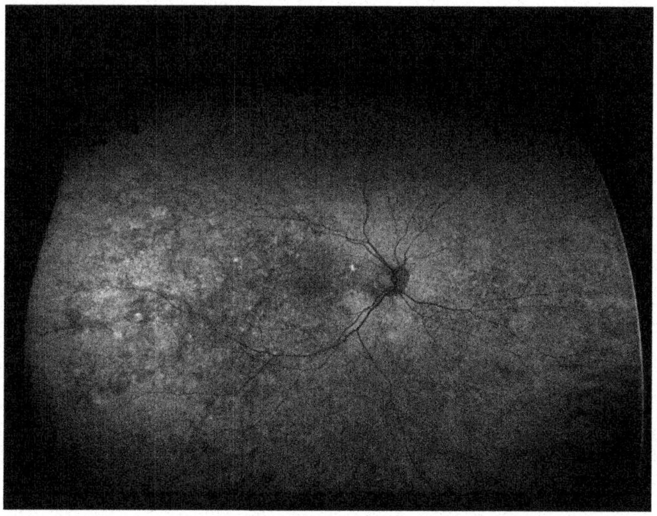

Fig. 11 Ubiquitous FAF changes in a patient with presumed choroideremia. Note the complete loss of normal background autofluorescence

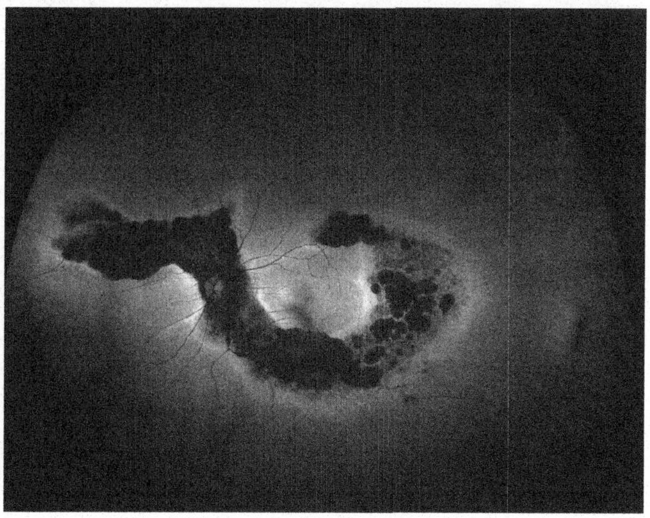

Fig. 12 This unique pattern of FAF changes was seen in a case with presumed pigmented paravenous chorioretinal atrophy

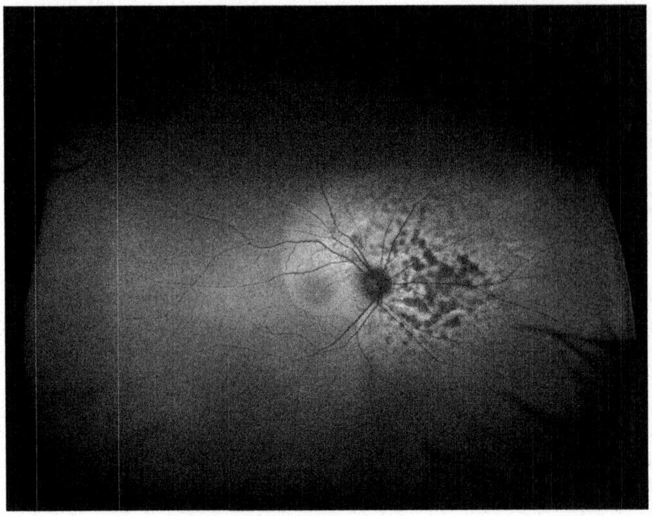

Fig. 13 A patient with a large peripapillary choroidal melanoma. The hyperfluorescence overlying the tumor can be a sign of orange pigment or chronic subretinal fluid accumulation

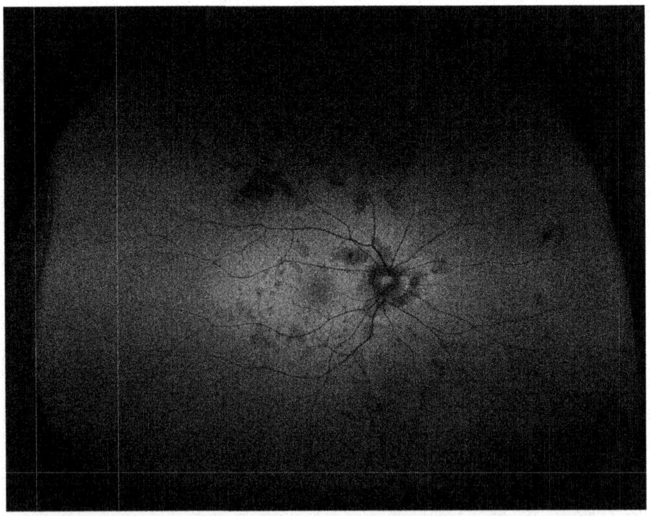

Fig. 14 Patchy loss of background FAF. In accordance with other clinical features, the diagnosis of atypical acute posterior multifocal placoid pigment epitheliopathy was made

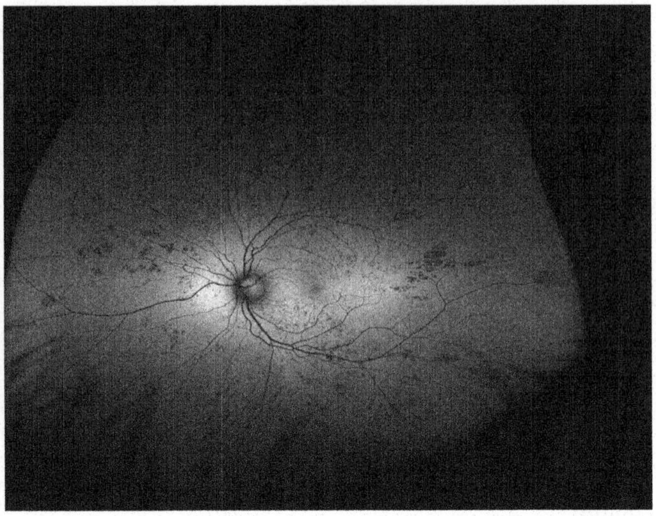

Fig. 15 Similar in appearance to the patient in Fig. 14, this patient had suffered from a central retinal vein occlusion. The dark areas are caused by retinal hemorrhages. This shows how important a correlation between FAF findings and funduscopy is

Ultra-wide Field

To date, most of the clinical and scientific work in FAF imaging has been restricted to the central 20–30° of the retinal fundus. This narrow focus on the posterior pole is likely rooted in hardware limitations that still pervade to this day. In principle, FAF acquisition is possible with almost any optical system. It requires an appropriate excitation light source and bandwidth filters for the emitted autofluorescent light in the acquisition module. Confocal scanning laser ophthalmoscopes and flash cameras are by far the most common devices used in FAF imaging. Both possess unique advantages but are typically generally limited by their field of view.

More recently, an ultra-wide-field scanning laser ophthalmoscope with FAF capability was introduced. Via a complex optical setup with ellipsoid mirrors, single-fundus images from posterior pole to ora serrata are possible. For one, this gives access to fundus areas that were previously inaccessible by FAF imaging. Initial reports revealed that diseases that were thought to be strictly macular presented with distinct peripheral changes on FAF [6]. The broader fundus view given by wide-field images can also help to discern logical patterns in the oftentimes confusing mix of FAF changes. For example, peripheral FAF abnormalities are very common in inflammatory diseases, such as Harada's disease [7]. But because the term "inflammatory diseases" brings together a very heterogeneous group of diseases, the FAF changes are manifold in variety. In cases like these, wide-field imaging can help practitioners to see the broader picture (Figs. 8, 9, 10, 11, and 12). So-called orange pigment in the often peripherally located choroidal melanoma lights up on autofluorescence, which enables a better differentiation from choroidal naevi (Fig. 13). A wide-field view is also of value in diseases such as central serous chorioretinopathy, where "gutter-like" disturbances in the RPE are easily revealed (Fig. 7) [8]. Retinal degenerative disorders represent another class of diseases in which FAF patterns can be diagnostic (Figs. 4, 5, and 6) [9]. Finally, various patterns of abnormal peripheral FAF appear to be more common in patients with advanced AMD (Fig. 16, 17, 18, 19, and 20) [10]. Larger, longitudinal studies, however, are required to fully define the clinical relevance of these observations. Regardless, one can expect that the importance of wide-field FAF imaging will continue.

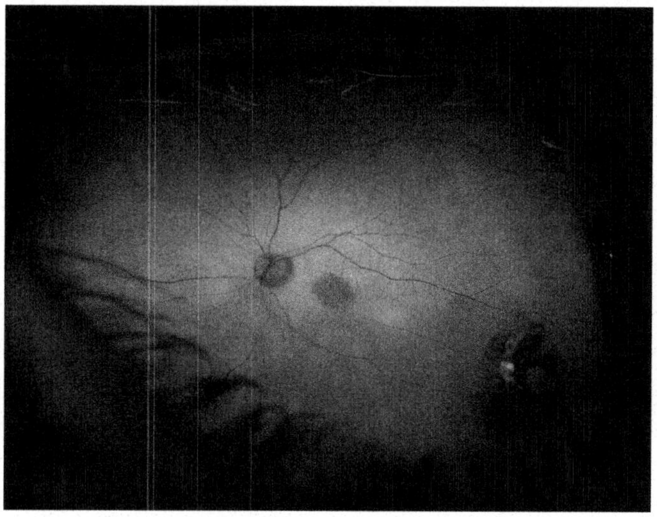

Fig. 16 This patient suffered from advanced dry AMD with central atrophy and noticed a further worsening of vision. Peripherally, a choroidal neovascularization (CNV) is visible. The heterogeneous FAF changes seen on the image are typical for CNV lesions. The overall image quality is reduced owing to a slight vitreous hemorrhage

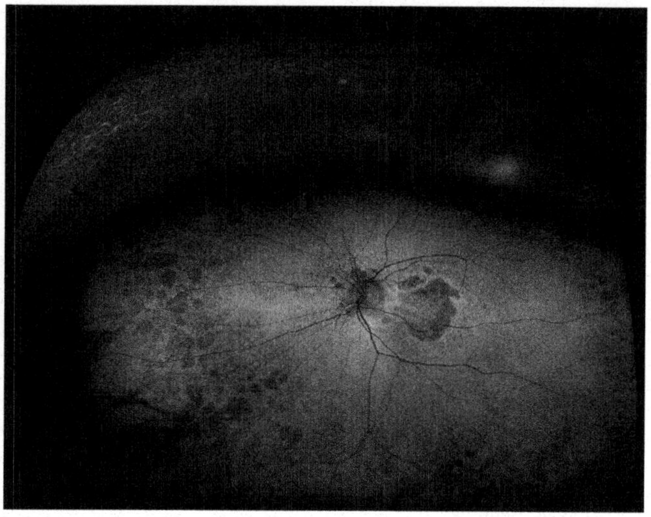

Fig. 17 The FAF image shows extensive areas of hypofluorescence, which coincide with areas of RPE atrophy. The patient had been diagnosed with advanced dry AMD with geographic atrophy. Remarkable is the extent of peripheral changes

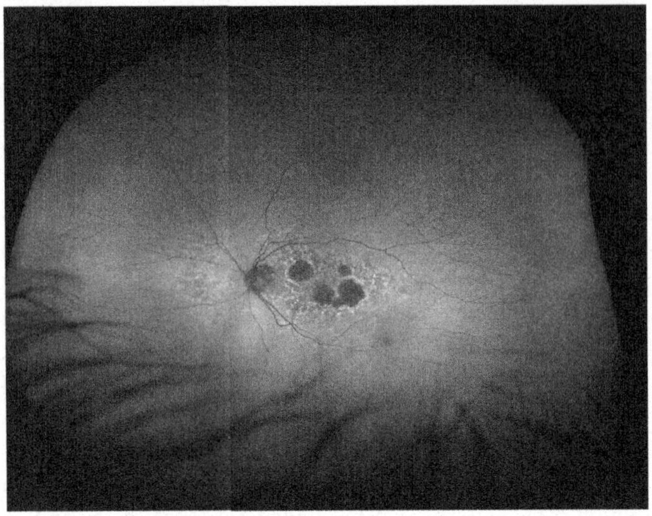

Fig. 18 Another case with geographic atrophy centrally. There are mid-peripheral changes nasal to the optic disc as well, but these are much more subtle than those shown in Fig. 17

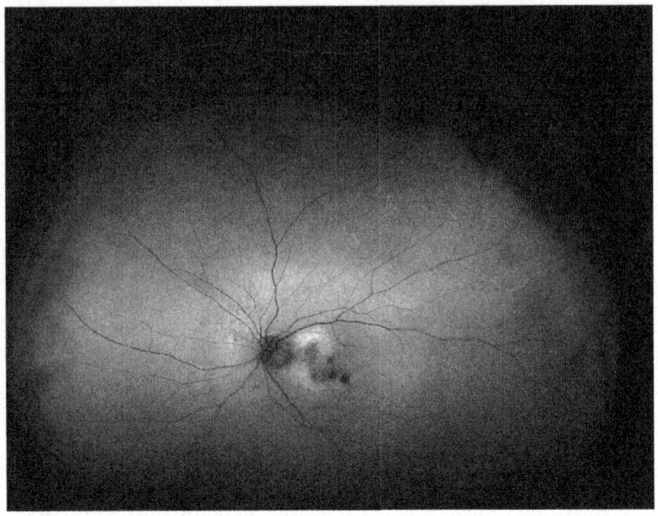

Fig. 20 A patient with neovascular AMD. Peripherally, there is an interesting pattern of lacelike hyperfluorescence with unclear clinical significance

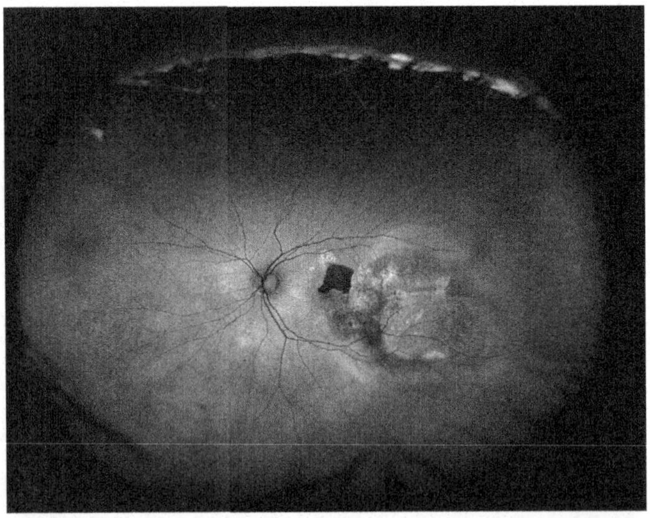

Fig. 19 This FAF image is from a patient with neovascular AMD. Centrally, there is very heterogeneous autofluorescence with mixed hyper- and hypofluorescence. The area of uniform hypofluorescence centrally could be blockage from a hemorrhage and requires funduscopic correlation

References

1. Delori FC, Dorey CK, Staurenghi G, Arend O, Goger DG, Weiter JJ. In vivo fluorescence of the ocular fundus exhibits retinal pigment epithelium lipofuscin characteristics. Invest Ophthalmol Vis Sci. 1995;36:718–29.
2. Schmitz-Valckenberg S, Holz FG, Bird AC, Spaide RF. Fundus autofluorescence imaging: review and perspectives. Retina. 2008;28:385–409.
3. Kellner U, Renner AB, Tillack H. Fundus autofluorescence and mfERG for early detection of retinal alterations in patients using chloroquine/hydroxychloroquine. Invest Ophthalmol Vis Sci. 2006;47:3531–8.
4. Schmitz-Valckenberg S, Brinkmann CK, Alten F, Herrmann P, Stratmenn NK, Göbel AP, et al. Semiautomated image processing method for identification and quantification of geographic atrophy in age-related macular degeneration. Invest Ophthalmol Vis Sci. 2011;52:7640–6.
5. Fleckenstein M, Schmitz-Valckenberg S, Martens C, Kosanetzky S, Brinkmann GK, Hageman GS, et al. Fundus autofluorescence and spectral-domain optical coherence tomography characteristics in a rapidly progressing form of geographic atrophy. Invest Ophthalmol Vis Sci. 2011;52:3761–6.
6. Heussen FM, Tan CS, Sadda SR. Prevalence of peripheral abnormalities on ultra-widefield greenlight (532 nm) autofluorescence imaging at a tertiary care center. Invest Ophthalmol Vis Sci. 2012;53:6526–31.
7. Heussen FM, Vasconcelos-Santos DV, Pappuru RR, Walsh AC, Rao NA, Sadda SR. Ultra-wide-field green-light (532-nm) autofluorescence imaging in chronic Vogt-Koyanagi-Harada disease. Ophthalmic Surg Lasers Imaging. 2011;42:272–7.
8. Pang CE, Shah VP, Sarraf D, Freund KB. Ultra-widefield imaging with autofluorescence and indocyanine green angiography in central serous chorioretinopathy. Am J Ophthalmol. 2014;158:362–71.e2.
9. Oishi A, Ogino K, Makiyama Y, Nakagawa S, Kurimoto M, Yoshimura N. Wide-field fundus autofluorescence imaging of retinitis pigmentosa. Ophthalmology. 2013;120:1827–34.
10. Tan CS, Heussen F, Sadda SR. Peripheral autofluorescence and clinical findings in neovascular and non-neovascular age-related macular degeneration. Ophthalmology. 2013;120:1271–7.

Wide-Field Retinal Imaging of Diabetic Retinopathy

5

J. Fernando Arevalo, Igor Kozak, and The KKESH Collaborative Retina Study Group*

Diabetic Retinopathy and Ultra-Wide-Field Fluorescein Angiography

Diabetic retinopathy (DR) is one of the diseases in which identifying pathology in the retinal periphery is of crucial importance. Posterior pole fluorescein angiography has been integral to the management of DR, in which it can reveal microaneurysms, nonperfusion, macular edema, and neovascularization. Because much of the abnormality in DR, especially nonperfusion, can occur in the mid periphery and periphery [1], ultra-wide-field imaging may be particularly useful in the evaluation of this condition. In a previous report, Wessel et al. [2] by overlaying a 7-standard field (7SF) template on the ultra-wide-field fluorescein angiography (UWFA) found that UWFA showed 3.2 times the amount of retinal area, 3.9 times the amount of retinal nonperfusion, 1.9 times the area of neovascularization, and 3.8 times the area of panretinal photocoagulation (PRP), compared with the simulated 7SF image. Another study showed that UWFA imaged significantly more retinal area and revealed more ischemia than fluorescein angiography using conventional digital acquisition systems [3]. It is not uncommon for DR patients with prior PRP to see on UWFA large fronds of neovascularization and peripheral ischemic retina, only part of which had previous laser treatment. Frequently, most of this is located outside the 7SF. On the basis of UWFA, patients may further undergo targeted PRP to the untreated peripheral ischemic areas (Figs. 1, 2, 3, 4, 5, 6, 7, 8, 9, 10, 11, 12, 13, 14, 15, 16, 17, and 18).

A small but significant proportion of patients (10 %) in the study by Wessel et al. [2] had normal 7SF fluorescein angiography with positive findings on UWFA, suggesting that UWFA may allow us to diagnose lesions previously missed by standard fluorescein angiography. Because the study was a retrospective review of all patients who underwent UWFA imaging, there may be a selection bias for patients more likely to exhibit peripheral abnormality, such that the true rate of missing abnormality with standard imaging may be lower in practice. Nevertheless, the study highlighted that UWFA demonstrates more abnormality than 7SF imaging and that the added retina visualized with UWFA can significantly change the qualitative assessment of the degree of retinopathy. The study suggested that UWFA expands our view of the periphery without significantly compromising the imaging of central abnormality because only 5.4 % of patients with clinically significant macular edema exhibited no macular edema on UWFA [2].

Prior studies suggest that mid-peripheral nonperfusion, as noted on standard fluorescein angiography, is associated with neovascularization [4]. More recently, Oliver and Schwartz [5] demonstrated that peripheral nonperfusion, which was present in 54 % of DR patients imaged by UWFA, was associated with increased risk of neovascularization, including neovascularization anterior to the equator and neovascularization posterior to the equator. Peripheral nonperfusion on UWFA was also associated with macular ischemia, although not macular edema. The group also noted a finding of late peripheral vascular leakage, which was associated both with peripheral nonperfusion and with neovascularization, especially posterior neovascularization. UWFA has been shown to demonstrate peripheral nonperfusion better

J.F. Arevalo, MD, FACS (✉)
Edmund F. and Virginia B. Ball Professor of Ophthalmology, Chairman, Department of Ophthalmology, Johns Hopkins Bayview Medical Center, Retina Division, Wilmer Eye Institute, The Johns Hopkins University School of Medicine, Baltimore, MD, USA
e-mail: arevalojf@jhmi.edu

I. Kozak, MD, PhD
Senior Academic Consultant, Vitreoretinal Division, King Khaled Eye Specialist Hospital, Riyadh, Kingdom of Saudi Arabia
e-mail: ikozak@kkesh.med.sa

I. Kozak, J.F. Arevalo (eds.), *Atlas of Wide-Field Retinal Angiography and Imaging*, DOI 10.1007/978-3-319-17864-6_5

than standard fluorescein angiography [6], and this, as well as the finding of peripheral vascular leakage, correlated to visually significant and treatable complications such as neovascularization [5]. UWFA may be useful in identifying patients who have not yet developed neovascularization or macular edema but are at increased risk to do so, based on the presence of extensive peripheral nonperfusion or vascular leakage. These patients may, in turn, warrant more frequent follow-up than might have been recommended using traditional fluorescein angiography imaging modalities.

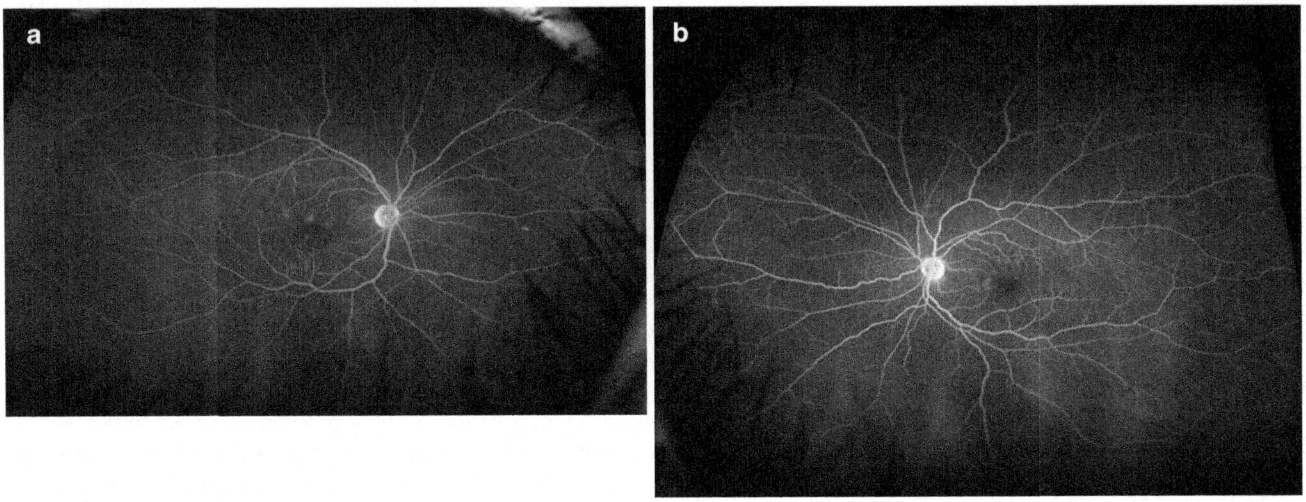

Fig. 1 (**a**) Mild nonproliferative DR. Wide-field fundus color images of the right eye of a 55-year-old woman with controlled type 2 diabetes shows few microaneurysms in the posterior pole and nasal mid periphery. (**b**) Mild nonproliferative DR. Wide-field fundus color images of the left eye of the same patient shows few microaneurysms in the posterior pole

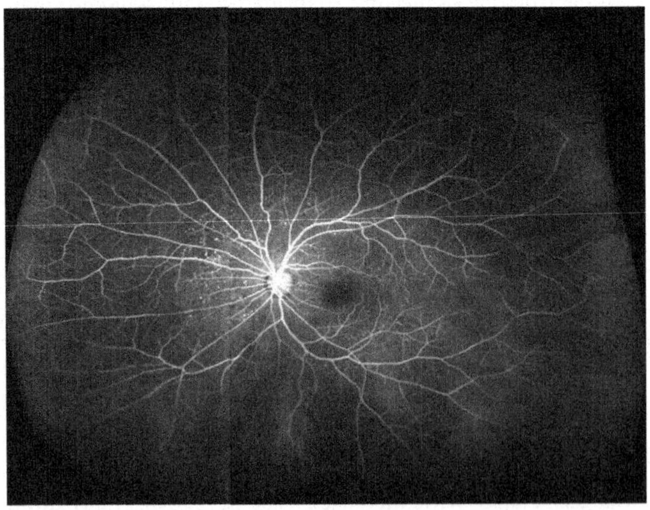

Fig. 2 Mild nonproliferative DR. Wide-field fundus color images of the right eye of a 60-year-old man with a history of primary open-angle glaucoma in both eyes shows scattered microaneurysms around the optic disc and outside the vascular arcades

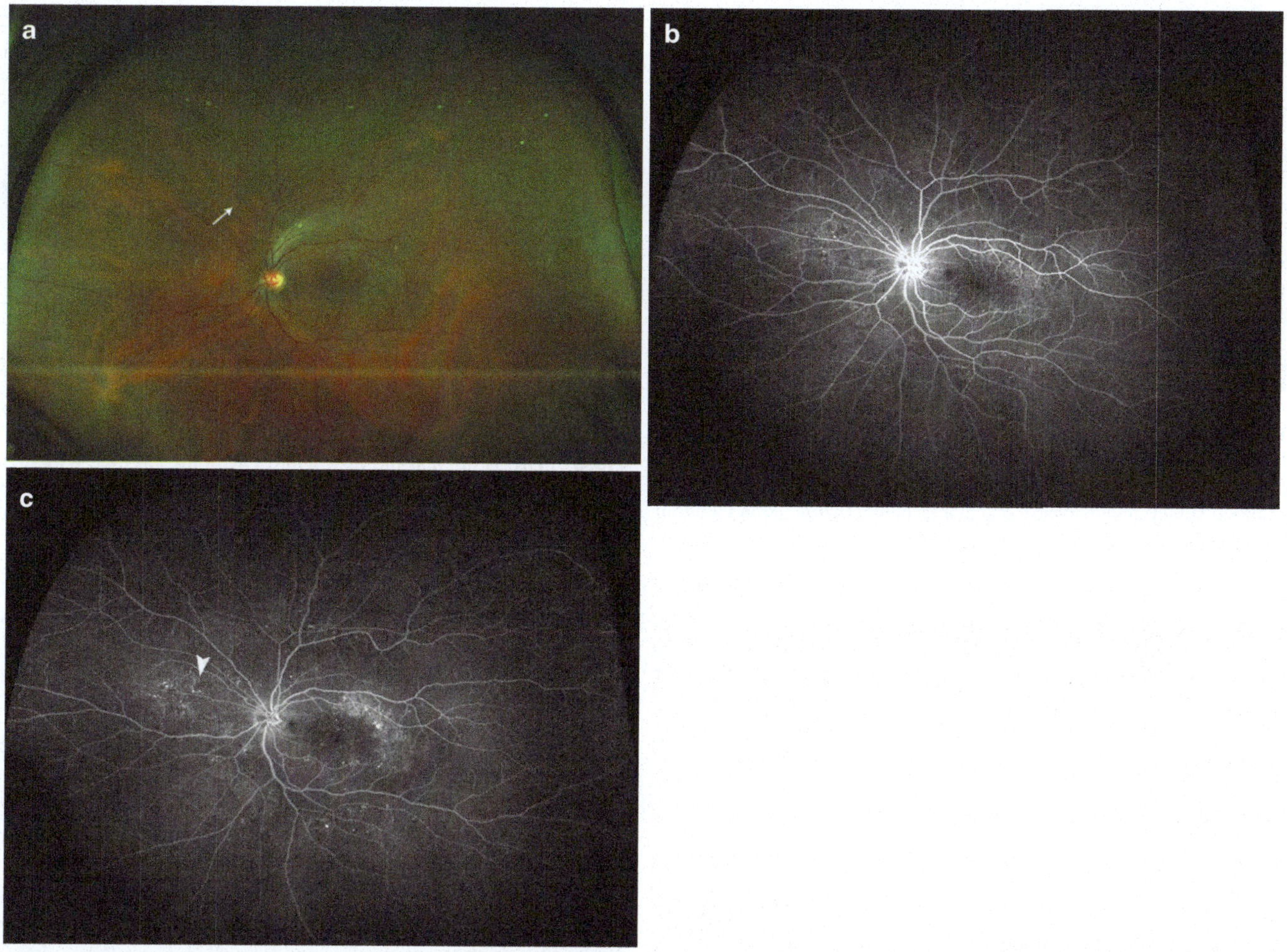

Fig. 3 (**a**) Moderate nonproliferative DR. A 56-year-old man with a history of DR and bevacizumab intravitreal injection for clinically significant macular edema in his left eye. Wide-field fundus color images of the left eye demonstrate several microaneurysms (*white arrow*). (**b**) Moderate nonproliferative DR. Wide-field early fundus fluorescein angiogram of the same eye demonstrates numerous microaneurysms and areas of capillary drop-out nasally. (**c**) Moderate nonproliferative DR. Wide-field late fundus fluorescein angiogram of the same eye demonstrates numerous microaneurysms, diffuse extramacular leak, and areas of capillary drop-out (*white arrowhead*)

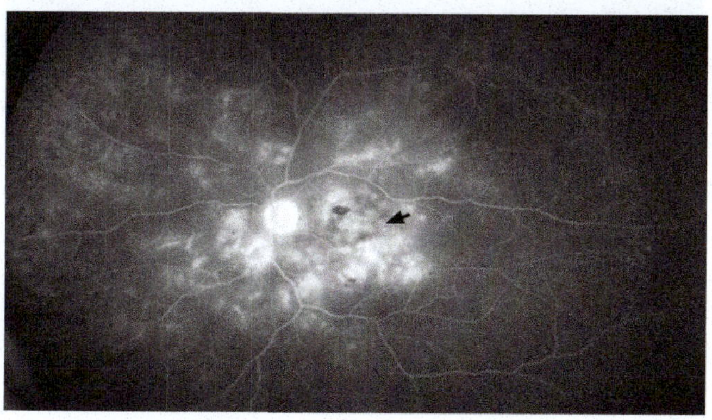

Fig. 4 Severe nonproliferative DR. A 73-year-old woman has a history of DR for 20 years and numerous intravitreal injections for clinically significant macular edema in her left eye. Wide-field fundus fluorescein angiogram of her left eye demonstrates areas of abnormal retinal pigment epithelium and severe macular edema (*black arrow*) but no neovascularization

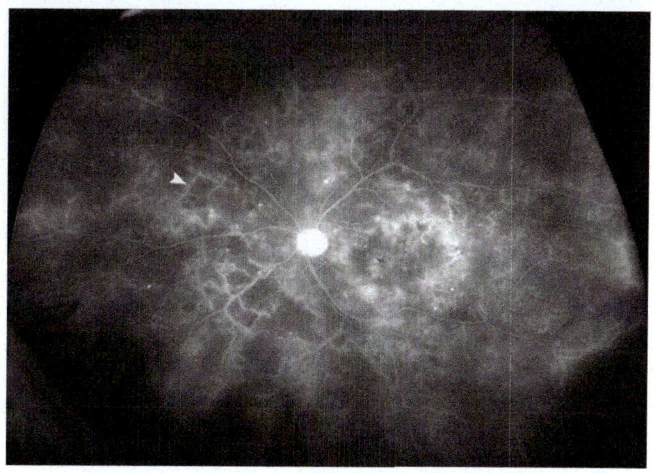

Fig. 5 Severe nonproliferative DR. A 38-year-old diabetic man with DR has slightly decreased vision in his left eye. Wide-field fundus fluorescein angiogram of his left eye demonstrates macular edema and extensive areas of retinal nonperfusion (*white arrow head*) in all quadrants but no neovascularization

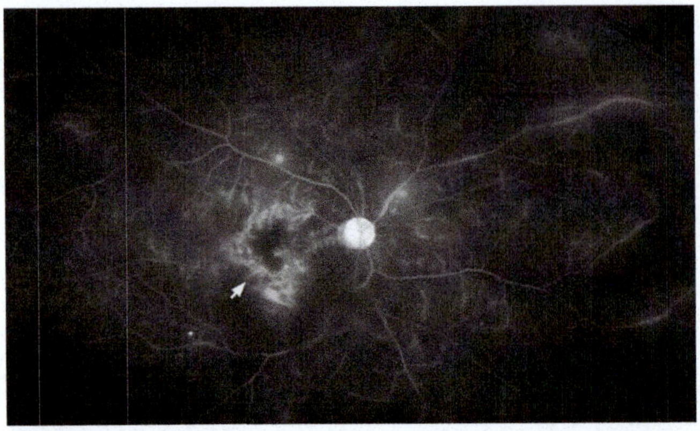

Fig. 6 Severe nonproliferative DR. A 48-year-old diabetic man has a history of DR and decreased visual acuity in his right eye. Wide-field fundus fluorescein angiogram of his right eye demonstrates sheathing of blood vessels and extensive macular ischemia (*white arrow*) without neovascularization

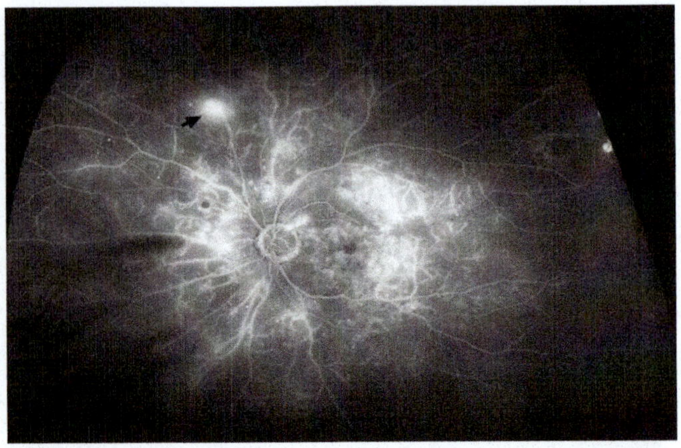

Fig. 8 PDR. A 60-year-old man with PDR in his left eye. Wide-field fundus fluorescein angiogram of his left eye demonstrates macular edema, areas of capillary nonperfusion nasally, and NVE (*black arrow*)

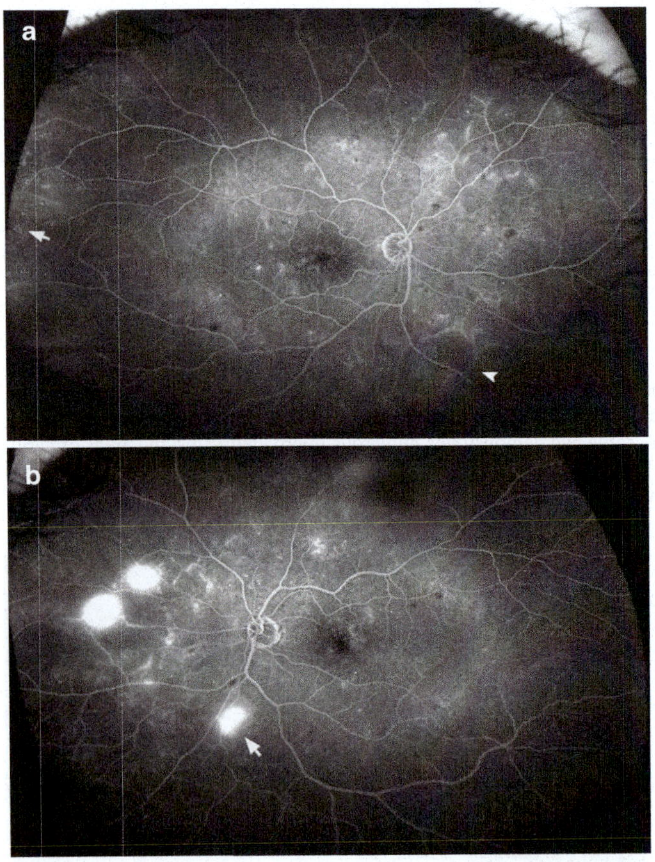

Fig. 7 (**a**) Bilateral DR. A 63-year-old diabetic man presented with DR in both eyes. Wide-field fundus fluorescein angiogram of the right eye demonstrates severe nonproliferative retinopathy with macular edema, capillary nonperfusion (*white arrowhead*), and numerous mid-peripheral and peripheral microaneurysms (*white arrow*) without neovascularization. (**b**) Bilateral DR. Wide-field fundus fluorescein angiogram of the left eye of the same patient demonstrates proliferative retinopathy with some macular edema and neovascularization elsewhere (NVE) (*white arrow*)

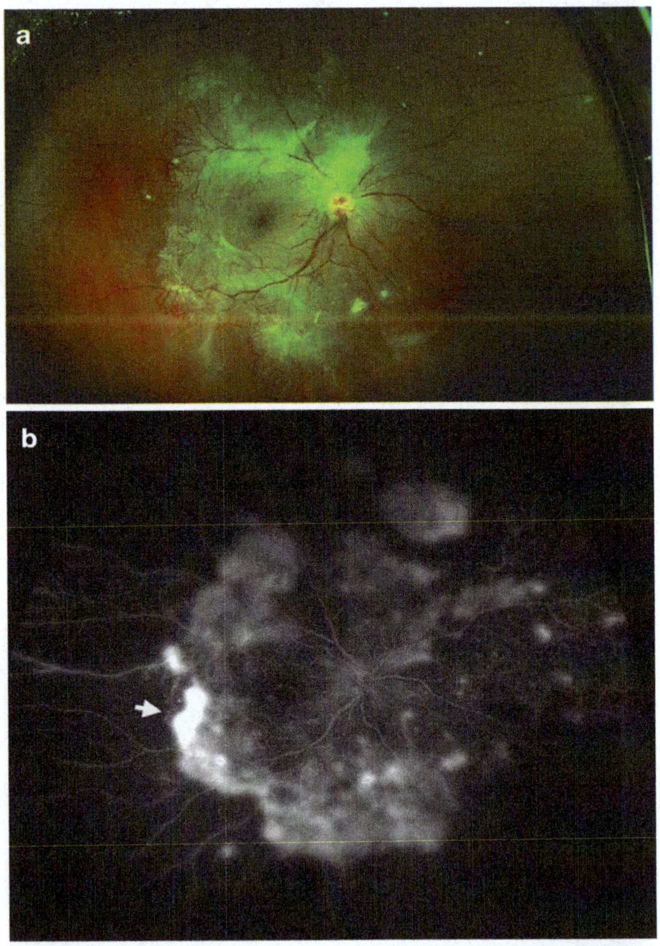

Fig. 9 (**a**) PDR. A 47-year-old diabetic woman with chronic PDR in her right eye. Wide-field fundus photography of her right eye demonstrates fibrovascular membrane with florid neovascularization. Visual acuity is 20/30. (**b**) PDR. Wide-field fundus fluorescein angiogram of the same eye demonstrates severe neovascularization (*white arrow*) and peripheral retinal nonperfusion

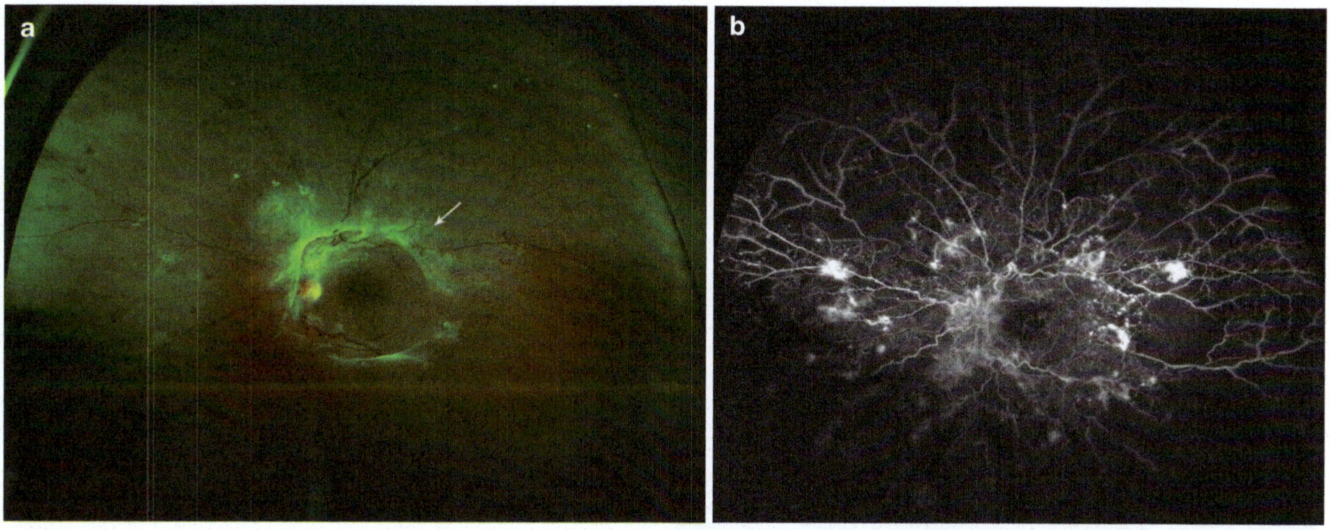

Fig. 10 (**a**) PDR. A 42-year-old diabetic woman with chronic PDR in her left eye. Wide-field fundus photography of her left eye demonstrates fibrovascular membrane with florid neovascularization (*white arrow*). Visual acuity is 2/200. (**b**) PDR. Wide-field fundus fluorescein angiogram of the same eye demonstrates severe widespread neovascularization, an island of macular ischemia, and large areas of retinal nonperfusion

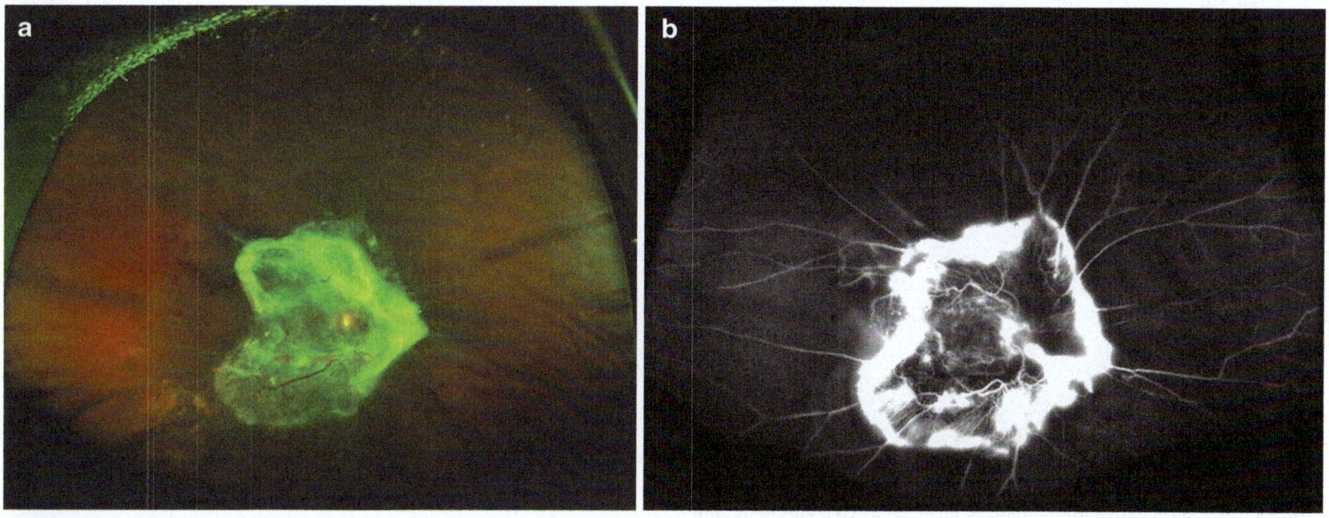

Fig. 11 (**a**) PDR with fibrovascular membrane. A 42-year-old woman with decompensated diabetes and PDR in her right eye. Wide-field fundus photography of her right eye demonstrates aggressive fibrovascular membrane and ischemic retinal vessels. (**b**) PDR with fibrovascular membrane. Wide-field fundus fluorescein angiogram of the same eye demonstrates severe neovascularization of the preretinal membrane, traction on retinal blood vessels, and extensive retinal ischemia

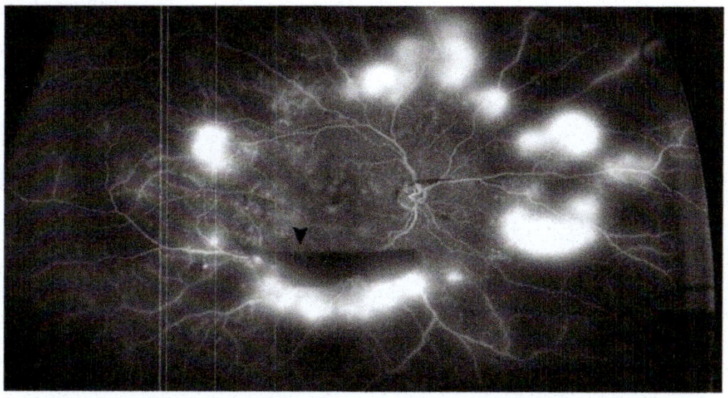

Fig. 12 Severe neovascularization with preretinal hemorrhage. A 58-year-old man with PDR in his right eye. Wide-field fundus fluorescein angiogram demonstrates extensive neovascularization with layered preretinal hemorrhage (*black arrowhead*)

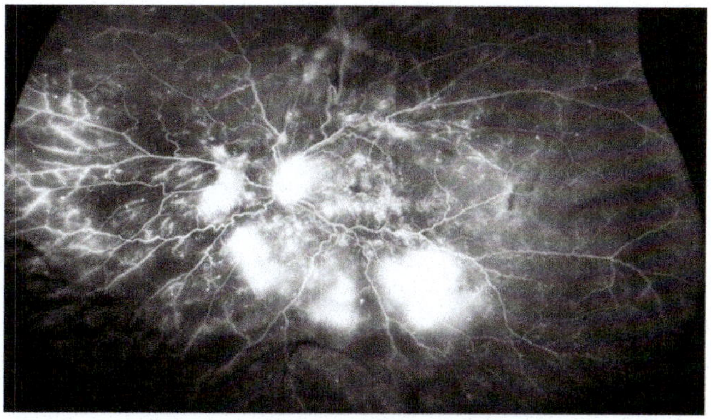

Fig. 13 Aggressive PDR. A 29-year-old woman with type 1 diabetes mellitus aggressive form of retinopathy shows neovascularization of disc (NVD), extensive NVE, and macular leakage

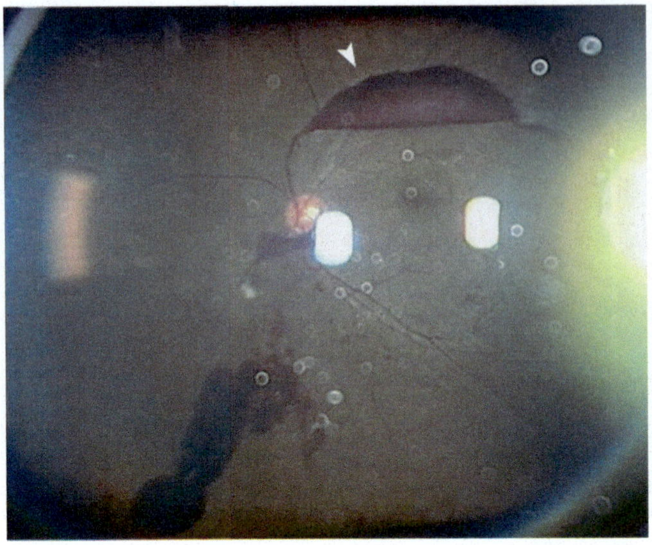

Fig. 14 Diabetic retinal hemorrhage. Wide-field biomicroscopic image of an eye with PDR and preretinal hemorrhage (*white arrowhead*). The image taken with a slit-lamp wide-field camera system is inverted

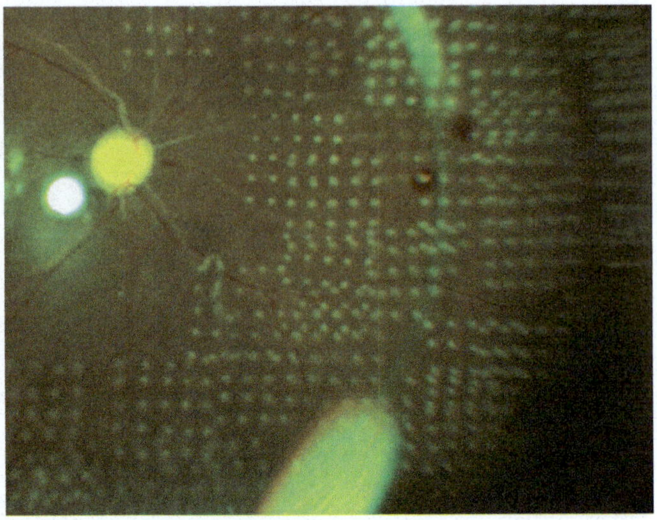

Fig. 16 PRP with navigated pattern laser. A 54-year-old man with PDR during photocoagulation with navigated laser delivery. Intraoperative view with wide-field laser contact lens shows pattern photocoagulation with 100-ms pulse duration

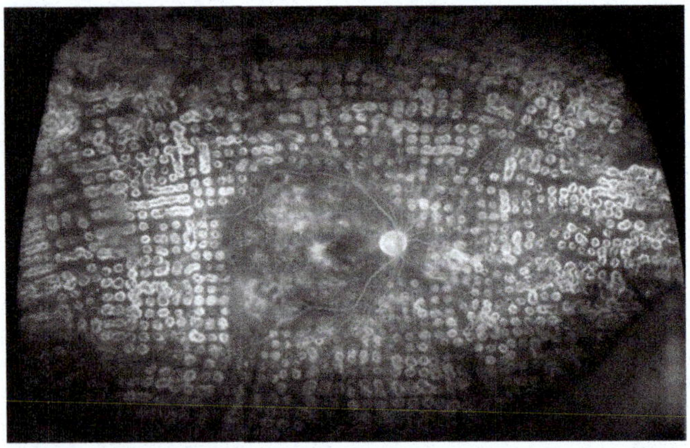

Fig. 15 PRP with conventional pattern laser. A 39-year-old man with a history of PDR after laser therapy. Wide-field fundus fluorescein angiogram of his right eye demonstrates photocoagulation spots with pattern laser

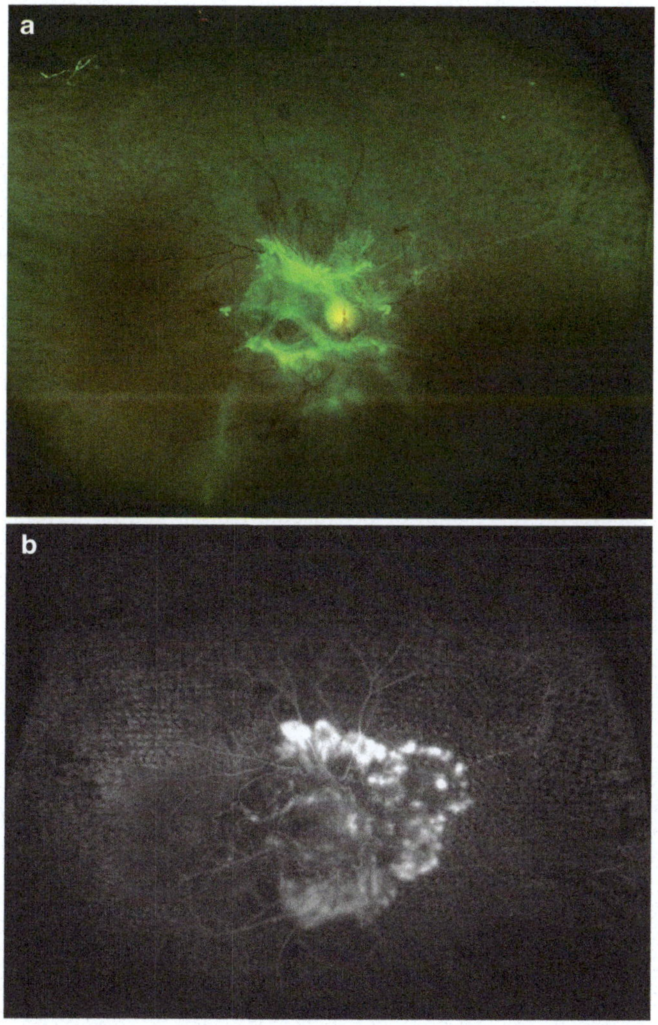

Fig. 17 (**a**) Persistent neovascularization. A 37-year-old man with PDR in both eyes. Wide-field color fundus photography of his right eye demonstrates fibrovascular membrane with persistent neovascularization in spite of previous full laser photocoagulation. (**b**) Persistent neovascularization. Wide-field fundus fluorescein angiogram of the same eye demonstrates dye leakage from persistent new vessels and old laser photocoagulation spots

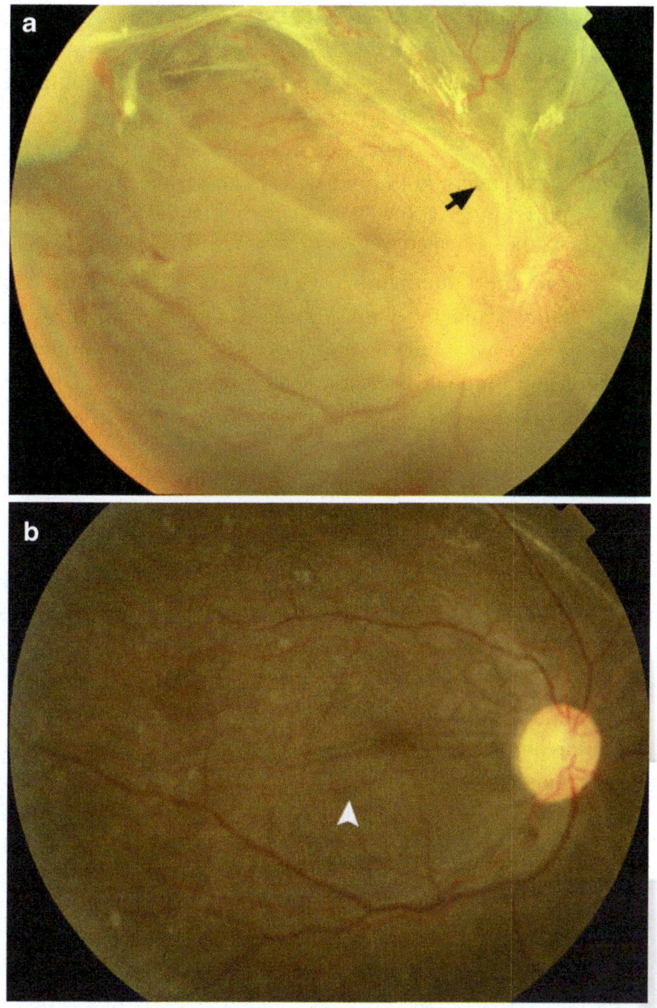

Fig. 18 (**a**) Surgical management of traction retinal detachment. A 38-year-old woman with type 1 diabetes mellitus and traction retinal detachment. Color fundus photography of her right eye demonstrates fibrovascular traction membrane with active neovascularization (*black arrow*). Visual acuity was 20/400. (**b**) Surgical management of traction retinal detachment. The same eye 1 year after pars plana vitrectomy, membrane peel, and gas tamponade shows a completely flat retina with residual internal limiting membrane wrinkling (*white arrowhead*) confirmed by optical coherence tomography (*not shown*). Visual acuity improved to 20/50

Detection and Classification of DR

Two studies have compared UWFA retinal imaging to dilated clinical funduscopic examination for the detection and classification of DR. Neubauer and colleagues [7] assessed DR severity level using both mydriatic stereoscopic funduscopy and nonmydriatic 200° UWFA images. DR and diabetic macular edema (DME) severity levels were determined based on the International Classification of Diabetic Retinopathy scale by 3 masked graders independently. In general, there was agreement between Optomap retinopathy grading and clinical assessment among the readers for the study. Sensitivity of 94 % and specificity of 100 % were demonstrated for all graders to detect more than mild DR. Grading of DME demonstrated only fair agreement between UWFA images and clinical examination.

Wilson and colleagues [8] compared UWFA images with both slit-lamp biomicroscopy examination and single- and dual-field mydriatic digital retinal photographs. Images were obtained and screened for "referable disease," defined as any of the following: ≥4 blot hemorrhages in 1 hemifield or quadrant, abnormalities of venous caliber, intraretinal microvascular abnormalities, retinal neovascularization, vitreous hemorrhage, or exudates or blot hemorrhage ≤1 disc diameter (DD) from the fovea. In comparison with slit-lamp biomicroscopy as the reference standard, UWFA images achieved a sensitivity of 83.6 % compared with 82.9 % for digital photography in the ability to identify referable disease.

One study reported at the 2011 Association for Research in Vision and Ophthalmology meeting has compared nonmydriatic UWFA retinal imaging with the Optos P200MA to clinical trial gold standard mydriatic Early Treatment of Diabetic Retinopathy Scale (ETDRS) protocol 7 standard field stereoscopic photographs [9]. The sensitivity of nonmydriatic UWFA images for detecting any DR and proliferative diabetic retinopathy (PDR) diagnosed on ETDRS photos were 99 and 73 %, respectively, with a specificity of 100 and 99 %, respectively. Despite the nonmydriatic acquisition of the UWFA images, the kappa values for agreement with ETDRS photos were similar to those reported between film and mydriatic digital images compared in multicenter clinical trials [10, 11]. There was excellent agreement between clinical-level DR severity grading on Optos 100° images and ETDRS photos as well as between grading of Optos images and results from clinical examination. Another study has demonstrated a substantial agreement for DME grading of Optos versus ETDRS images as well [12]. However, in this study, 9.3 % of 100° UWFA images were ungradable for level of DR severity.

UWFA-Guided Targeted PRP

UWFA may also directly guide the treatment of patients undergoing panretinal photocoagulation. The Diabetic Retinopathy Study (DRS) showed complications of PRP in that 10 % of patients suffer a decrease in vision after PRP and 5 % develop constriction of their visual field. Complications further included macular edema, hemorrhage, choroidal detachment, angle-closure glaucoma, and decrease in color vision and contrast [13]. By targeting PRP directly to the areas of ischemia, rather than broadly throughout the retina, we may be able to spare healthy retinal tissue and reduce the side effects of PRP while directly treating those areas most likely contributing to the hypoxic drive. Original case series of UWFA-guided targeted PRP in PDR described successful regression of neovascularization and no adverse effects [6]. Subsequent studies have reported on safety and efficacy of targeted PRP using a pattern laser delivery system [14, 15] and computer-assisted navigated laser delivery [16].

DR remains one of the most evidence-guided diseases in the field of retina. As such, it is important to note that seminal studies in DR such as the DRS and the ETDRS were conducted before the advent of UWFA. This raises important questions regarding how and when we can apply older studies toward the management of patients in an age in which we are able to visualize and image far more retinal abnormality than was previously possible. For example, PRP is generally not indicated for patients with retinopathy in the absence of neovascularization. However, our newfound ability to visualize specific areas of peripheral nonperfusion as well as to apply targeted PRP through UWFA may shift the scales regarding the risk-benefit ratio of prophylactic PRP prior to the development of neovascularization or macular edema; this remains to be investigated. Moreover, as ischemia likely drives macular edema, targeted PRP to areas of peripheral nonperfusion may also prove useful as an adjunctive therapy for macular edema; studies investigating this modality are currently under way. In general, studies comparing targeted PRP with true "panretinal" photocoagulation are necessary.

Acknowledgment *The following investigators belong to The King Khaled Eye Specialist Hospital (KKESH) Collaborative Retina Study Group: J. Fernando Arevalo, MD, FACS (PI), Saba Al Rashaed, MD, Eman Al Kahtani, MD, Sawsan Nowilaty, MD, Hassan A. Al-Dhibi, MD, Yahya A. Al-Zahrani, MD, Igor Kozak, MD, PhD, Sulaiman Al-Sulaiman, MD, Patrik Schatz, MD, Abdulelah Al-Abdullah, MD, Khalid Al Rubaie, MD, Yousef Al Dhafiri, MD, Badr Al Ahmadi, MD, Abdulaziz Al Hadlaq, MD, Majed Al Harbi, MD, Abdulaziz Al Oreany, MD, Adel Al-Akeely, MD, Mohammad Hazzazi, MD, Mohammed Talea, MD, Ghazai Al-Thobaiti, MD.

References

1. Shimizu K, Kobayashi Y, Muraoka K. Mid-peripheral fundus involvement in diabetic retinopathy. Ophthalmology. 1981;88:601–12.
2. Wessel MM, Aaker GD, Parlitsis G, Cho M, D'Amico DJ, Kiss S. Ultra-wide-field angiography improves the detection and classification of diabetic retinopathy. Retina. 2012;32:785–91.
3. Friberg TR, Gupta A, Yu J, Huang L, Suner J, Puliafito CA, et al. Ultrawide angle fluorescein angiographic imaging: a comparison to conventional digital acquisition system. Ophthalmic Surg Lasers Imaging. 2008;39:304–11.
4. Shimizu K, Muraoka K. Diabetic retinopathy. Is it a maculopathy? A super-wide fluorescein angiographic evaluation. Dev Ophthalmol. 1981;2:235–42.
5. Oliver SCN, Schwartz SD. Peripheral vessel leakage (PVL): a new angiographic finding in diabetic retinopathy identified with ultra wide-field fluorescein angiography. Semin Ophthalmol. 2010;25:27–33.
6. Reddy S, Shwartz SD. Ultra wide field fluorescein angiography guided targeted retinal photocoagulation. Semin Ophthalmol. 2009;29:9–14.
7. Neubauer AS, Kernt M, Haritoglou C, et al. Nonmydriatic screening for diabetic retinopathy by ultra-widefield scanning laser ophthalmoscopy (Optomap). Graefes Arch Clin Exp Ophthalmol. 2008;246:229–35.
8. Wilson PJ, Ellis JD, MacEwen CJ, Priglinger SG, Kampik A, Ulbig MW. Screening for diabetic retinopathy: a comparative trial of photography and scanning laser ophthalmoscopy. Ophthalmologica. 2010;224:251–7.
9. Noble J, Silva PS, Cavallerano JD, Sun JK, Aiello LM, Aiello LP. Comparison of nonmydriatic Optos® fundus imaging with mydriatic Early Treatment Diabetic Retinopathy Study (ETDRS) 7-standard field stereo photography and clinical grading. Paper presented at the annual meeting of the Association for Research in Vision and Ophthalmology, Fort Lauderdale; May 2011, 1283/A33.
10. Hubbard LD, Sun W, Cleary PA, Danis RP, Hainsworth DP, Peng Q, et al. Comparison of digital and film grading of diabetic retinopathy severity in the Diabetes Control and Complications Trial/Epidemiology of Diabetes Interventions and Complications Study. Arch Ophthalmol. 2011;129:718–26.
11. Gangaputra S, Almukhtar T, Glassman AR, Aiello LP, Bressler N, Bressler SB, et al. Comparison of film and digital fundus photographs in eyes of individuals with diabetes mellitus. Invest Ophthalmol Vis Sci. 2011;52:6168–73.
12. Boucher MC, Gresset JA, Angioi K, Olivier S. Effectiveness and safety of screening for diabetic retinopathy with two nonmydriatic digital images compared with the seven standard stereoscopic photographic fields. Can J Ophthalmol. 2003;38:557–68.
13. The Diabetic Retinopathy Study Research Group. Photocoagulation treatment of proliferative diabetic retinopathy: clinical application of Diabetic Retinopathy Study (DRS) findings. DRS report number 8. Ophthalmology. 1981;88:583–600.
14. Muqit MM, Young LB, McKenzie R, John B, Marcellino GR, Henson DB, et al. Pilot randomized clinical trial of Pascal TargETEd Retinal versus variable fluence PANretinal 20 ms laser in diabetic retinopathy: PETER PAN study. Br J Ophthalmol. 2013;97:220–7.
15. Muqit MM, Marcellino GR, Henson DB, Young LB, Patton N, Charles SJ, et al. Optos-guided pattern scan laser (Pascal)-targeted retinal photocoagulation in proliferative diabetic retinopathy. Acta Ophthalmol. 2013;91:251–8.
16. Kozak I, Arevalo JF, Gupta V, Chhablani J, Kim JS. Navigated targeted panretinal photocoagulation for diabetic retinopathy (paper on demand). Paper presented at the 32nd annual meeting of the American Society of Retina Specialists (ASRS), San Diego; 9–13 Aug 2014.

Wide-Field Retinal Imaging of Branch Retinal Vein Occlusions

6

Pradeep S. Prasad and Irena Tsui

Branch retinal vein occlusion (BRVO) is a significant cause of vision loss and, after diabetic retinopathy, is the second most common type of retinal vascular disease. Risk factors for BRVO include advancing age as well as cardiovascular risk factors such as hypertension, diabetes, and hyperlipidemia. Systemic conditions including hypercoagulability syndromes and behavioral factors such as cigarette smoking can also increase the risk of BRVO. BRVO can be categorized as major (affecting a major venous arcade) or minor (affecting a smaller venous tributary). Additionally, BRVO can be categorized as ischemic or nonischemic. Visually significant sequelae typically occur in association with major and ischemic BRVO. These sequelae include macular edema, macular ischemia, neovascularization, vitreous hemorrhage, neovascular glaucoma, and tractional retinal detachment. Treatment options include intravitreal injection of anti-vascular endothelial growth factor (anti-VEGF) and corticosteroid medications, laser photocoagulation, and vitreoretinal surgery.

Epidemiology and Risk Factors

Retinal venous occlusive disease is a common cause of vision loss affecting approximately 16 million people worldwide with an incidence of 5.2 per 1000 people. BRVO is approximately four to six times more prevalent than central retinal vein occlusion (CRVO) and is more common among Latinos and Asians than non-Latino blacks and whites. Advanced age, particularly age older than 65, significantly increases the risk of BRVO. There is no evidence for gender predilection in BRVO [1–5].

Hypertension is the most common systemic condition associated with BRVO. Other risk factors for BRVO include hyperlipidemia, diabetes, peripheral arterial disease, increased body mass index, and smoking [6–8]. Meta-analysis of patients with BRVO indicates odds ratios of 3.0, 2.3, and 1.1 in patients with hypertension, hyperlipidemia, and diabetes, respectively [9]. The same risk factors have also been identified in patients younger than 50 with BRVO [10].

In patients for whom no underlying cardiovascular risk factor can be identified, other causative systemic conditions can be considered including hypercoagulable state, use of medications that can increase the risk of thromboembolic event (e.g., oral contraceptive use), malignancy, systemic inflammatory disease, and hyperviscosity syndromes [11, 12]. Typically, evaluation for these conditions should be reserved for young patients, on in patients with a suspicious clinical history and performed in consultation with an internist or hematologist-oncologist.

Pathophysiology and Clinical Findings

BRVOs most often occur at arteriovenous crossing sites [13]. Anatomically, retinal arteries and veins can share a common adventitial sheath at their crossing sites and it has been proposed that systemic diseases that thicken retinal arteries may promote occlusion of the associated veins [14]. The location of the occlusion determines the extent of retinal involvement with occlusion proximal to the disc affecting a quadrant or up to half of the retinal vasculature (major BRVO and hemi-central retinal vein occlusion [HRVO], respectively). Alternatively, occlusions distal to the nerve, particularly those affecting small tributaries in the macula (minor or

P.S. Prasad, MD (✉) • I. Tsui, MD
Retina Division, Jules Stein Eye Institute,
University of California, Los Angeles,
Los Angeles, CA, USA
e-mail: Prasad@jsei.ucla.edu; itsui@jsei.ucla.edu

I. Kozak, J.F. Arevalo (eds.), *Atlas of Wide-Field Retinal Angiography and Imaging*, DOI 10.1007/978-3-319-17864-6_6

macular BRVO) may affect only a small wedge-shaped area of the retina and, therefore, may be associated with minimal or no symptoms [15, 16]. Similarly, location distal to macular vascular distribution or in the nasal quadrants may escape early detection as visual changes can be minimal.

Visual symptoms associated with acute onset of BRVO typically include blurred vision with visual field defects correlating with the location of the affected vein. Later visual sequelae may include blurred vision associated with perfusion abnormalities such as ischemia, macular edema, or neovascularization. Floaters associated with vitreous hemorrhage or vitreoretinal interface abnormalities can occur [17]. Clinical findings in the acute state include retinal venous tortuosity and intraretinal hemorrhage distal to the site of occlusion. Macular edema may be present, although the presence of intraretinal hemorrhage may obscure adequate visualization. Other retinal vascular changes include the formation of microaneurysms and telangiectasias associated with the shunting of blood through patent veins. Depending on the location of the BRVO, telangiectatic shunts may be seen extending across the horizontal raphe.

Evaluation and Management

Evaluation of patients with BRVO should include examination of the anterior chamber with attention to the formation of rubeosis iridis and neovascularization of the angle. Funduscopic examination allows for classification of the BRVO and evaluation for retinal neovascularization and macular edema, although adequate visualization may be limited by the presence of hemorrhage. Optical coherence tomography (OCT), particularly in the presence of dense hemorrhage, can be useful in to evaluate for the presence of cystoid macular edema [18]. Fluorescein angiography can also assist in identifying angiographic macular edema as well as areas of capillary nonperfusion if not blocked by hemorrhage [19]. Wide-field fluorescein angiography can both assess the macular vascular issues as well as aid in identifying peripheral capillary nonperfusion, neovascularization, or vascular abnormalities [20].

Treatable complications of BRVO include macular edema and neovascularization. Both the Branch Retinal Vein Occlusion Study (BVOS), utilizing standard fluorescein angiography, and more recent studies utilizing wide-field fluorescein angiography have identified the presence of capillary nonperfusion as a risk factor for the development of neovascularization [21]. Laser photocoagulation to nonperfused retina has been shown to decrease the risk of neovascularization, although it is unclear if treatment prior to the development of neovascularization is indicated [22]. Likewise, capillary nonperfusion on wide-field angiography has been associated with the presence of macular edema in patients with major BRVO. It has been postulated that increased production of VEGF and other growth factors by nonperfused retina may cause macular edema via a growth factor-mediated increase in capillary permeability [23]. It is unknown if targeted photocoagulation of peripheral nonperfusion can play an adjunct role in the treatment of BRVO-associated macular edema, although early studies suggest this to be the case.

Current treatments for macular edema include intravitreal injection of anti-VEGF medications, intravitreal injection of corticosteroid preparations and grid macular photocoagulation [24]. Intravitreal injection of anti-VEGF medications is currently the preferred first-line treatment given the risk of glaucoma and cataract formation associated with intravitreal steroids [25–29]. Macular photocoagulation can also be considered as an adjunct or rescue treatment in patients with recalcitrant macular edema [30, 31].

Vitreoretinal surgery is typically reserved for patients with persistent or recurrent vitreous hemorrhage associated with retinal neovascularization. Vitrectomy has also been shown to be of benefit in patients with recalcitrant macular edema [32]. The mechanism for this is unclear but may be related to increased oxygen tension within the vitreous cavity or decreased vitreomacular adhesion following vitrectomy.

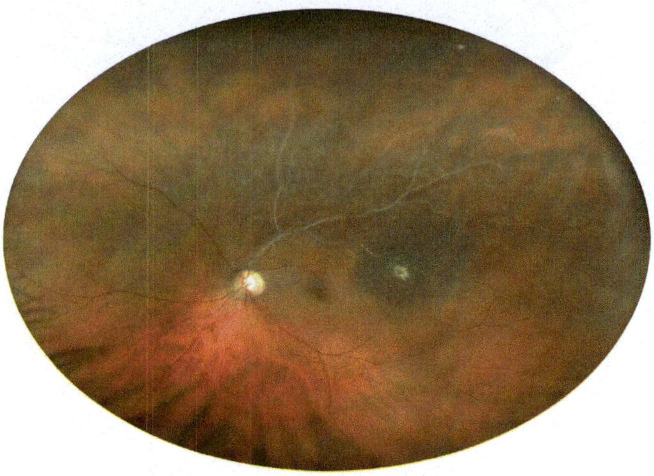

Fig. 1 Color fundus photo of the left eye demonstrates a chronic superotemporal BRVO with venous sclerosis, temporal macular microaneurysms, and exudates

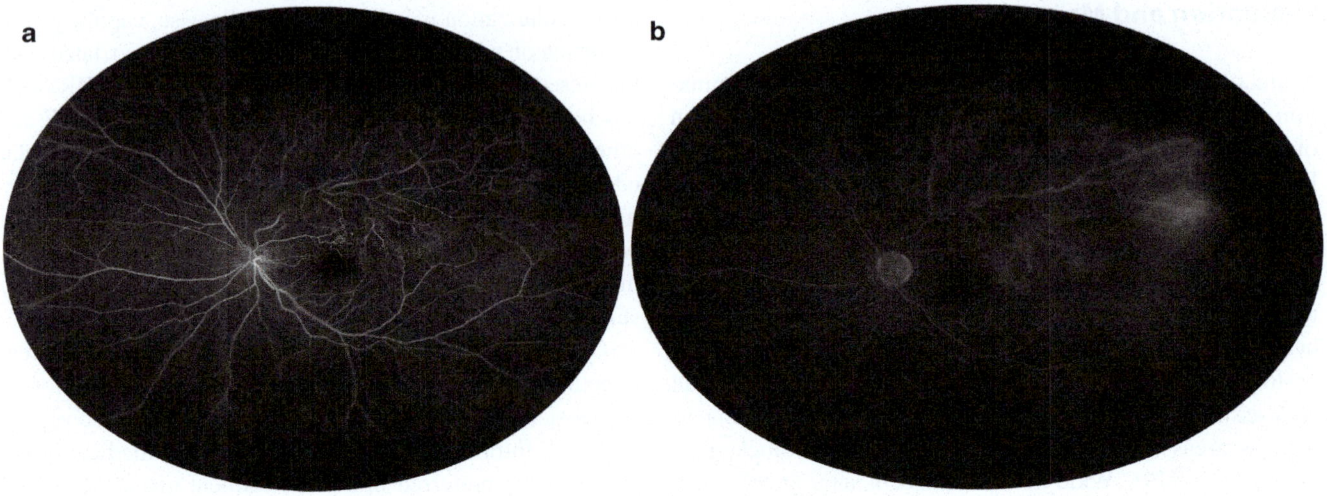

Fig. 2 (**a**) Wide-field fluorescein angiogram of the left eye highlights superotemporal BRVO with venous tortuosity, superotemporal capillary nonperfusion, and collateral venous flow across the horizontal raphe. (**b**) Late-phase wide-field angiogram of left eye demonstrates late venous staining and leakage

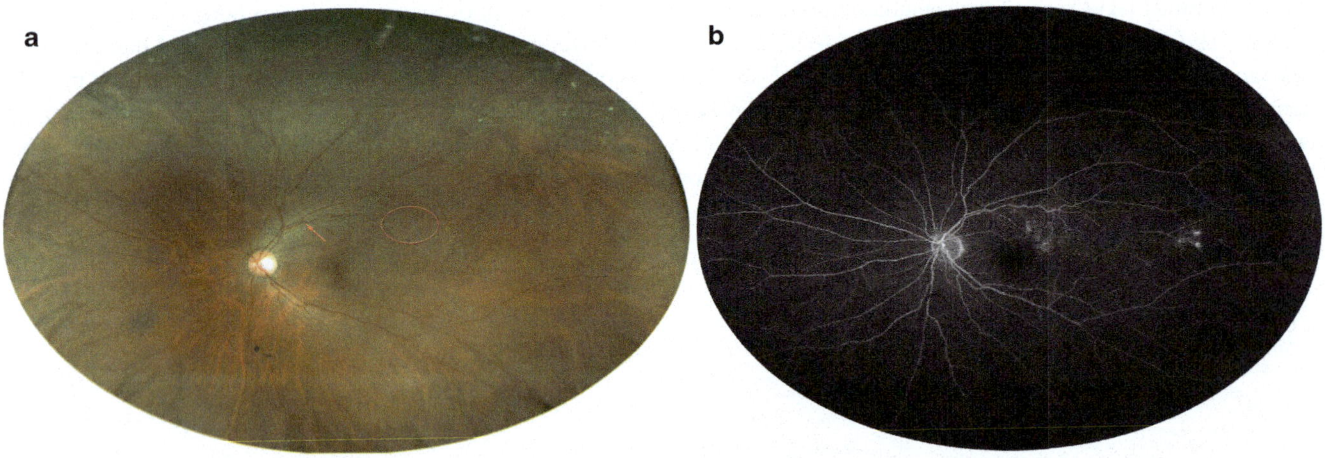

Fig. 3 (**a**) Superotemporal BRVO in the left eye with subtle venous tortuosity distal to arteriovenous crossing site (*arrow*) and collateral formation (*circle*). (**b**) Fluorescein angiogram demonstrates angiographic macular edema, grid photocoagulation in the macula, and temporal bulbs of early neovascularization

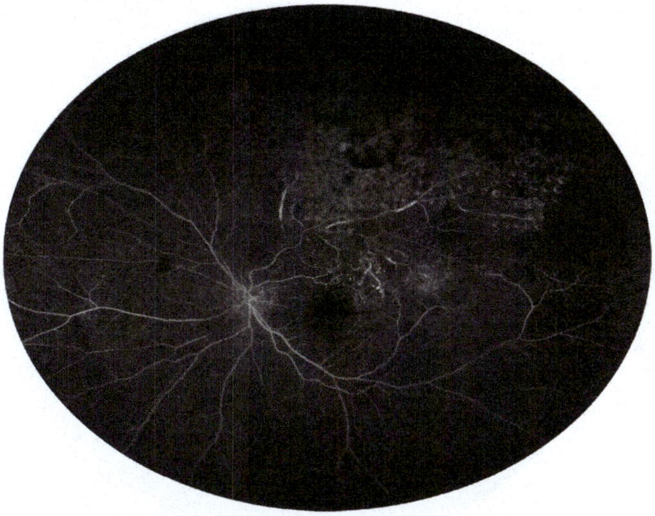

Fig. 4 Superotemporal ischemic BRVO with macular and superotemporal peripheral nonperfusion. Quadratic scatter photocoagulation scars can be seen in the superotemporal periphery with untreated capillary nonperfusion in the temporal periphery

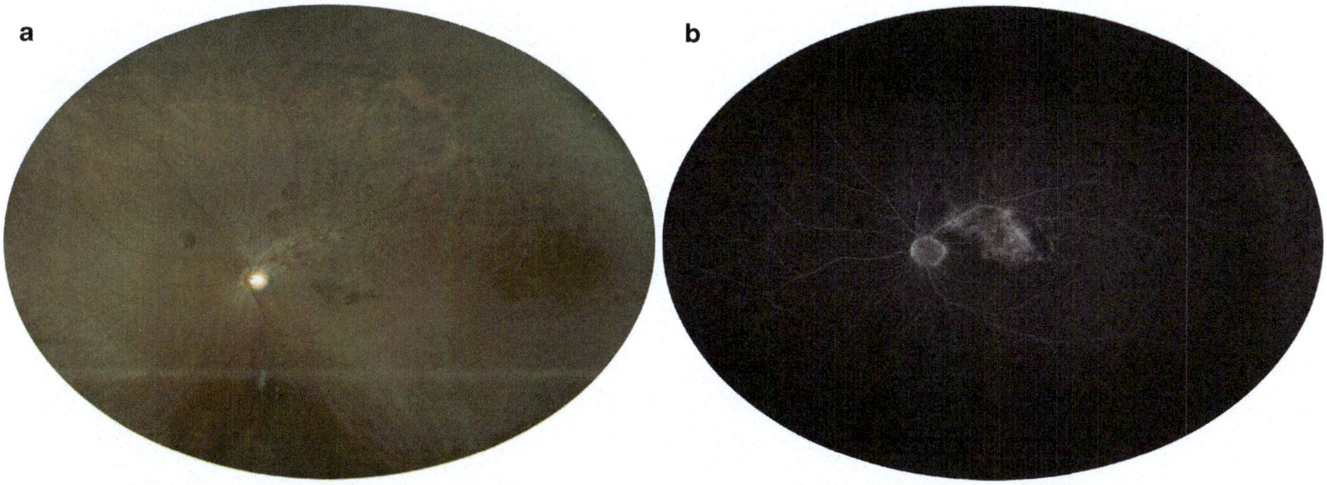

Fig. 5 (**a**) Superotemporal BRVO with occlusion site proximal to the optic disc. Intraretinal hemorrhages extend to the superotemporal periphery. Cotton-wool spots along the superotemporal arcade can be seen in the superior macula. (**b**) Late-phase wide-field fluorescein angiogram demonstrates intense angiographic leakage in the macula with capillary nonperfusion in the superotemporal far periphery

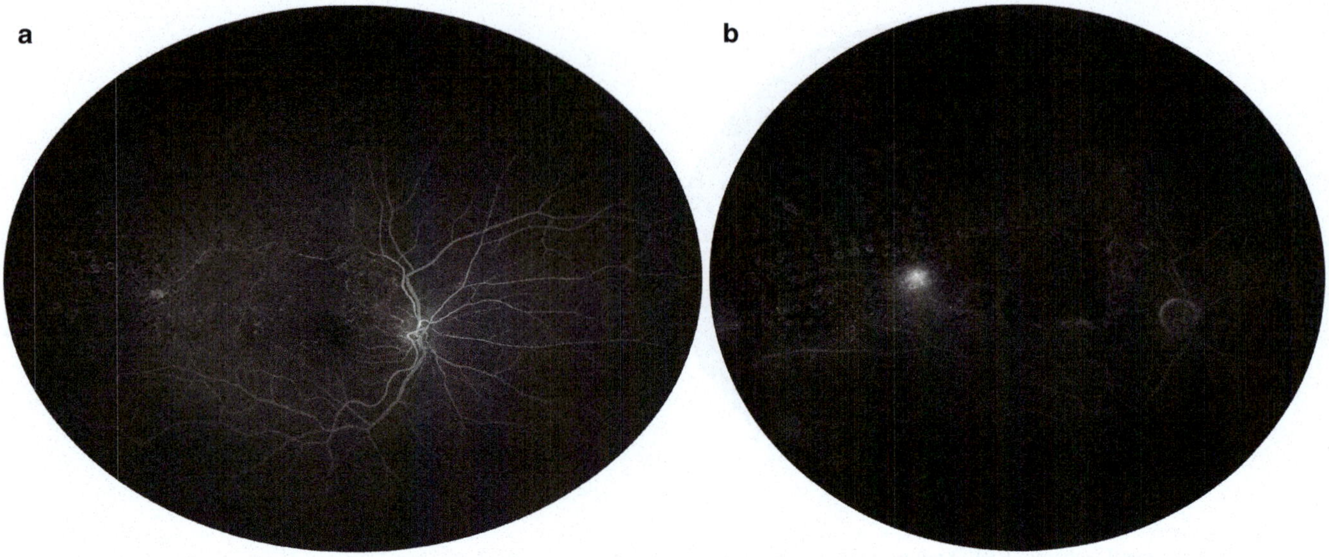

Fig. 6 (**a**) Transit-phase, wide-field angiogram of a superotemporal ischemic BRVO of the right eye with quadratic scatter photocoagulation. (**b**) Late-phase wide-field angiogram of the same eye demonstrates neovascularization at the border between treated and untreated capillary nonperfusion

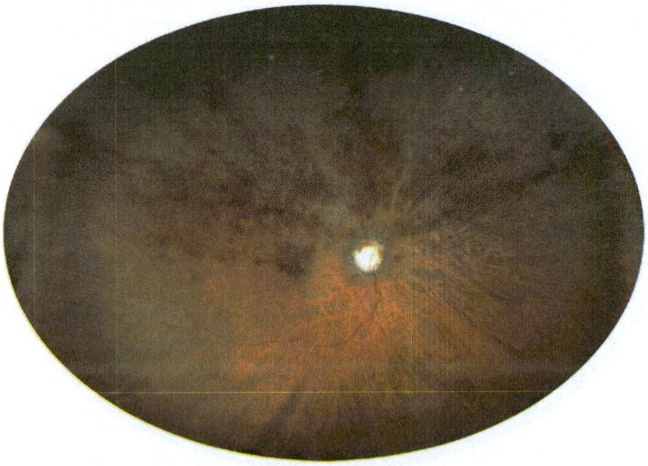

Fig. 7 HCVO of the right eye associated with superior hemisphere intraretinal hemorrhages and superior disc collaterals

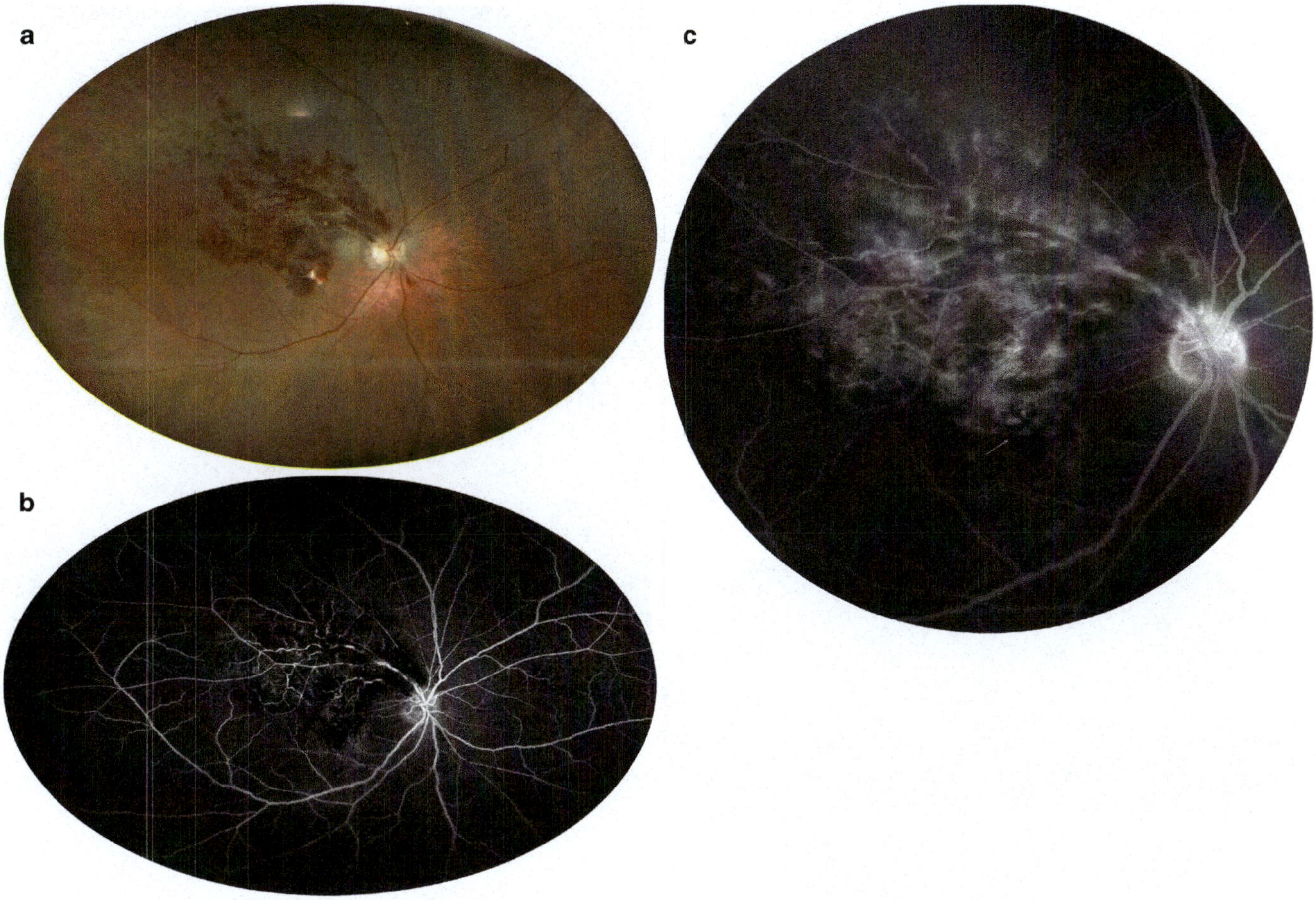

Fig. 8 (**a**) Superotemporal BRVO of the right eye with intraretinal hemorrhages extending inferior to the horizontal raphe. (**b**) Intraretinal hemorrhages associated with blocking defects in the transit phase of the angiogram. (**c**) Later phases of the angiogram are associated with venous staining, leakage, and petalloid macular edema (*arrow*)

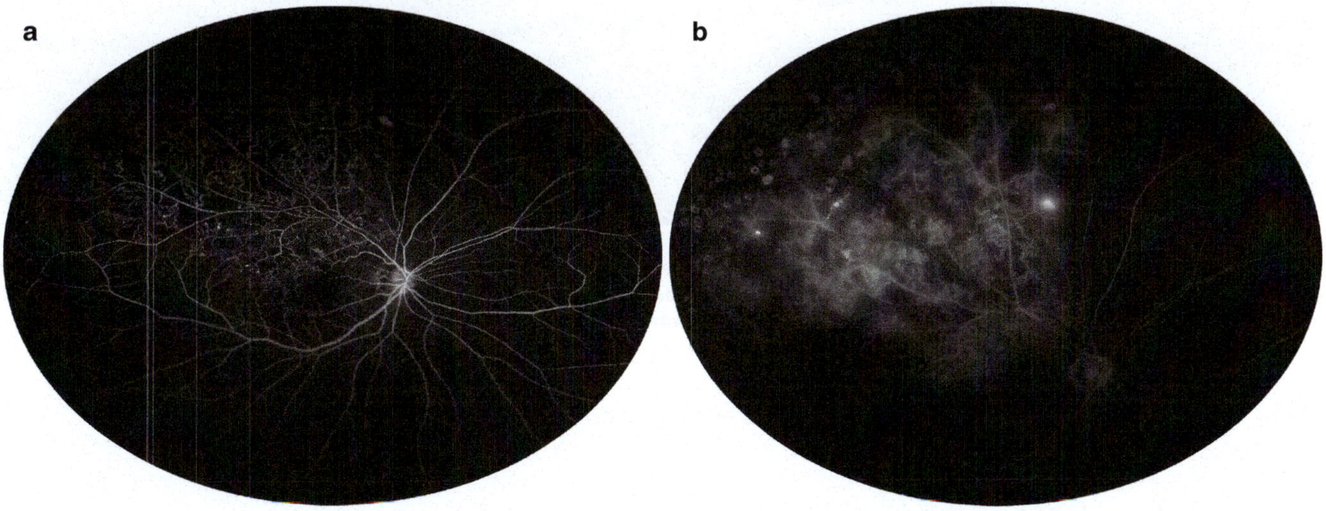

Fig. 9 (**a**) Superotemporal BRVO with significant capillary nonperfusion and vascular pruning. (**b**) Limited scatter photocoagulation can be seen in the periphery. Note the intense vascular leakage and the bulb of neovascularization superiorly

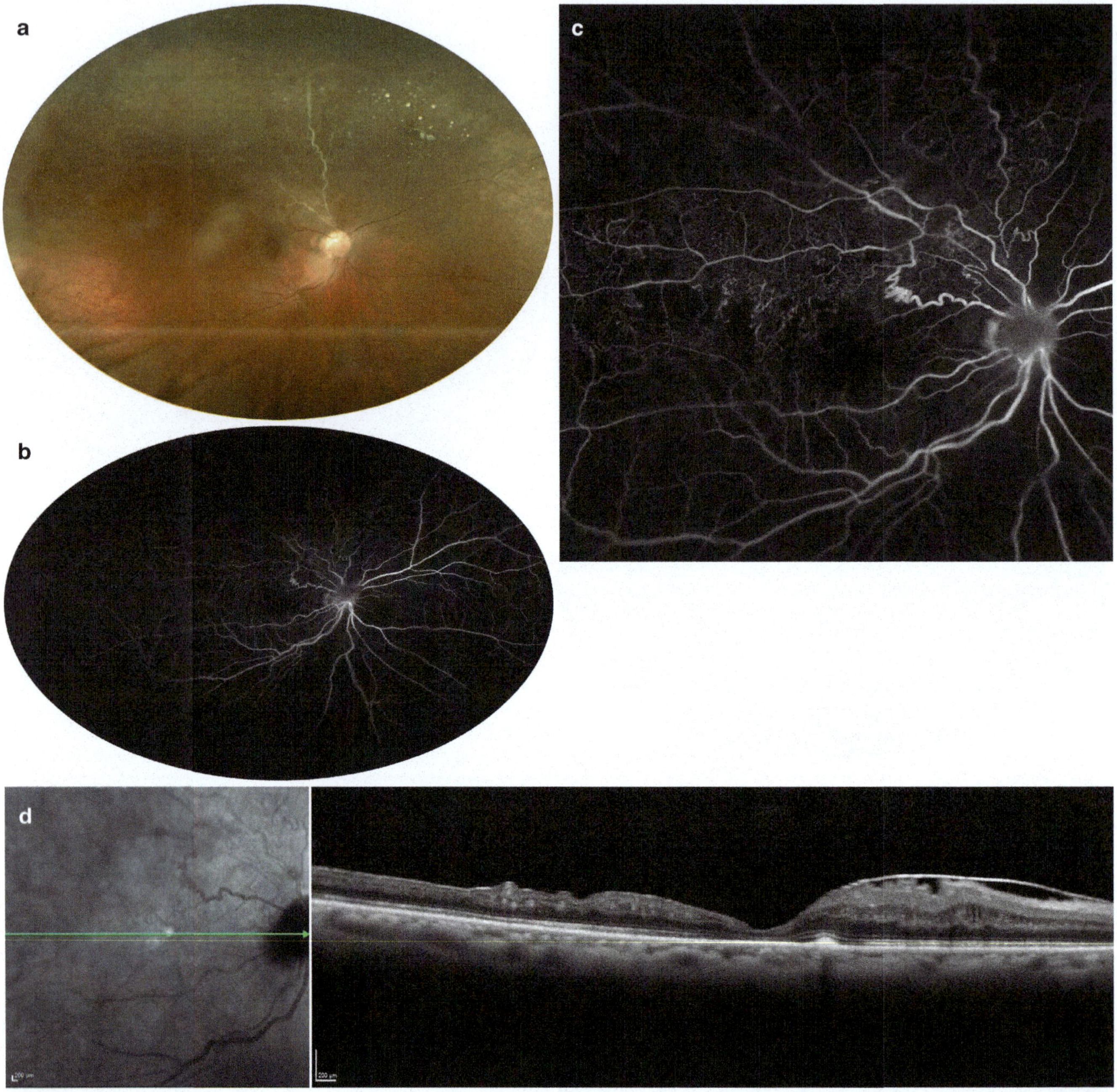

Fig. 10 (a) Superotemporal BRVO with venous sclerosis and adjacent collateral formation. (b) Wide-field fluorescein angiography demonstrates widespread capillary nonperfusion. (c) High-resolution imaging of the macula demonstrates temporal macular ischemia. (d) Spectral domain OCT of the macula demonstrates foveal and temporal inner retinal atrophy corresponding to areas of capillary nonperfusion

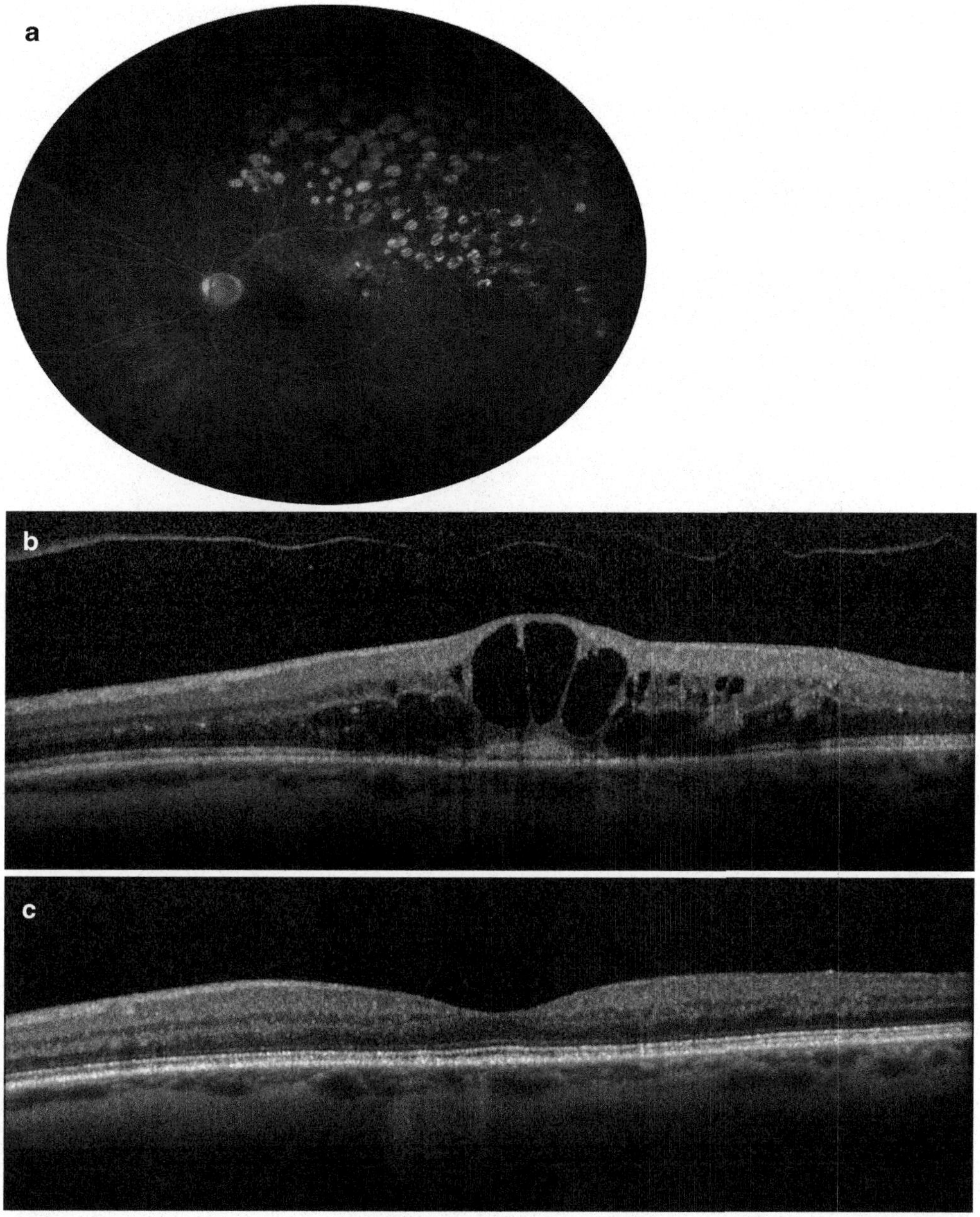

Fig. 11 (**a**) Ischemic BRVO with angiographic macular edema and superotemporal scatter photocoagulation scars. (**b**) Spectral domain OCT demonstrates cystoid macular edema and posterior hyaloid separation. (**c**) Spectral domain OCT demonstrates resolution of cystoid macular edema following intravitreal injection of ranibizumab

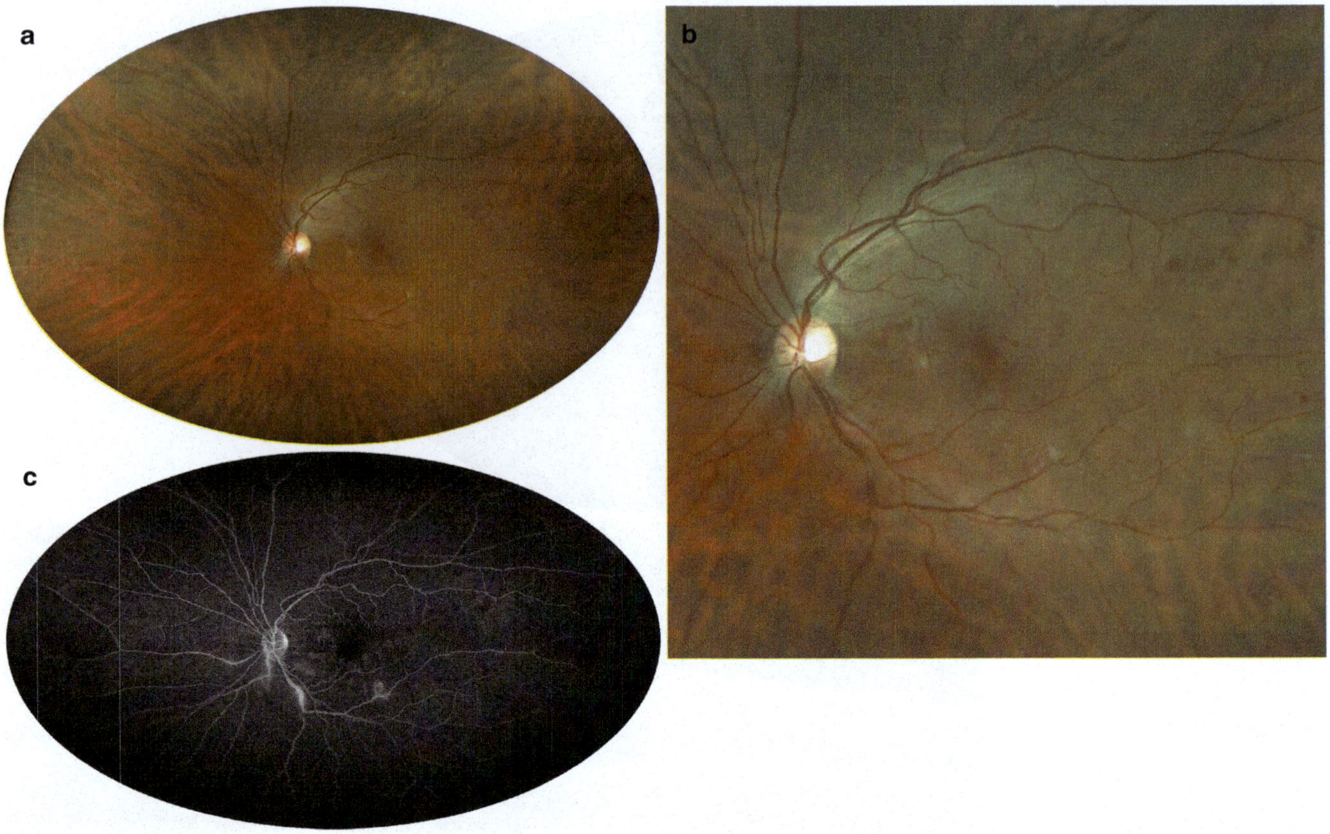

Fig. 12 (**a**) Inferior HRVO with intraretinal hemorrhages along the horizontal raphe and nasal vascular sclerosis. (**b**) Inferior disc collaterals associated with the HRVO. (**c**) Late-phase wide-field angiogram demonstrates venous staining, collateral formation across the horizontal raphe temporal and nasal to the optic disc, and a wedge-shaped area of capillary nonperfusion nasally

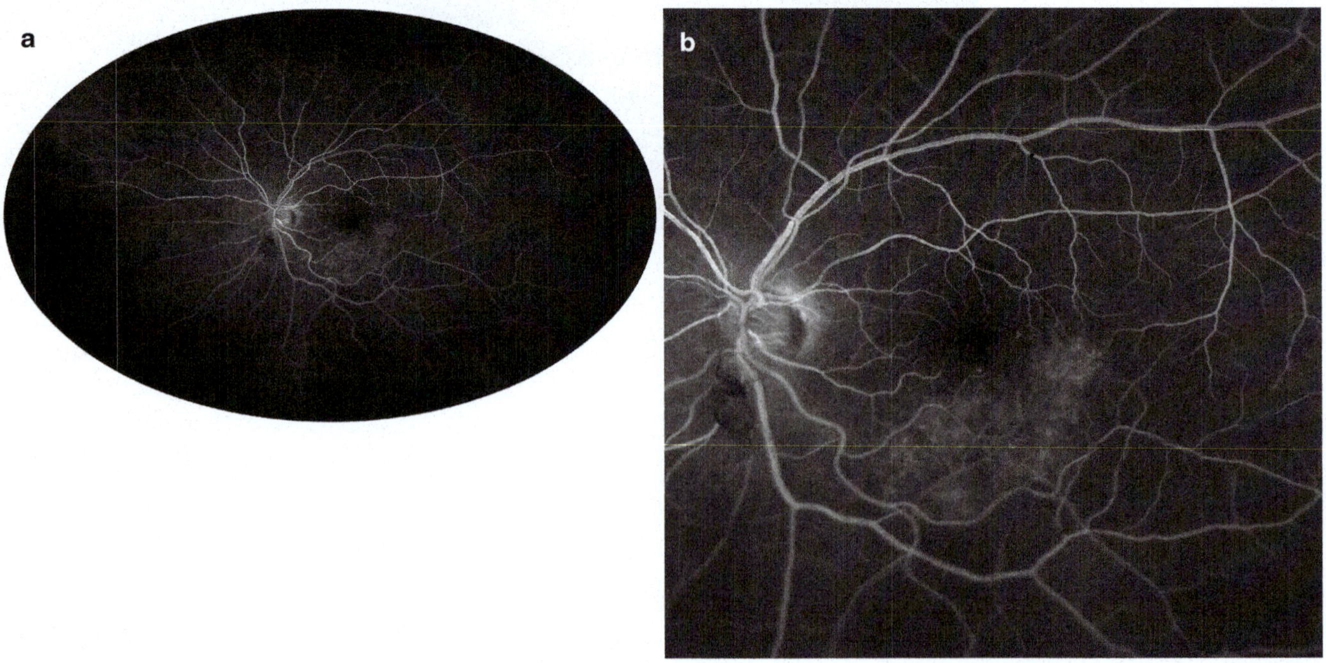

Fig. 13 (**a**) Wide-field fluorescein angiogram of an Inferotemporal macular BRVO. (**b**) Grid laser photocoagulation has been applied in the area of angiographic edema

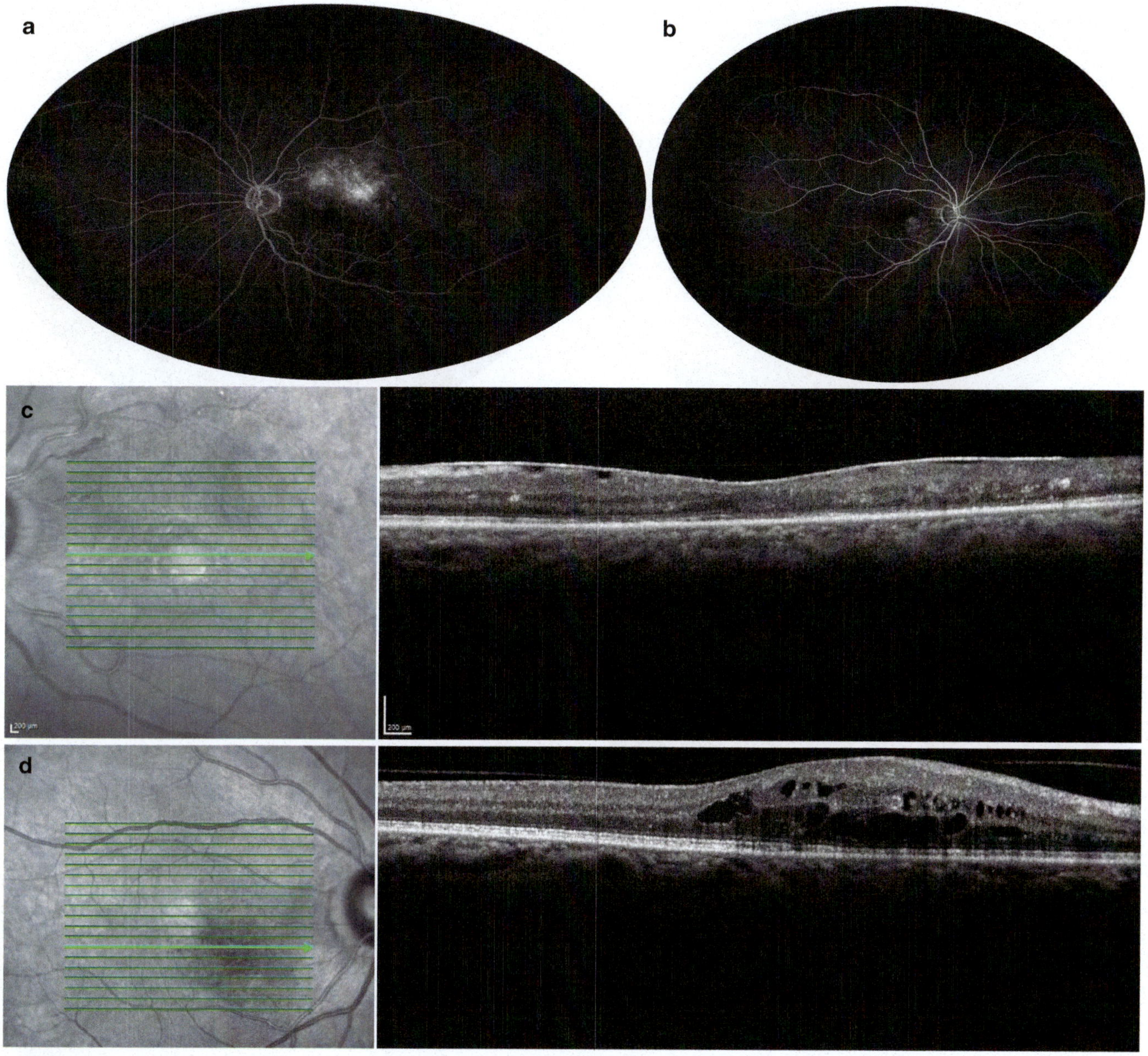

Fig. 14 (**a**) Major BRVO of the left eye associated with intense angiographic macular edema. (**b**) Macular BRVO of the right eye associated with angiographic macular edema. (**c**) OCT demonstrates an epiretinal membrane without cystoid macular edema, despite the presence of leakage on fluorescein angiography. (**d**) OCT with cystoid macular edema of the right eye

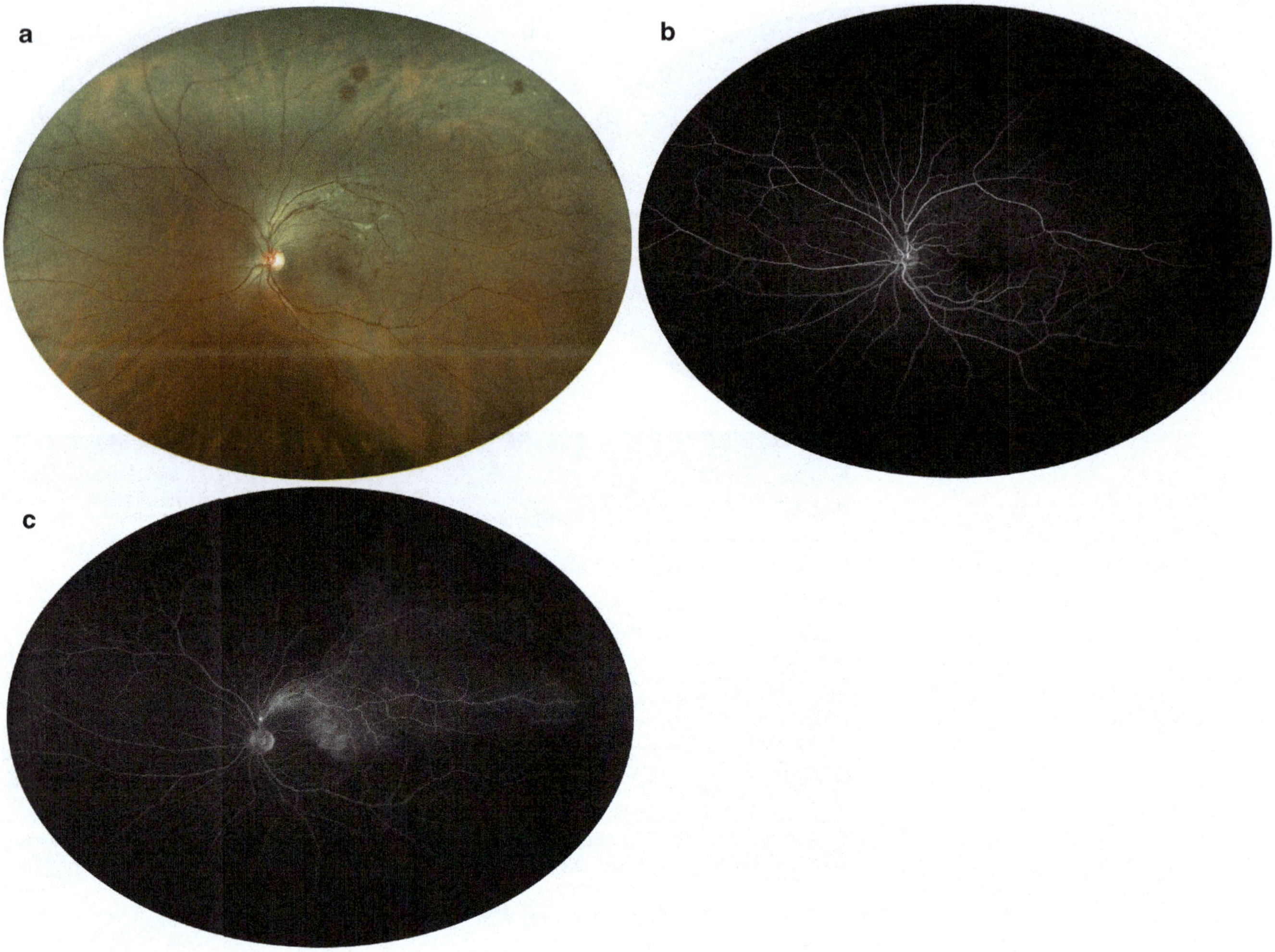

Fig. 15 (**a**) Superotemporal BRVO with intraretinal hemorrhage, macular collaterals, and peripheral venous tortuosity. (**b**) Laminar phase of wide-field fluorescein angiogram highlights areas of delayed venous filling and capillary nonperfusion in superotemporal quadrant. (**c**) Late phase of wide-field fluorescein angiography demonstrates angiographic leakage and late perfusion of the superotemporal periphery

References

1. Rogers S, McIntosh RL, Cheung N, Lim L, Wang JJ, Mitchell P, et al. The prevalence of retinal vein occlusion: pooled data from population studies from the United States, Europe, Asia, and Australia. Ophthalmology. 2010;117:313–9.
2. Cugati S, Wang JJ, Rochtchina E, Mitchell P. Ten-year incidence of retinal vein occlusion in an older population: the Blue Mountains Eye Study. Arch Ophthalmol. 2006;124:726–32.
3. Hayreh SS, Zimmerman MB, Podhajsky P. Incidence of various types of retinal vein occlusion and their recurrence and demographic characteristics. Am J Ophthalmol. 1994;117:429–41.
4. Klein R, Klein BEK, Moss SE, Meuer SM. The epidemiology of retinal vein occlusion: the Beaver Dam Eye Study. Trans Am Ophthalmol Soc. 2000;98:133–43.
5. Klein R, Moss SE, Meuer SM, Klein BE. The 15-year cumulative incidence of retinal vein occlusion: the Beaver Dam Eye Study. Arch Ophthalmol. 2008;126:513–8.
6. Kolar P. Risk factors for central and branch retinal vein occlusion: a meta-analysis of published clinical data. J Ophthalmol. 2014;2014:724780.
7. Jaulim A, Ahmed B, Khanam T, Chatziralli IP. Branch retinal vein occlusion: epidemiology, pathogenesis, risk factors, clinical features, diagnosis, and complications. An update of the literature. Retina. 2013;33:901–10.
8. Eye Disease Case–control Study Group. Risk factors for branch retinal vein occlusion. Am J Ophthalmol. 1993;116:286–96.
9. O'Mahoney PR, Wong DT, Ray JG. Retinal vein occlusion and traditional risk factors for atherosclerosis. Arch Ophthalmol. 2008;126:692–9.
10. Lam HD, Lahey JM, Kearney JJ, Ng RR, Lehmer JM, Tanaka SC. Young patients with branch retinal vein occlusion: a review of 60 cases. Retina. 2010;30:1520–3.
11. Cahill MT, Stinnett SS, Fekrat S. Meta-analysis of plasma homocysteine, serum folate, serum vitamin B12, and thermolabile MTHFR genotype as risk factors for retinal vascular occlusive disease. Am J Ophthalmol. 2003;136:1136–50.
12. Janssen MC, den Heijer M, Cruysberg JR, Wollersheim H, Bredie SJ. Retinal vein occlusion: a form of venous thrombosis or a complication of atherosclerosis? A meta-analysis of thrombophilic factors. Thromb Haemost. 2005;93:1021–6.
13. Zhao J, Sastry SM, Sperduto RD, Chew EY, Remaley NA. Arteriovenous crossing patterns in branch retinal vein occlusion. The Eye Disease Case–control Study Group. Ophthalmology. 1993;100:423–8.
14. Christoffersen NL, Larsen M. Pathophysiology and hemodynamics of branch retinal vein occlusion. Ophthalmology. 1999;106(11): 2054–62.
15. Kumar B, Yu DY, Morgan WH, Barry CJ, Constable IJ, McAllister IL. The distribution of angioarchitectural changes within the vicinity of the arteriovenous crossing in branch retinal vein occlusion. Ophthalmology. 1998;105:424–7.
16. Joffe L, Goldberg RE, Magargal LE, Annesley WH. Macular branch vein occlusion. Ophthalmology. 1980;87:91–8.
17. Hayreh SS, Zimmerman MB. Branch retinal vein occlusion: natural history of visual outcome. JAMA Ophthalmol. 2014;132:13–22.
18. Spaide RF, Lee JK, Klancnik Jr JK, Gross NE. Optical coherence tomography of branch retinal vein occlusion. Retina. 2003;23: 343–7.
19. Hayreh SS, Rojas P, Podhajsky P, Montague P, Woolson RF. Ocular neovascularization with retinal vascular occlusion—III. Incidence of ocular neovascularization with retinal vein occlusion. Ophthalmology. 1983;90:488–506.
20. Tsui I, Bajwa A, Franco-Cardenas V, Pan CK, Kim HY, Schwartz SD. Peripheral fluorescein angiographic findings in fellow eyes of patients with branch retinal vein occlusion. Int J Inflam. 2013;2013:464127.
21. Prasad PS, Oliver SC, Coffee RE, Hubschman JP, Schwartz SD. Ultra wide-field angiographic characteristics of branch retinal and hemicentral retinal vein occlusion. Ophthalmology. 2010;117:780–4.
22. Branch Vein Occlusion Study Group. Argon laser scatter photocoagulation for prevention of neovascularization and vitreous hemorrhage in branch vein occlusion. A randomized clinical trial. Arch Ophthalmol. 1986;104:34–41.
23. Noma H, Minamoto A, Funatsu H, Tsukamoto H, Nakano K, Yamashita H, et al. Intravitreal levels of vascular endothelial growth factor and interleukin-6 are correlated with macular edema in branch retinal vein occlusion. Graefes Arch Clin Exp Ophthalmol. 2006;244:309–15.
24. Chatziralli IP, Jaulim A, Peponis VG, Mitropoulos PG, Moschos MM. Branch retinal vein occlusion: treatment modalities: an update of the literature. Semin Ophthalmol. 2014;29:85–107.
25. Campochiaro PA, Heier JS, Feiner L, Gray S, Saroj N, Rundle AC, et al. Ranibizumab for macular edema following branch retinal vein occlusion: six-month primary end point results of a phase III study. Ophthalmology. 2010;117:1102–12.
26. Hikichi T, Higuchi M, Matsushita T, Kosaka S, Matsushita R, Takami K, et al. Two-year outcomes of intravitreal bevacizumab therapy for macular oedema secondary to branch retinal vein occlusion. Br J Ophthalmol. 2014;98:195–9.
27. Figueroa MS, Contreras I, Noval S, Arruabarrena C. Results of bevacizumab as the primary treatment for retinal vein occlusions. Br J Ophthalmol. 2010;94:1052–6.
28. Scott IU, Ip MS, VanVeldhuisen PC, Oden NL, Blodi BA, Fisher M, et al. A randomized trial comparing the efficacy and safety of intravitreal triamcinolone with standard care to treat vision loss associated with macular edema secondary to branch retinal vein occlusion: the Standard Care vs Corticosteroid for Retinal Vein Occlusion (SCORE) study report 6. Arch Ophthalmol. 2009;127:1115–28.
29. Haller JA, Bandello F, Belfort R, Blumenkranz MS, Gillies M, Heier J, et al. Dexamethasone intravitreal implant in patients with macular edema related to branch or central retinal vein occlusion twelve-month study results. Ophthalmology. 2011; 118:2453–60.
30. Branch Vein Occlusion Study Group. Argon laser photocoagulation for macular edema in branch vein occlusion. Am J Ophthalmol. 1984;98:271–82.
31. Farese E, Cenamo G, Velotti N, Traversi C, Rinaldi M, De Crecchio G. Intravitreal bevacizumab combined with grid photocoagulation in recurrent macular edema secondary to retinal vein occlusion. Eur J Ophthalmol. 2014;24:761–70.
32. Saika S, Tanaka T, Miyamoto T, Ohnishi Y. Surgical posterior vitreous detachment combined with gas/air tamponade for treating macular edema associated with branch retinal vein occlusion: retinal tomography and visual outcome. Graefes Arch Clin Exp Ophthalmol. 2001;239:729–32.

7 Wide-Field Retinal Imaging of Central Retinal Vein Occlusions

Irena Tsui and Pradeep S. Prasad

Central retinal vein occlusion (CRVO) is a significant cause of vision loss occurring about three times less frequently than branch retinal vein occlusion. Systemic risk factors for CRVO include age older than 55 years as well as cardiovascular risk factors such as hypertension, diabetes, and hyperlipidemia. Glaucoma is associated with CRVO because of increased vulnerability of the central retinal vein at the lamina cribosa. Clinically, CRVOs are classified as nonischemic versus ischemic based on visual acuity, afferent pupillary defect status, and fluorescein angiography. The prognoses for ischemic versus nonischemic CRVO are different, and there are various degrees of ischemia in CRVO. This chapter illustrates the heterogeneous patterns of retinal nonperfusion in CRVO using wide-field fluorescein angiography. Visually significant sequelae of CRVO include macular edema, macular ischemia, neovascularization, vitreous hemorrhage, and neovascular glaucoma. Treatment options include intravitreal injection of anti–vascular endothelial growth factor (anti-VEGF), corticosteroids, laser photocoagulation, and vitreoretinal surgery.

Epidemiology and Risk Factors

CRVOs occur three times less commonly than branch retinal vein occlusion, and the cumulative 15-year incidence of CRVO is reported to be 0.5 % [1]. Ninety-percent of CRVO patients are older than 55 years, but they occur in younger patients as well. There is no known racial predilection, and CRVO occurs more frequently in males.

Common systemic risk factors for CRVO include hypertension, diabetes, and high cholesterol [2]. Hypercoagulable states and autoimmune and inflammatory conditions are less commonly associated conditions [3]. CRVOs can also be secondary to structural changes such as glaucomatous cupping, optic nerve swelling, or space-occupying orbital lesions [4].

I. Tsui, MD (✉) • P.S. Prasad, MD
Retina Division, Department of Ophthalmology,
Jules Stein Eye Institute, University of California, Los Angeles,
Los Angeles, CA, USA
e-mail: itsui@jsei.ucla.edu; Prasad@jsei.ucla.edu

Pathophysiology and Clinical Findings

The exact pathogenesis of CRVO is unknown, but one commonly cited theory is that arteriosclerotic changes of the central retinal artery cause compression of the central retinal vein at the lamina cribosa, resulting in blood stasis and thrombus formation. CRVO results in increased resistance and stagnation of blood flow from the retina. Subsequent ischemic damage increases VEGF in the vitreous cavity [5].

Traditionally, CRVO has been divided into ischemic, nonischemic, or indeterminate with approximately 80 % of indeterminate eyes progressing to the ischemic type, although wide-field angiography is poised to change this classification scheme as very few eyes are classified as indeterminate with WFA. A significant number of eyes can progress from a perfused state to a non-perfused state as the retinal vascular damage evolves [6]. Impending CRVO is an ill-defined term that refers to milder signs and symptoms; it may resolve or progress to a complete CRVO. The presentation of CRVO is variable from asymptomatic to severely decreased vision. Transient visual obscurations with gradual and progressive vision loss over days to weeks are often reported. Sudden and severe loss of vision is seen with ischemic CRVOs.

Eyes with nonischemic CRVOs typically present with visual acuity of 20/200 or better. Other distinguishing factors between nonischemic and ischemic CRVOs include the presence or absence of afferent pupillary defect, a rosette of dense cotton wool patches surrounding the optic nerve head, massive intraretinal hemorrhage, and fluorescein angiographic findings. Fundus

I. Kozak, J.F. Arevalo (eds.), *Atlas of Wide-Field Retinal Angiography and Imaging*, DOI 10.1007/978-3-319-17864-6_7

examination is notable for dilated, torturous veins and a variable amount of intraretinal hemorrhage in all four quadrants; optic nerve edema can also be present [7]. Cotton-wool spots can be seen, often associated with hypertension. Over 3 years' time, approximately one third of nonischemic CRVOs progress to the ischemic type. In later stages of ischemic CRVO, vitreous hemorrhage and neovascular glaucoma can develop. Chronically, disc collaterals and pigmentary changes in the macular form occur.

Evaluation and Management

Ischemic CRVO has been defined as greater than ten disc diameters (DD) of nonperfusion detected with non-wide-field or traditional fluorescein angiography. However, with the routine use of wide-field fluorescein angiography, peripheral patterns of nonperfusion with much greater than ten DD of nonperfusion are being detected (Figs. 1, 2, 3, 4, 5, and 6) and extrapolation of posterior angiographic data to the entire retinal circulation is no longer necessary. Careful anterior segment examination, including gonioscopy, should be performed to evaluate for anterior segment neovascularization. Thirty percent of patients with ischemic CRVO develop neovascular glaucoma, an important ocular morbidity. Optical coherence tomography should also be done at each visit to evaluate for macular edema.

Management of CRVO has changed and improved markedly. Treatable complications are macular edema, nonperfusion, and subsequent neovascularization [8]. For over a decade, since the Central Vein Occlusion Study (CVOS) was published in the mid-1990s [9], the standard of care for CRVO was laser photocoagulation after development of 2 clock-hours of anterior segment neovascularization. Wide-field fluorescein angiography has increased the detection of peripheral nonperfusion and subsequent ischemia in eyes with CRVO, enabling earlier and targeted laser photocoagulation. The CVOS also recommended against treating macular edema in CRVO with grid laser [10].

Anti-VEGF agents are considered first-line therapy to treat macular edema in CRVO. Multiple, well-executed, prospective, randomized clinical trials have demonstrated the utility of pharmacotherapy. In the CRUISE Study (Treatment of Macular Edema following Central Retinal Vein Occlusion: Evaluation of Efficacy and Safety) [11], almost 50 % of eyes treated with anti-VEGF improved by 3 lines of vision. In 2009, dexamethasone implant was the first U.S. Food and Drug Administration (FDA)–approved agent to treat macular edema in CRVO. In the GENEVA Study (Global Evaluation of Implantable Dexamethasone in Retinal Vein Occlusion with Macular Edema) [12], almost 20 % of eyes treated with dexamethasone implant improved by 3 lines of vision at 6 months. In the SCORE (Standard vs Corticosteroid for Retinal Vein Occlusion) Study [13], over 25 % of eyes treated with intravitreal triamcinolone acetonide improved by 3 lines of vision at 1 year. Steroids carry the additional risk of cataract formation and glaucoma.

There is increasingly a trend toward combination therapies (i.e., anti-VEGF, steroid, peripheral laser) in order to maximize patient-centered outcomes [14, 15]. Pars plana vitrectomy is reserved for complications such as vitreous hemorrhage and epiretinal membranes in the absence of severe ischemia. Radial optic neurotomy is no longer recommended for treatment of CRVO.

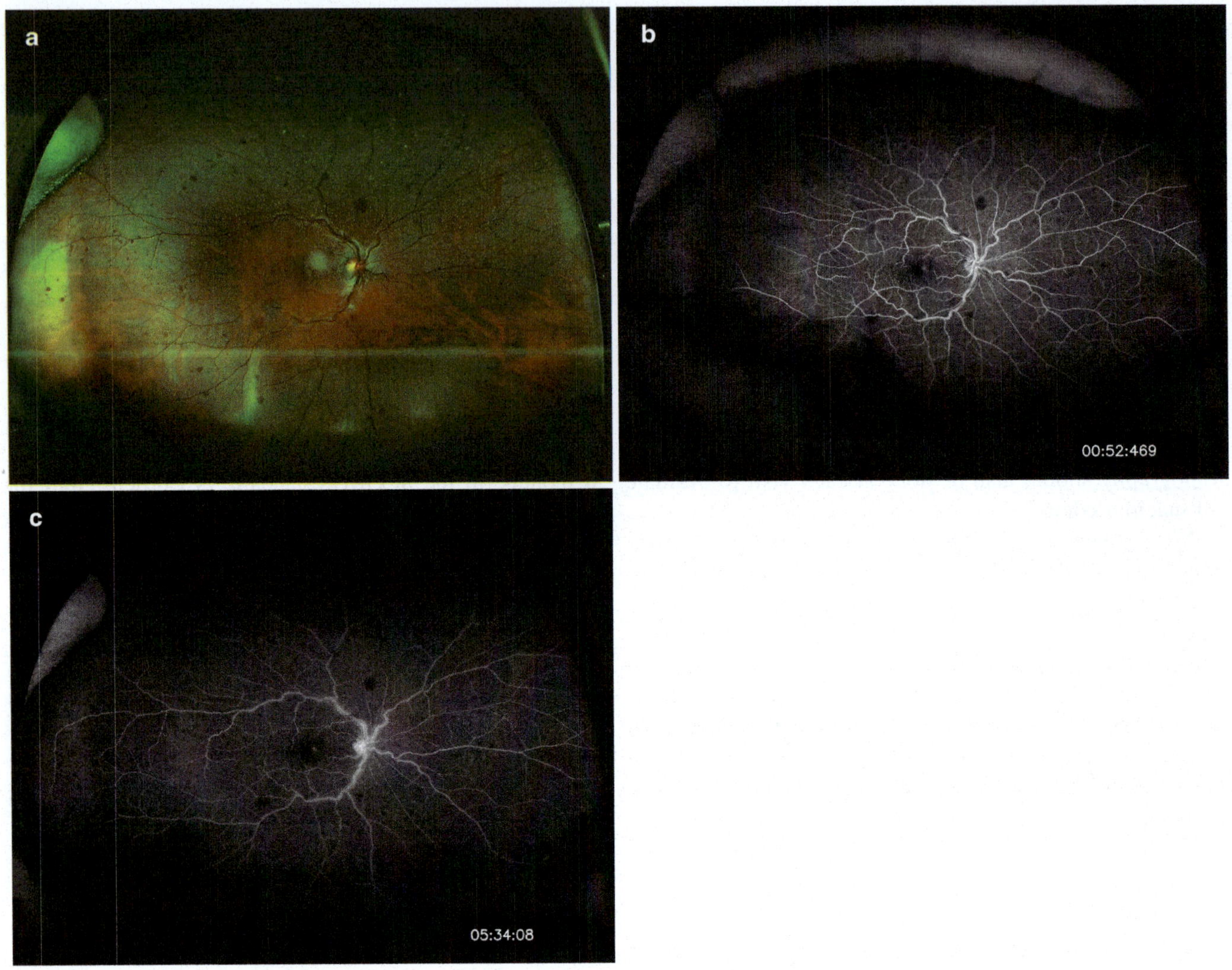

Fig. 1 (**a**) Color fundus photograph shows engorged veins and mild four-quadrant dot blot hemorrhage. (**b**) Fluorescein angiography in mid phase shows blocking defects and delayed filling of peripheral venous vasculature. (**c**) Fluorescein angiography in late phase shows with blocking defects and staining of large vessel venous vasculature

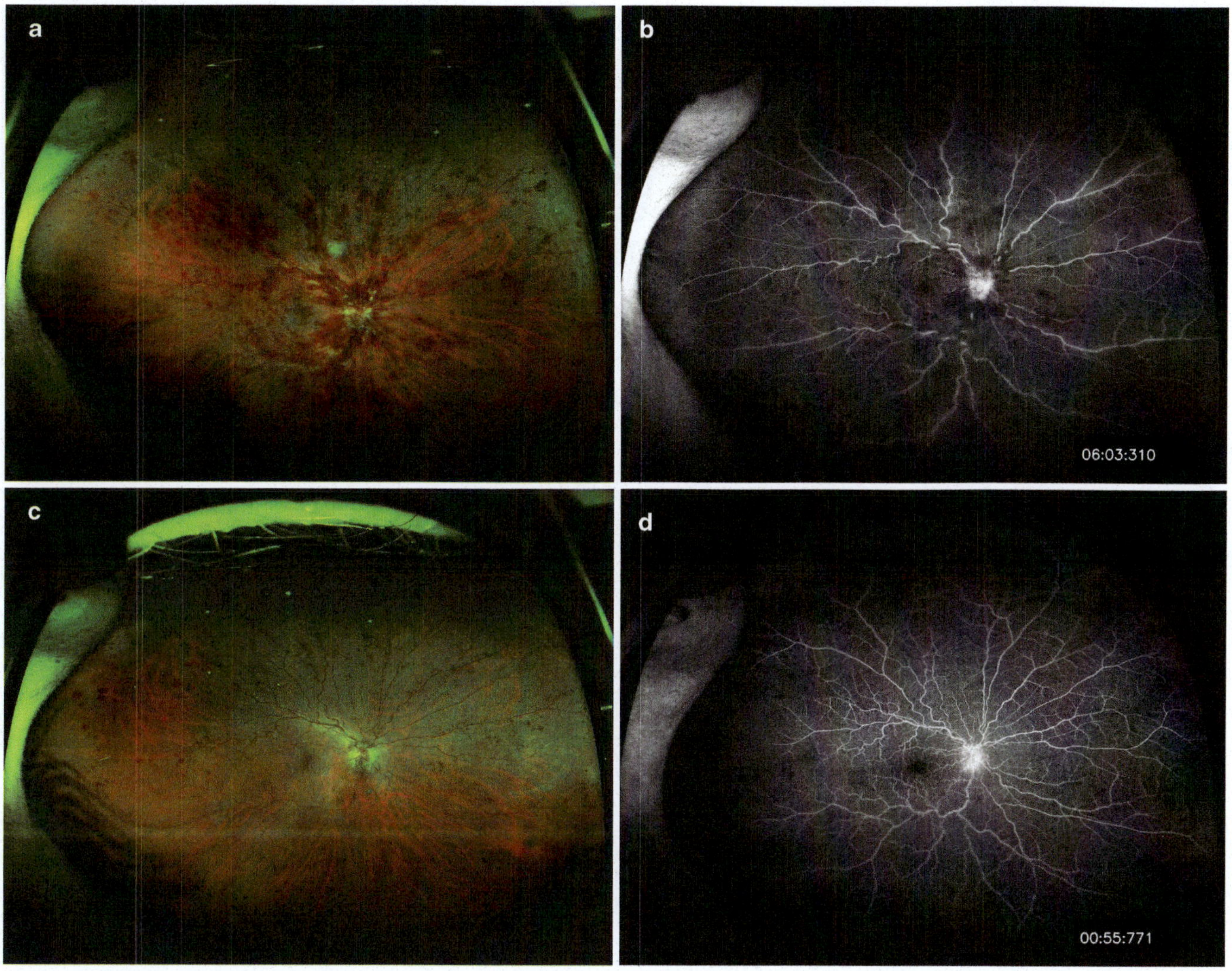

Fig. 2 (**a**) Color fundus photograph shows hemorrhagic CRVO with prominent optic nerve swelling. (**b**) Fluorescein angiography in late phase shows blocking defects, optic nerve head leakage, and staining of large vessel venous vasculature. (**c**) Nine months later, after anti-VEGF therapy, intraretinal hemorrhages have largely resolved. (**d**) Mid-phase fluorescein angiography shows delayed filling of peripheral veins temporally

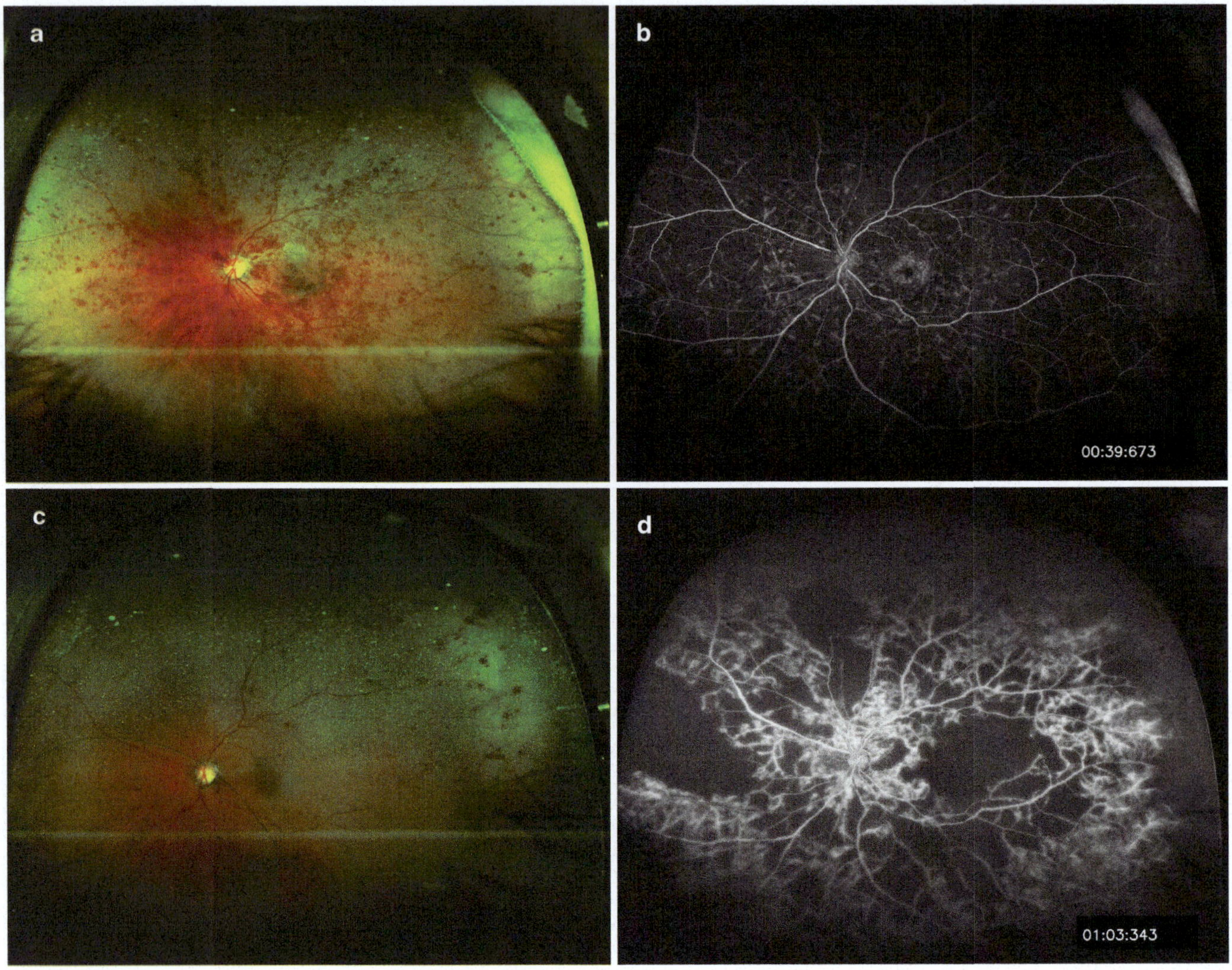

Fig. 3 (**a**) Color fundus photograph shows hemorrhagic CRVO. (**b**) Fluorescein angiography shows leakage of small vessels. (**c**) Nine months later, after anti-VEGF therapy, intraretinal hemorrhages have largely resolved. (**d**) However, fluorescein angiography reveals progression to profound and widespread nonperfusion

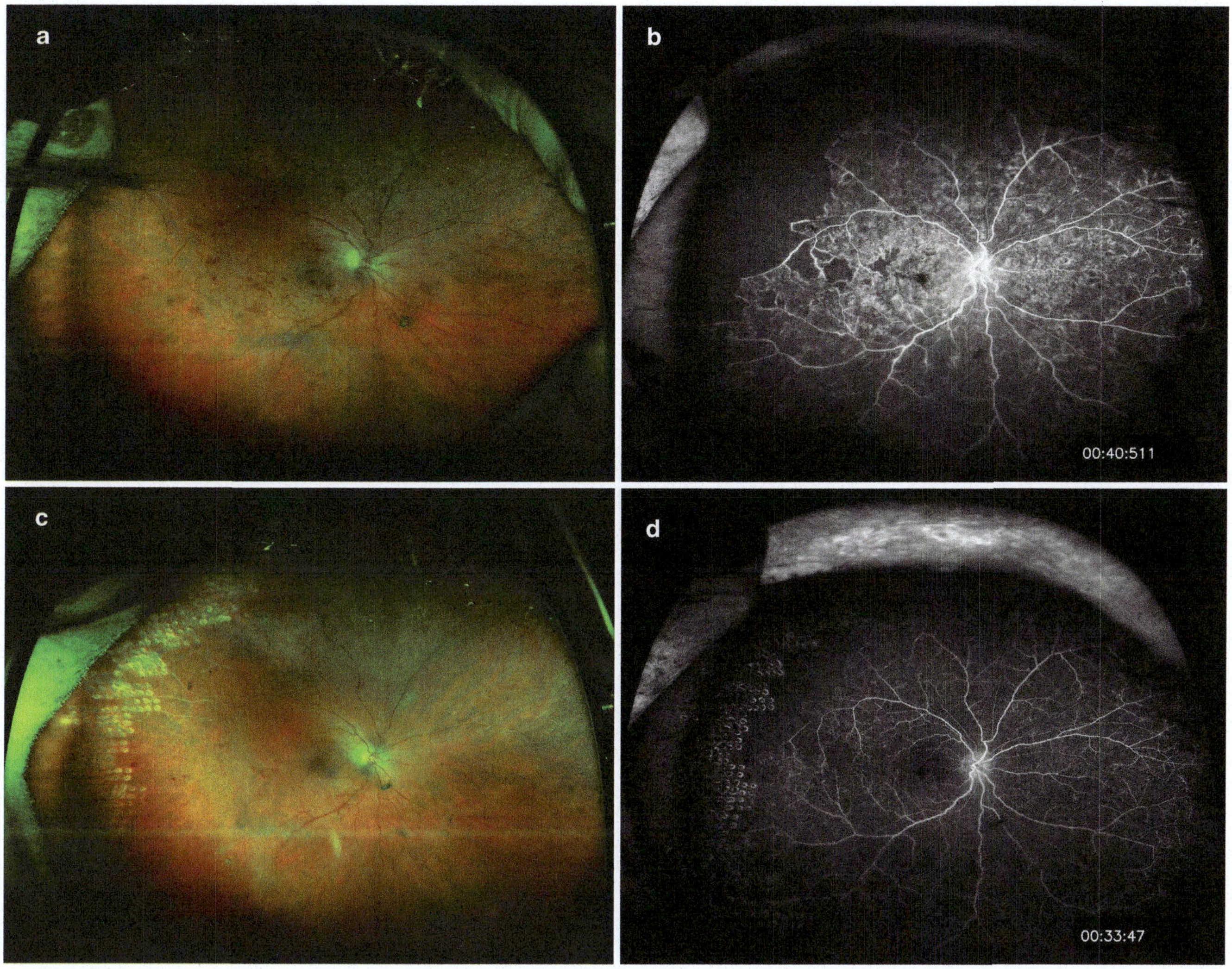

Fig. 4 (**a**) Color fundus photograph shows intraretinal hemorrhage, mostly in the posterior pole, with ischemic vessels in the superotemporal periphery. (**b**) Fluorescein angiography shows temporal nonperfusion extending into the macula. (**c**) Six months later, color fundus photograph shows targeted laser photocoagulation. (**d**) Fluorescein angiography shows residual areas of untreated nonperfusion temporally

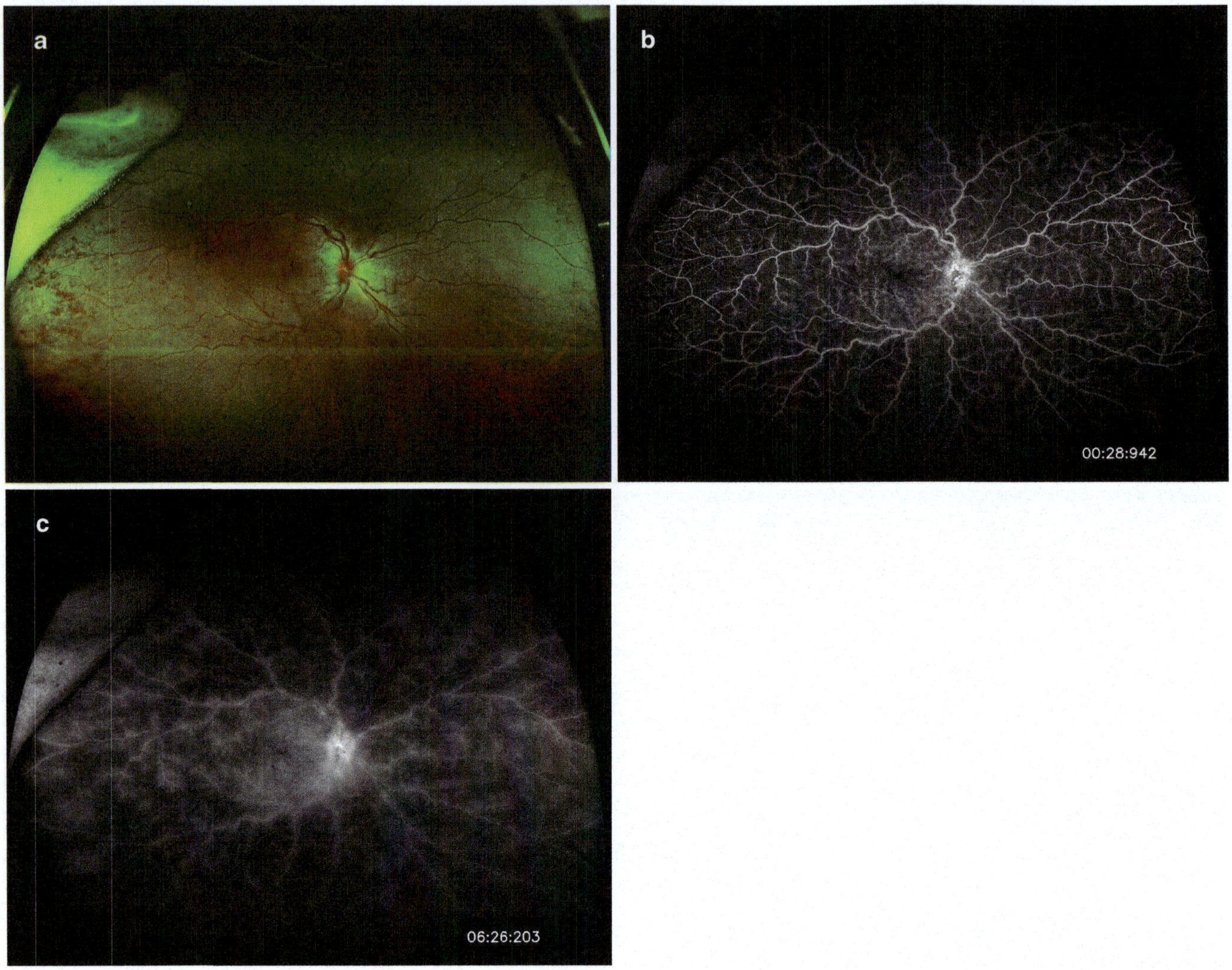

Fig. 5 (**a**) Color fundus photograph shows mild optic nerve swelling, engorged veins, and intraretinal hemorrhage, mostly in the periphery. (**b**) Fluorescein angiography shows staining of large venous vessels and capillary nonperfusion throughout the fundus. (**c**) Fluorescein angiography in late phase shows leakage of both small and large vessels

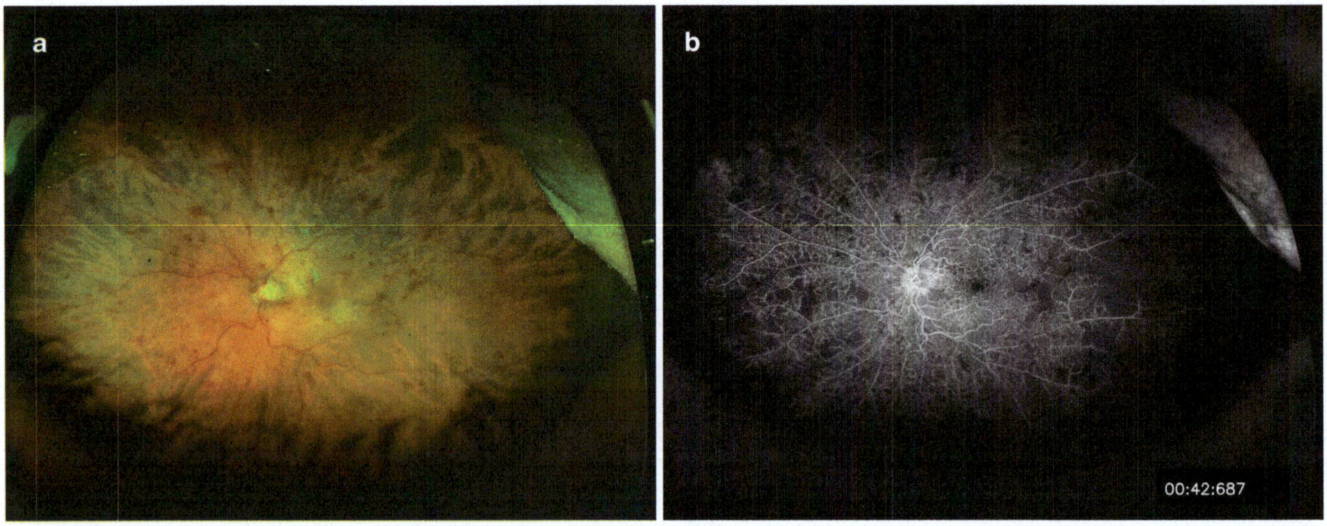

Fig. 6 (**a**) Color fundus photograph shows optic nerve cupping, increased venous tortuosity, and mild-moderate four-quadrant dot blot hemorrhage. (**b**) Fluorescein angiography shows widespread nonperfusion and leakage of small vessels

References

1. Klein R, Moss SE, Meuer SM, Klein BE. The 15-year cumulative incidence of retinal vein occlusion: the Beaver Dam Eye Study. Arch Ophthalmol. 2008;126:513–8.
2. Hayreh SS, Zimmerman B, McCarthy MJ, Podhajsky P. Systemic diseases associated with various types of retinal vein occlusion. Am J Ophthalmol. 2001;131:61–77.
3. Lahey JM, Kearney JJ, Tunc M. Hypercoagulable states and central retinal vein occlusion. Curr Opin Pulm Med. 2003;9:385–92.
4. Hayreh SS, Zimmerman MB, Beri M, Podhajsky P. Intraocular pressure abnormalities associated with central and hemicentral retinal vein occlusion. Ophthalmology. 2004;111:133–41.
5. Noma H, Funatsu H, Mimura T, Harino S, Hori S. Vitreous levels of interleukin-6 and vascular endothelial growth factor in macular edema with central retinal vein occlusion. Ophthalmology. 2009;116:87–93.
6. The Central Vein Occlusion Study Report. Baseline and early natural history. Arch Ophthalmol. 1993;111:1087–95.
7. Hayreh SS, Zimmerman MB. Fundus changes in central retinal vein occlusion. Retina. 2015;35:29–42.
8. Hayreh SS, Podhajsky PA, Zimmerman MB. Natural history of visual outcome in central retinal vein occlusion. Ophthalmology. 2011;118:119–33.e1–2.
9. The Central Vein Occlusion Study Group N report. A randomized clinical trial of early panretinal photocoagulation for ischemic central vein occlusion. Ophthalmology. 1995;102:1434–44.
10. The Central Vein Occlusion Study Group M report. Evaluation of grid pattern photocoagulation for macular edema in central vein occlusion. Ophthalmology. 1995;102:1425–33.
11. Brown DM, Campochiaro PA, Singh RP, Li Z, Gray S, Saroj N, et al. Ranibizumab for macular edema following central retinal vein occlusion: six-month primary end point results of a phase III study. Ophthalmology. 2010;117:1124–33.e1.
12. Haller JA, Bandello F, Belfort Jr R, Blumenkranz MS, Gillies M, Heier J, et al. Dexamethasone intravitreal implant in patients with macular edema related to branch or central retinal vein occlusion twelve-month study results. Ophthalmology. 2011; 118:2453–60.
13. Ip MS, Scott IU, VanVeldhuisen PC, Oden NL, Blodi BA, Fisher M, et al. A randomized trial comparing the efficacy and safety of intravitreal triamcinolone with observation to treat vision loss associated with macular edema secondary to central retinal vein occlusion: the Standard Care vs Corticosteroid for Retinal Vein Occlusion (SCORE) study report 5. Arch Ophthalmol. 2009; 127:1101–14.
14. Singer M, Tan CS, Bell D, Sadda SR. Area of peripheral retinal nonperfusion and treatment response in branch and central retinal vein occlusion. Retina. 2014;34:1736–42.
15. Rehak M, Tilgner E, Franke A, Rauscher FG, Brosteanu O, Wiedemann P. Early peripheral laser photocoagulation of nonperfused retina improves vision in patients with central retinal vein occlusion (results of a proof of concept study). Graefes Arch Clin Exp Ophthalmol. 2014;252:745–52.

8 Wide-Field Retinal Imaging of Other Retinal Vascular Diseases

Igor Kozak, J. Fernando Arevalo, and The KKESH Collaborative Retina Study Group*

Recent advances in wide-field imaging have helped to document and monitor retinovascular diseases of the retinal periphery. This is of utmost importance in order to observe behavior of the lesions. These lesions include vascular tumors, aneurysms, or vasculitides of inflammatory and infectious etiology. Ultra-wide-field imaging can also assist in directing laser photocoagulation in the treatment of both adult and pediatric retinal diseases. Following are some examples encountered in clinical practice.

I. Kozak, MD, PhD (✉)
Senior Academic Consultant, Vitreoretinal Division, King Khaled Eye Specialist Hospital, Riyadh, Kingdom of Saudi Arabia
e-mail: ikozak@kkesh.med.sa

J.F. Arevalo, MD, FACS
Edmund F. and Virginia B. Ball Professor of Ophthalmology, Chairman, Department of Ophthalmology,
Johns Hopkins Bayview Medical Center, Retina Division, Wilmer Eye Institute, The Johns Hopkins University School of Medicine, Baltimore, MD, USA
e-mail: arevalojf@jhmi.edu

I. Kozak, J.F. Arevalo (eds.), *Atlas of Wide-Field Retinal Angiography and Imaging*, DOI 10.1007/978-3-319-17864-6_8

Coats Disease

Coats disease is an idiopathic, retinal vascular abnormality of young males characterized by telangiectatic retinal vessels with aneurysms. Abnormal permeability of these vessels leads to exudative retinal detachment and subretinal lipid deposits. Often subfoveal exudation leading to permanent severe vision loss occurs prior to presentation. The severe forms of the disease often involve neovascular glaucoma and phthisis bulbi [1, 2]. Ultra-wide-field fundus photography and angiography can be used successfully as an outpatient procedure in the pediatric patient population without the necessity of examination under anesthesia and can aid the physician in the documentation and evaluation of Coats disease (Figs. 1, 2, 3, and 4) [3].

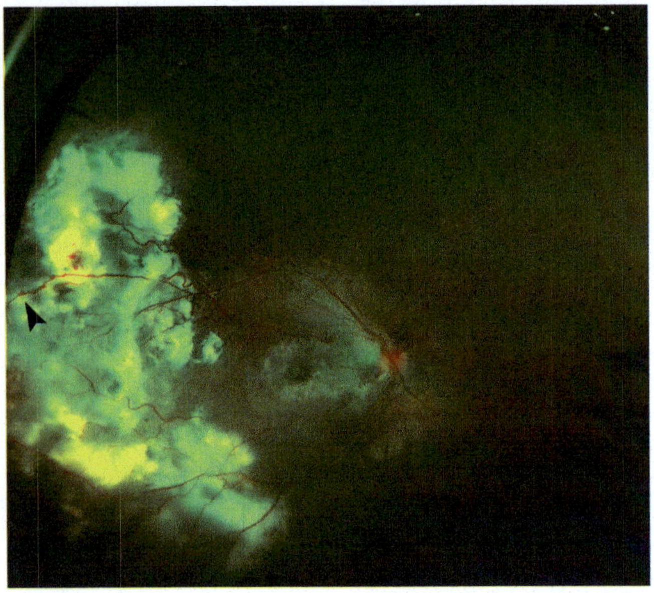

Fig. 1 Coats disease. Wide-field color fundus image of a 15-year-old boy with unilateral peripheral lesion in the temporal retina. The image shows extensive subretinal exudation and teleangiectatic retinal vessels (*black arrowhead*)

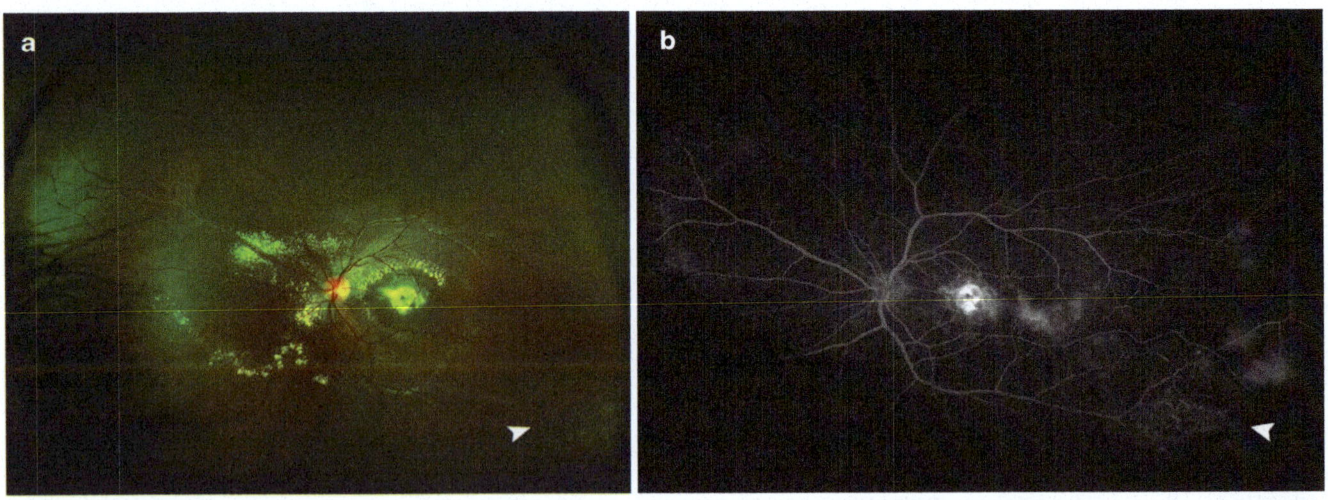

Fig. 2 (**a**) Coats disease. Wide-field fundus color image of a 15-year-old boy shows subretinal exudates in the posterior pole and around the optic disc with peripheral vascular lesion inferotemporally (*white arrowhead*). Visual acuity due to macular lesion was 20/400. (**b**) Wide-field fundus fluorescein angiogram of the same eye shows staining of the macular scar, (peri-) macular leakage, and leaking peripheral teleangiectatic retinal blood vessels

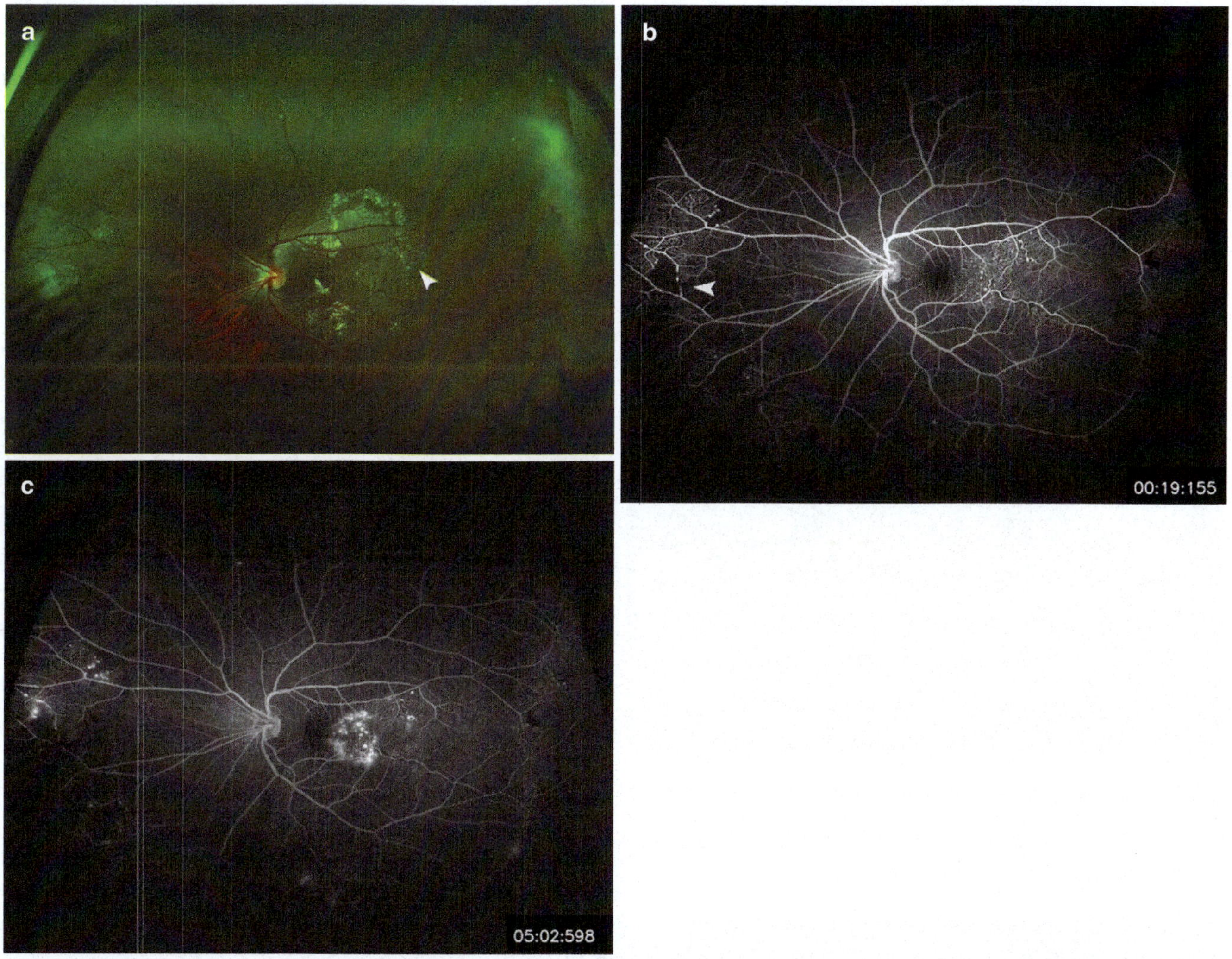

Fig. 3 (**a**) Coats disease. Wide-field fundus color image of an 18-year-old male patient with hard exudates throughout the posterior pole with teleangiectatic blood vessels temporal to the macula (*white arrowhead*) and in the nasal periphery. (**b**) Wide-field early fundus fluorescein angiogram of the same eye shows teleangiectatic blood vessels temporal to the macula and in the nasal periphery (*white arrowhead*) along with areas of capillary drop-out. (**c**) Wide-field late fundus fluorescein angiogram of the same eye shows leakage from teleangiectatic blood vessels both temporal to the macula and in the nasal periphery

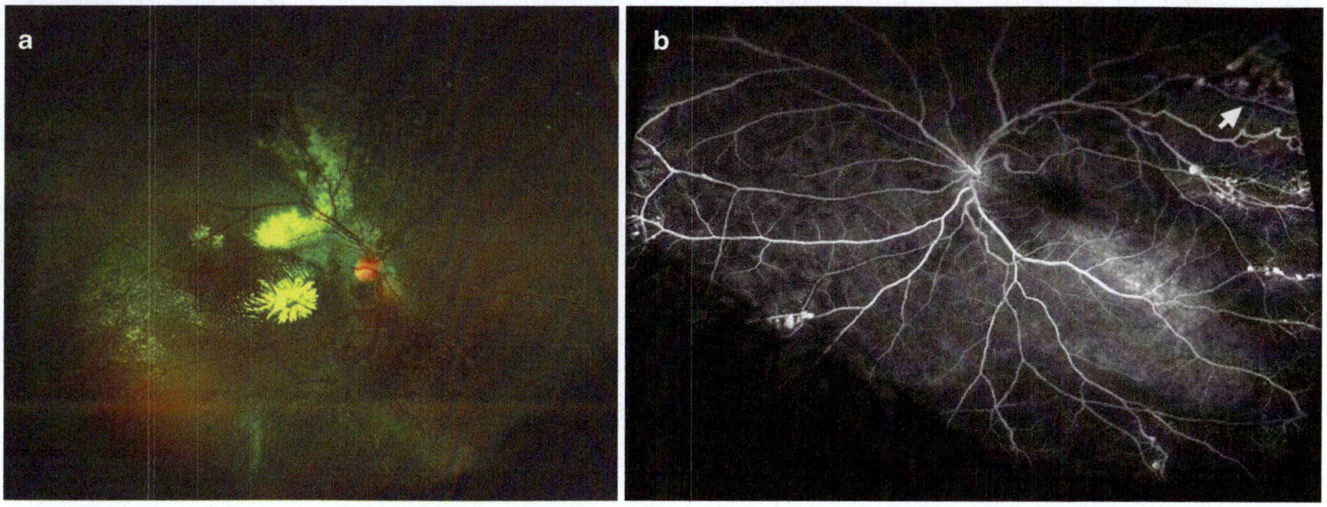

Fig. 4 (**a**) Bilateral Coats disease. Wide-field fundus color image of right eye of a 21-year-old man with macular star and hard exudates throughout the posterior pole and outside of the vascular arcades. (**b**) Wide-field fundus fluorescein angiogram of the left eye of the same patient shows teleangiectatic blood vessels in the retinal periphery and mid periphery temporally (*white arrow*)

Von Hippel–Lindau Disease

Von Hippel–Lindau Disease (VHL) is an autosomal dominant inherited systemic cancer syndrome that gives rise to cystic and highly vascularized tumors in many organs, including the eye [4]. Patients with VHL are at increased risk of developing central nervous system and retinal hemangioblastomas, clear cell renal carcinoma, pheochromocytomas, neuroendocrine tumors and cysts of the pancreas, endolymphatic sac tumors, or papillary cystadenomas of the epididymis and broad ligament [5]. Retinal hemangioblastomas, present in up to 85 % of individuals with VHL, are the most common lesion of VHL disease (Figs. 5, 6, and 7) [6].

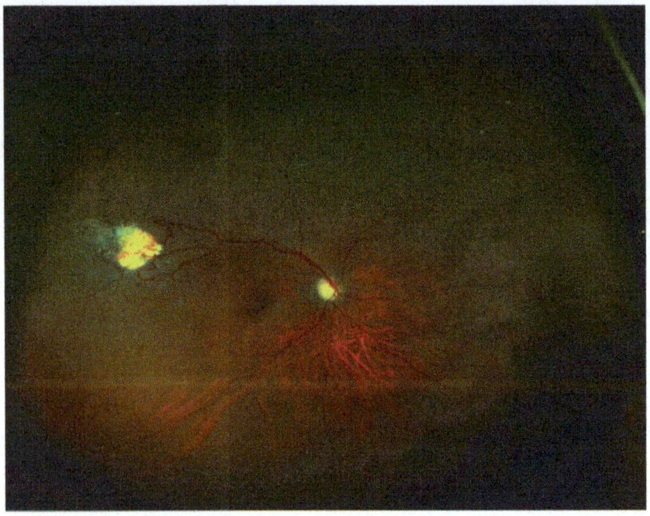

Fig. 5 VHL disease. Wide-field fundus color image of right eye of a 74-year-old woman with history of primary open-angle glaucoma and VHL disease. The image shows increased cup-to-disc ratio and vascular tumor along the superior vascular arcade

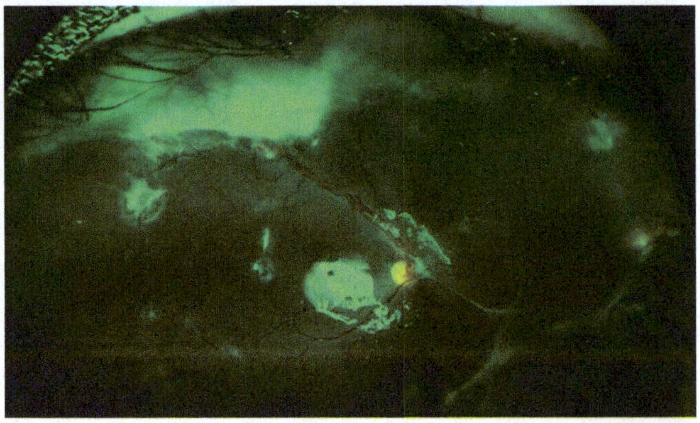

Fig. 6 VHL disease. Wide-field fundus color image of right eye of a 22-year-old woman with history of retinal hemangioblastomas. The right eye underwent removal of large superior hemangioblastoma followed by silicone oil tamponade. The other eye is lost to VHL disease

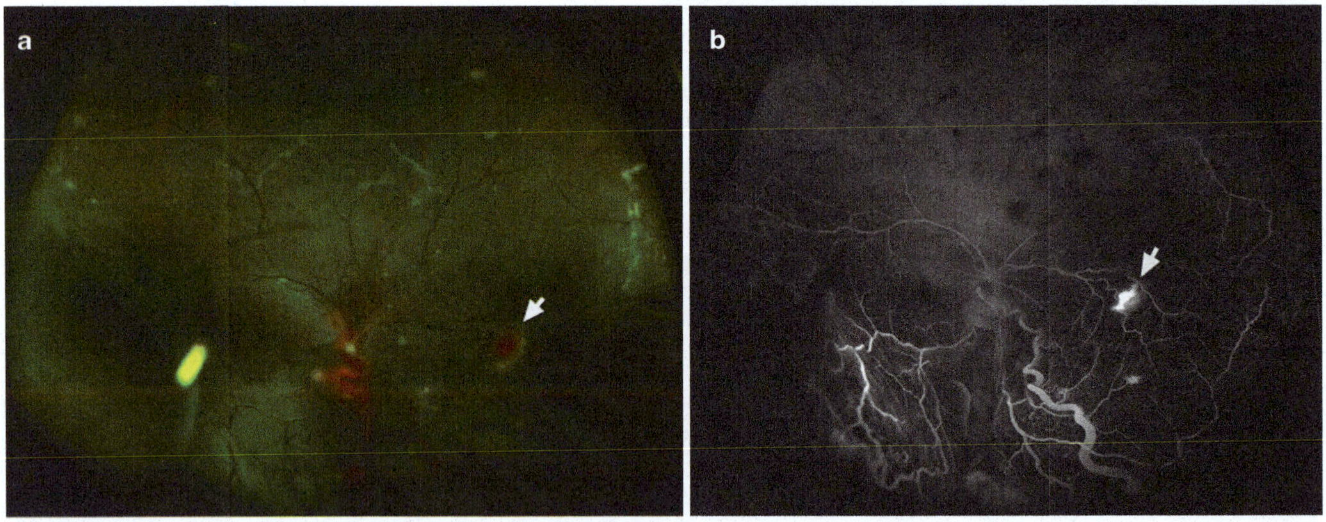

Fig. 7 (**a**) VHL disease. Wide-field fundus color image of the right eye of a 17-year-old boy who underwent external drainage, Ozurdex implant, and cryotherapy for extensive subretinal exudation due to VHL disease. The image demonstrates residual inferotemporal exudative detachment and vascular lesion nasally (*white arrow*). (**b**) Wide-field fundus fluorescein angiogram of the same eye shows prominent retinal vessels and dye leakage from the vascular lesion (*white arrow*)

Familial Retinal Arterial Macroaneurysms

Familial retinal arterial macroaneurysms (FRAM), a rare progressive recessive phenotype of familial retinal arterial macroaneurysms with supravalvular pulmonary stenosis, has been described in a total of eight Saudi Arabian families from different regions of the country [7]. Homozygosity mapping-guided genetic analysis for these families revealed that a single common homozygous founder mutation in IGFBP7 (4q12 MIM 602,867) underlies the phenotype [8]. The fact that recessive mutation in this insulin-like growth factor–binding protein causes FRAM with supravalvular pulmonary stenosis suggests that the normally encoded protein has a role in formation and/or maintenance of the cardiovascular system (Figs. 8, 9, and 10) [9].

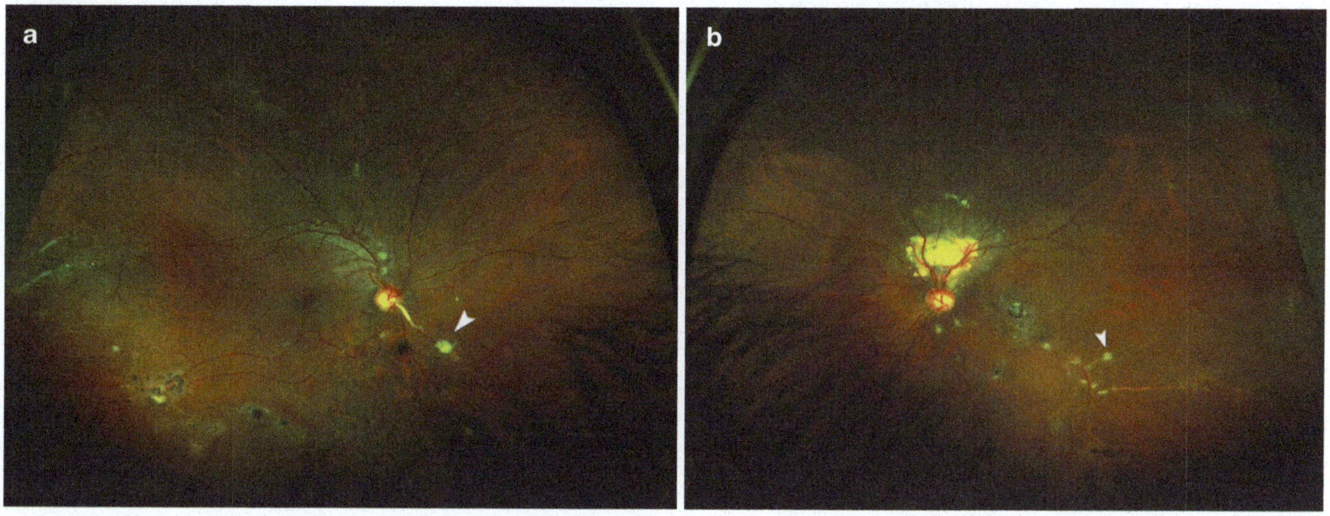

Fig. 8 (**a**) FRAM. Wide-field fundus color image of the right eye of a 22-year-old man diagnosed with FRAM and cardiac abnormalities demonstrates old vascular lesions post–focal laser photocoagulation (*white arrowhead*). Visual acuity is 20/25. (**b**) Wide-field fundus color image of the left eye of the same patient demonstrates peripapillary exudation and old aneurysms (*white arrowhead*). Visual acuity is 20/125

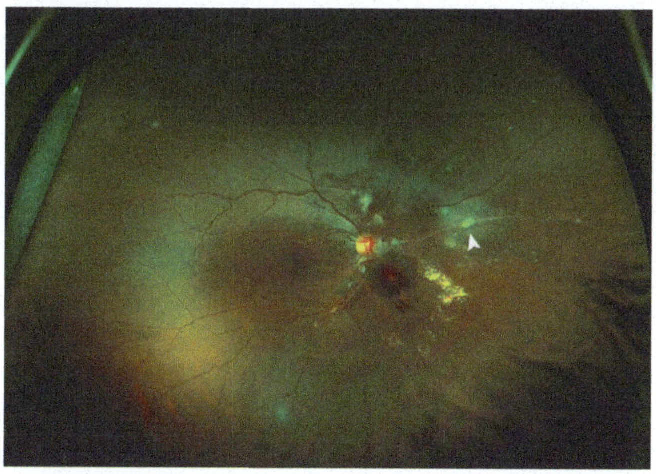

Fig. 9 FRAM. Wide-field fundus color image of the right eye of a 29-year-old woman diagnosed with FRAM demonstrates peripapillary subretinal hemorrhage with hard exudates and old macroaneurysm (*white arrowhead*)

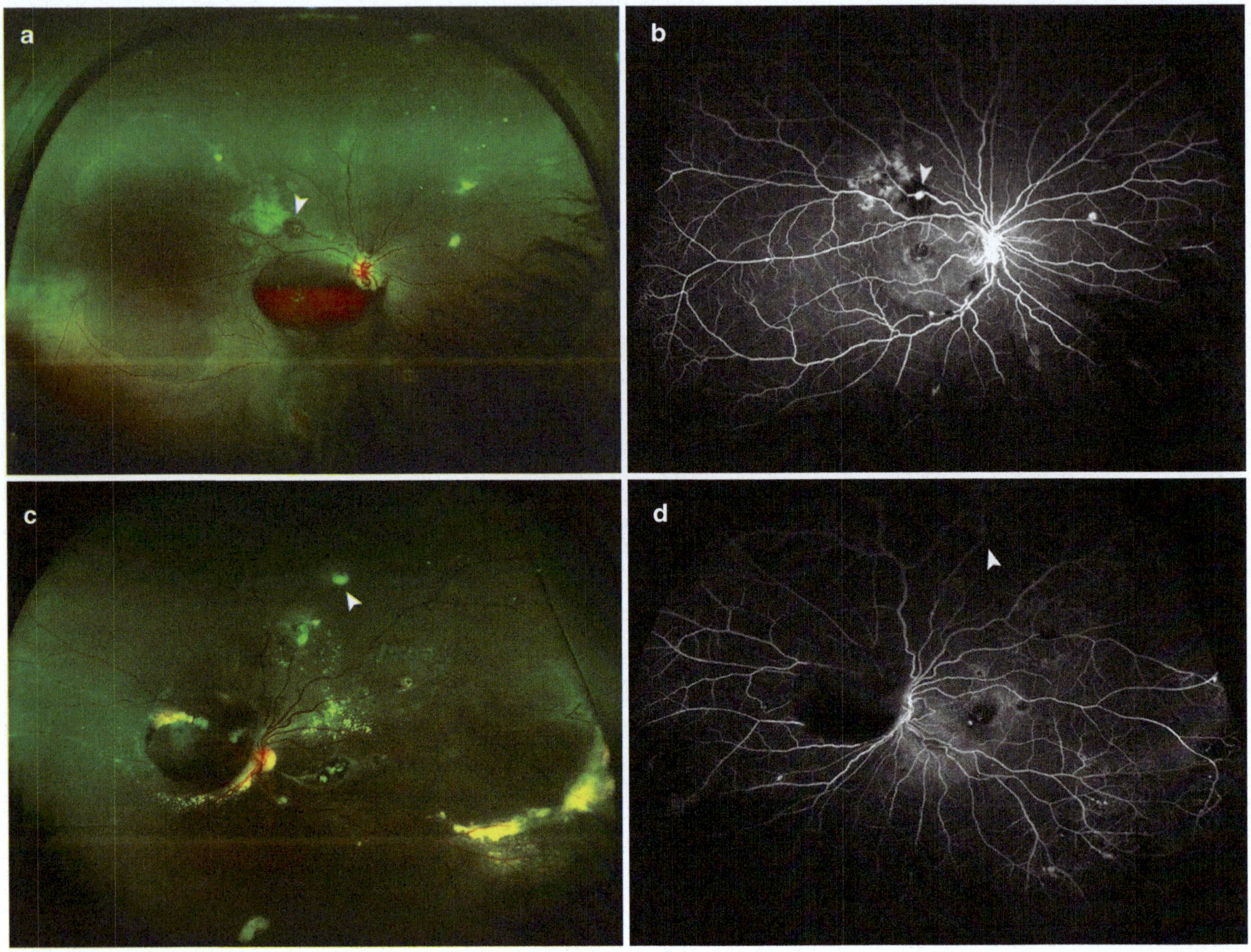

Fig. 10 (**a**) FRAM. Wide-field fundus color image of the right eye of a 16-year-old boy with FRAM and cardiac abnormalities demonstrates old aneurysms (*white arrowhead*) and premacular hemorrhage, which is located under the internal limiting membrane (ILM) by optical coherence tomography (OCT). (**b**) Wide-field fundus fluorescein angiogram of the same eye after resolution of sub-ILM hemorrhage shows numerous macroaneurysms (*white arrowhead*). (**c**) Wide-field fundus color image of the left eye of the same boy shows sub-ILM cyst, hard exudates, and macroaneurysms (*white arrowhead*). (**d**) Wide-field fundus fluorescein angiogram of the left eye shows numerous aneurysms (*white arrowhead*)

Retinal Macroaneurysm

Retinal arterial macroaneurysms are acquired saccular dilatations of the large arterioles of the retina, usually within the first three orders of bifurcation. Macroaneurysms are mostly monocular, usually affect females and elderly people, and are commonly associated with systemic hypertension [10, 11]. No genetic predisposition has been identified so far (Fig. 11). Ultra-wide imaging technology assists in documenting pathology in numerous other retinovascular diseases (Figs. 12, 13, 14, and 15).

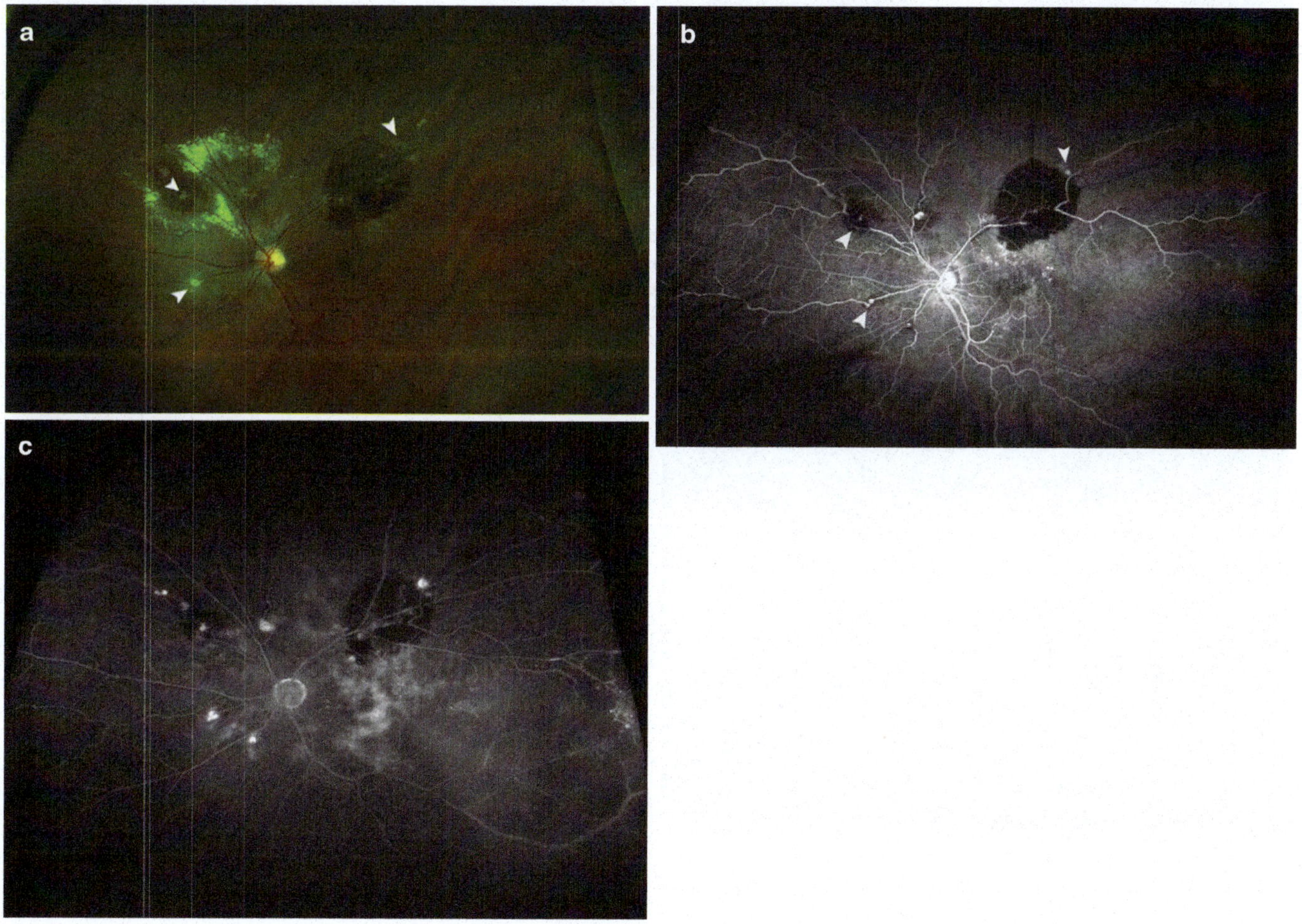

Fig. 11 (**a**) Retinal arterial macroaneurysms. Wide-field fundus color image of the left eye of a 59-year-old hypertensive man with no mutations shows multiple aneurysms (*white arrowheads*) associated with subretinal hemorrhage and exudation. The other eye had hypertensive retinopathy with no aneurysms. (**b**) Wide-field early fundus fluorescein angiogram of the same eye shows multiple aneurysms (*white arrowheads*) and blockage from hemorrhage. (**c**) Wide-field late fundus fluorescein angiogram of the same eye shows macular leakage and nonperfusion in the temporal retinal periphery

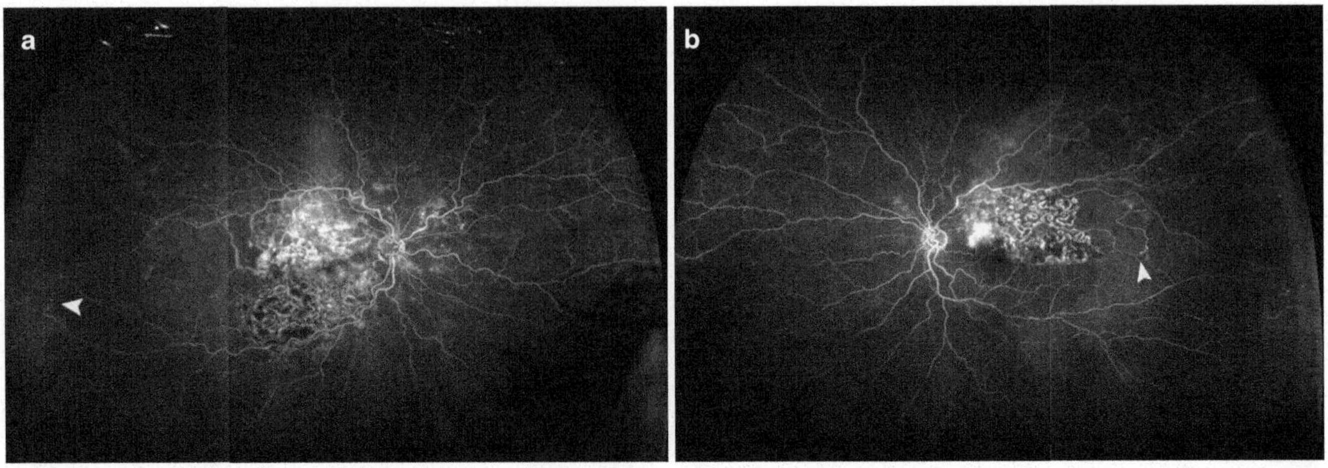

Fig. 12 (**a**) Bilateral vein occlusion with peripheral nonperfusion. A 62-year-old woman with primary open-angle glaucoma and a history of branch retinal vein occlusion in both eyes underwent grid laser photocoagulation for associated macular edema. Wide-field fundus fluorescein angiogram of her right eye shows laser photocoagulation spots in the posterior pole and collateral blood vessels (*white arrowhead*) and areas of capillary drop-out in the temporal periphery. (**b**) Wide-field fundus fluorescein angiogram of her left eye shows laser photocoagulation spots superior to the macula, collateral blood vessels (*white arrowhead*), and areas of capillary drop-out in the superotemporal periphery

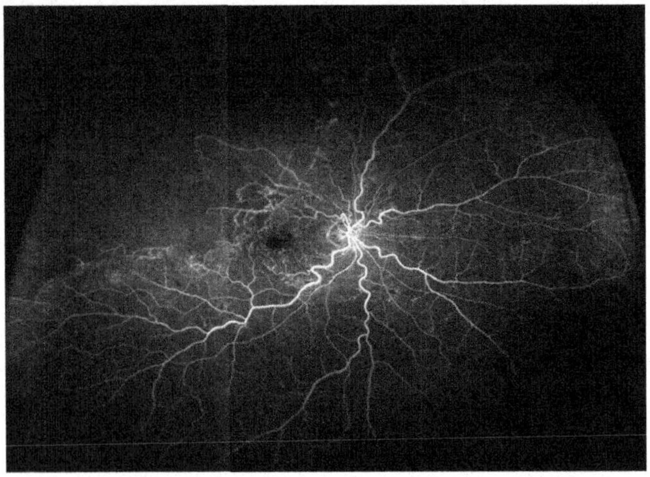

Fig. 13 Peripheral retinal ischemia. Wide-field fundus fluorescein angiogram of the right eye of a 51-year-old hypertensive woman shows extensive peripheral retinal ischemia. No history of vascular occlusion could be elicited

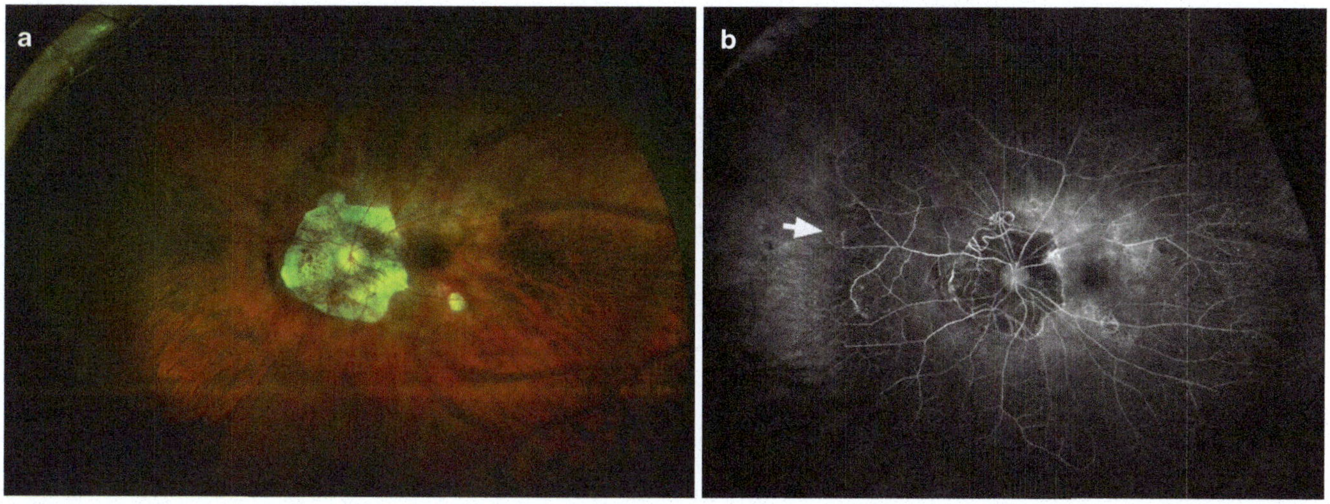

Fig. 14 (**a**) Myopic peripheral nonperfusion. Wide-field fundus color image of the left eye of a 59-year-old woman with degenerative myopia and a history of glaucoma in both eyes shows severe peripapillary atrophy. (**b**) Wide-field fundus fluorescein angiogram of the same eye shows retinal pigment epithelium defect around the optic nerve head and circular peripheral retinal nonperfusion (*white arrow*)

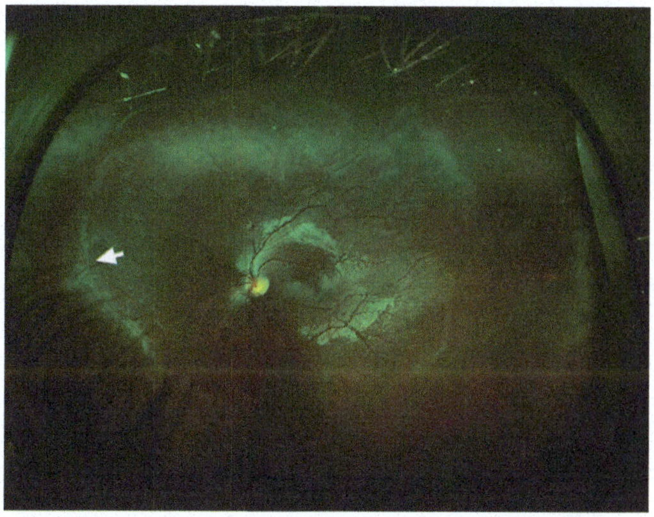

Fig. 15 Vasculopathy of retinopathy of prematurity. Wide-field fundus color image of the left eye of a 29-year-old woman with a history of retinopathy of prematurity demonstrates a remnant of an old vascular ridge without any traction or neovascularization (white arrow)

Acknowledgment *The following investigators belong to The King Khaled Eye Specialist Hospital (KKESH) Collaborative Retina Study Group: J. Fernando Arevalo, MD, FACS (PI), Saba Al Rashaed, MD, Eman Al Kahtani, MD, Sawsan Nowilaty, MD, Hassan A. Al-Dhibi, MD, Yahya A. Al-Zahrani, MD, Igor Kozak, MD, PhD, Sulaiman Al-Sulaiman, MD, Patrik Schatz, MD, Abdulelah Al-Abdullah, MD, Khalid Al Rubaie, MD, Yousef Al Dhafiri, MD, Badr Al Ahmadi, MD, Abdulaziz Al Hadlaq, MD, Majed Al Harbi, MD, Abdulaziz Al Oreany, MD, Adel Al-Akeely, MD, Mohammad Hazzazi, MD, Mohammed Talea, MD, Ghazai Al-Thobaiti, MD.

References

1. Do DV, Haller JA. Coats disease. In: Ryan SJ, Schachat AP, editors. Retina. Philadelphia: Elsevier; 2006. p. 1417–27.
2. Shields JA, Shields CL, Honavar SG, Demirci H. Clinical variations and complications of coats disease in 150 cases: the 2000 Sanford Gifford Memorial Lecture. Am J Ophthalmol. 2001;131: 561–71.
3. Kang KB, Wessel MM, Tong J, D'Amico DJ, Chan RV. Ultra-widefield imaging for the management of pediatric retinal diseases. J Pediatr Ophthalmol Strabismus. 2013;50:282–8.
4. Haddad NM, Cavallerano JD, Silva PS. Von Hippel-Lindau disease: a genetic and clinical review. Semin Ophthalmol. 2013;28:377–86.
5. Maher ER. Von Hippel-Lindau disease. Curr Mol Med. 2004;4:833–42.
6. Chew EY. Ocular manifestations of von Hippel-Lindau disease: clinical and genetic investigations. Trans Am Ophthalmol Soc. 2005;103:495–511.
7. Abu-Safieh L, Abboud EB, Alkuraya H, Shamseldin H, Al-Enzi S, Al-Abdi L, et al. Mutation of IGFBP7 causes upregulation of BRAF/MEK/ERK pathway and familial retinal arterial macroaneurysms. Am J Hum Genet. 2011;89:313–9.
8. Dhindsa HS, Abboud EB. Familial retinal arterial macroaneurysms. Retina. 2002;22:607–15.
9. Khan AO. Ocular genetic disease in the Middle East. Curr Opin Ophthalmol. 2013;24:369–78.
10. Robertson DM. Macroaneurysms of the retinal arteries. Trans Am Acad Ophthalmol Otolaryngol. 1973;77:OP55–67.
11. Abdel-Khalek MN, Richardson J. Retinal macroaneurysm: natural history and guidelines for treatment. Br J Ophthalmol. 1986;70:2–11.

Wide-Field Imaging of Retinal Dystrophies

9

Pradeep S. Prasad and David Sarraf

Hereditary degenerations of the retina, choroid, and vitreous are a heterogeneous group of disorders with variable age of onset and a diverse spectrum of symptoms, signs, inheritance patterns, and systemic associations. Wide-field imaging can serve as an important resource in the diagnosis and management of these challenging conditions. This chapter reviews the various dystrophies of the retina, choroid, and vitreous with particular attention to the application of wide-field photography, fluorescein angiography, and autofluorescence imaging in the evaluation of these disorders.

Dystrophies of the Retina and Retinal Pigment Epithelium

Retinitis Pigmentosa

Retinitis pigmentosa (RP) refers to a group of retinal diseases characterized by hereditary loss and dysfunction of rods more than cones and can be categorized based on the absence or presence of associated systemic disease (nonsyndromic and syndromic RP, respectively). In addition, a number of noninherited conditions affecting the retina can phenotypically resemble RP, termed pseudoretinitis pigmentosa. Typical or nonsyndromic RP can be inherited in an autosomal recessive, autosomal dominant, or X-linked recessive fashion, with the autosomal recessive mode of inheritance being the most common and the X-linked recessive mode associated with earlier age of onset and more pronounced vision loss.

Clinical symptoms of typical RP include nyctalopia, photopsia, progressive loss of peripheral vision, and in some cases, loss of central vision. Funduscopic findings include vascular attenuation, retinal pigment epithelial (RPE) mottling, and peripheral pigment migration (bone spicules). Waxy pallor of the optic disc is a late finding. Wide-field color fundus photography and autofluorescence can be particularly useful to document the extent of RPE mottling and bone spicule formation and can be used as an objective surveillance tool for disease progression. In very early stages of the disease, mid-peripheral and peripheral fundus autofluorescence changes may be seen on wide-field imaging that precede manifestations in the posterior pole. Local complications of disease include posterior subcapsular cataract, vitreous cell, cystoid macular edema (CME), epiretinal membrane (ERM) formation, and rarely, Coats-like retinal exudation.

Numerous systemic conditions may be associated with RP, the most common being Usher syndrome, characterized by variable degrees of congenital deafness (type 1 more severe than type 2) and vestibular dysfunction. Like Usher syndrome, Laurence-Moon-Bardet-Biedl syndrome is a retinal ciliopathy (mutations that involve microtubule defects present in cilia of the outer segments and the inner ear) characterized by RP and deafness as well as obesity, polydactyly, renal disease, and/or hypogonadism. Systemic conditions with RP and associated inborn errors of metabolism include hereditary abetalipoproteinemia (Bassen-Kornzweig syndrome), phytanic acid oxidase deficiency (Refsum disease), neuronal ceroid lipofuscinosis (Batten disease), mucopolysaccharide storage disorders, and some mitochondrial syndromes.

Dystrophies of the Choroid

Gyrate Atrophy

Gyrate atrophy results from an autosomal recessive deficiency of ornithine aminotransferase and is diagnosed by elevated levels of serum ornithine. Confluent peripheral chorioretinal atrophy is very characteristic and the atrophic lesions have a sharply demarcated "scalloped" appearance

P.S. Prasad, MD (✉)
Department of Ophthalmology, Jules Stein Eye Institute, University of California, Los Angeles, Los Angeles, CA, USA
e-mail: Prasad@jsei.ucla.edu

D. Sarraf, MD
Jules Stein Eye Institute, David Geffen School of Medicine, University of California, Los Angeles, Los Angeles, CA, USA
e-mail: dsarraf@ucla.edu

I. Kozak, J.F. Arevalo (eds.), *Atlas of Wide-Field Retinal Angiography and Imaging*, DOI 10.1007/978-3-319-17864-6_9

that is diagnostic and may progress in later stages to involve the posterior pole. Clinical features include nyctalopia and visual field constriction. Wide-field fluorescein angiography may reveal hyperfluorescence at the scalloped margins of the lesion with variable degrees of window defect owing to progressive loss of the RPE and choriocapillaris.

Choroideremia

Choroideremia is an X-linked recessive disorder associated with poor dark adaptation, nyctalopia, and visual field constriction. "Salt and pepper" pigmentary mottling affecting the retinal mid periphery can be seen early in the disease, which eventually progresses to patchy chorioretinal atrophy extending toward the posterior pole. Choriocapillaris loss and scalloped atrophy can be seen late in the disease, making the condition difficult to distinguish from gyrate atrophy. Female carriers are typically asymptomatic and may exhibit only peripheral RPE mottling and/or reticular degeneration and, rarely, peripheral chorioretinal atrophy. Wide-field color fundus photography can be used to document peripheral disease progression, the pattern of which may be useful in distinguishing choroideremia from gyrate atrophy.

Vitreoretinal Dystrophies

Stickler and Wagner Syndromes

Stickler syndrome is a chondrodysplasia resulting from a mutation in the gene encoding either type II or type XI collagen, important constituents of the vitreous. Ocular findings include high myopia, optically empty vitreous, vitreous bands, radial perivascular retinal pigmentary degeneration, and lattice degeneration, which can often be appreciated and documented on wide-field color fundus photography. Stickler syndrome patients are at particularly high risk for retinal detachment (RD), and prophylactic barricade laser retinopexy of high-risk lesions may be indicated to prevent vision loss due to RD. Systemic features include mid-face dysplasia, cleft palate, bifid uvula, hearing loss, marfanoid body habitus, and early-onset arthropathy.

Wagner syndrome results from defects in the gene encoding versican protein, a proteoglycan found in the vitreous. Clinical findings are very similar to those of Stickler and again include myopia, optically empty vitreous, vitreoretinal bands, and perivascular pigmentary changes and a high risk for retinal detachment. Unlike Stickler syndrome, ocular abnormalities can include anterior segment dysgenesis, foveal ectopia, and RPE atrophy. Wagner syndrome is not associated with craniofacial abnormalities or arthropathy.

X-Linked Retinoschisis

X-linked retinoschisis is caused by an X-linked recessive mutation of the retinoschisin gene (*RS1*) resulting in bilateral macular schisis at the level of the nerve fiber layer. Peripheral retinoschisis, occurring in approximately 50 % of individuals and typically located inferotemporally, can be seen and documented on wide-field color fundus photography. Vision loss may result from foveal retinoschisis, which can have a characteristic radial spokelike appearance. Vitreous hemorrhage and retinal detachment are common complications of this disorder. Unlike other causes of cystoid changes in the macula, fluorescein angiography does not result in leakage in the macula in X-linked retinoschisis. Electroretinogram (ERG) testing demonstrates an electronegative waveform in which the a-wave is normal and the b-wave is significantly reduced. Female carriers are typically unaffected.

Enhanced S-Cone Syndrome

Enhanced S-cone syndrome (Goldmann-Favre syndrome) is an autosomal recessive disorder that can be complicated by macular and peripheral retinal schisis and is, therefore, similar to X-linked juvenile schisis. This rare disorder is caused by a defect in the *NR2E3* gene resulting in overexpression of short-wavelength cones. ERG analysis shows an extinguished rod response but, because of overpopulation of S cones, the maximal response is similar in morphology to the photopic flash response. Symptoms include early-onset nyctalopia and visual field constriction. Wide-field funduscopic features include optically empty vitreous and a very characteristic distribution of pigmentary degeneration and dense subretinal clumping sharply concentric to the posterior pole.

Familial Exudative Vitreoretinopathy

Familial exudative vitreoretinopathy (FEVR) is an inherited disorder of the retina characterized by peripheral ischemia and retinal vascular abnormalities including shunt formation, neovascularization, and exudative leakage, which can phenotypically resemble retinopathy of prematurity. The condition is typically inherited in an autosomal dominant fashion, although other modes of inheritance (e.g., X-linked transmission via the Norrie disease protein [*NDP*] gene) have been reported and systemic associations can occur with select mutations. FEVR can be associated with subretinal and preretinal hemorrhage in the later stages of the disease resulting in retinal folds, macular dragging, and tractional retinal detachment; panretinal laser therapy as guided by wide-field fluorescein angiography may aid in preventing these complications.

Macular Dystrophies

Stargardt Disease

Stargardt disease is the most common macular dystrophy, typically inherited as an autosomal recessive mutation in the *ABCA4* gene. Autosomal dominant transmission is also possible (*ELOVL4* gene). The clinical appearance can be variable and may include macular atrophy in a bull's-eye or geographic pattern. Other typical findings include a "beaten bronze" sheen of the fovea, peripheral or central flecks in a pisciform or triradiate configuration with peripapillary sparing, and a dark or "silent" choroid on wide-field fluorescein angiography due to excessive accumulation of lipofuscin in the RPE. Wide-field autofluorescence can be particularly useful in later stages of the disease to document peripheral retinal involvement and to monitor for progression. Vision impairment is typically central and progressive and begins in the first or second decades of life.

Best Macular Dystrophy

Best macular dystrophy, or Best disease, is an autosomal dominant condition associated with mutation in the Best 1 gene encoding bestrophin. The condition is characterized by abnormal accumulation of lipofuscin in the subretinal space. The natural history of the disease classically begins as a yellow, homogeneous, dome-shaped lesion in the fovea resembling an egg yolk (vitelliform stage). The lesion is typically solitary but may be multifocal. The vitelliform material may layer in the subretinal space (pseudohypopyon stage); later, the lesion becomes less homogeneous taking on a "scrambled-egg" appearance (vitelliruptive stage). Visual function is typically preserved until later stages of the disease associated with chorioretinal atrophy, choroidal neovascular membrane formation, and subretinal fibrosis. Electro-oculogram (EOG) testing is diagnostic (with an Arden ratio close to 1.0), whereas scotopic and photopic ERG responses are preserved.

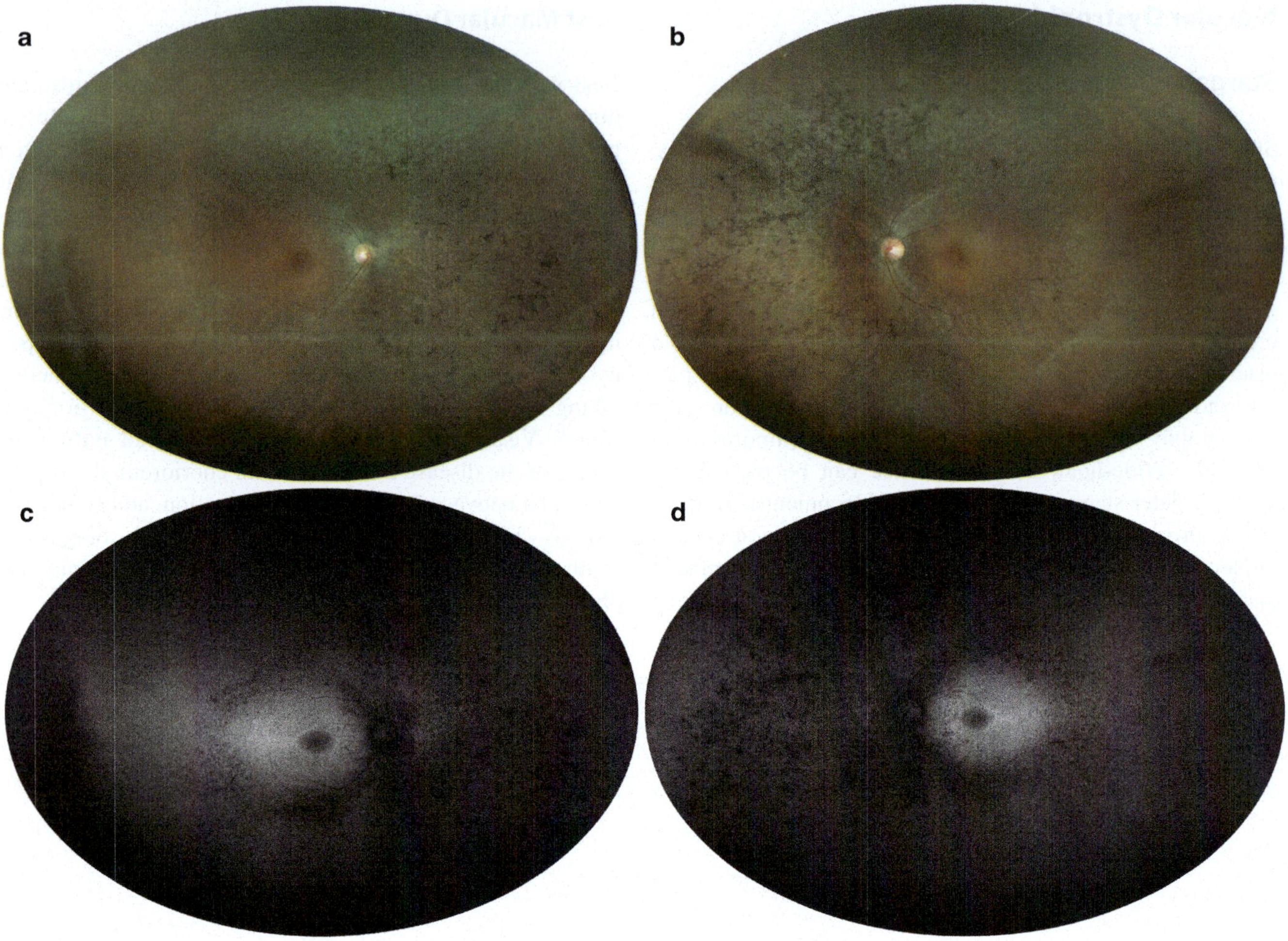

Fig. 1 Multimodal wide-field imaging of RP. (**a, b**) Wide-field color fundus photography. There is mild pallor of the optic disc and vascular attenuation. Bone spicule formation is primarily localized to the nasal periphery. (**c, d**) Wide-field fundus autofluorescence. Areas of punctate hypoautofluorescence correspond to bone spicule deposition in the color photos. A hypoautofluorescent ring is apparent along the major vascular arcades and around the macula. There is a hyperautofluorescent ring in the macula of each eye. This is referred to as the "Robson Holder ring". (**e, f**) High-magnification autofluorescence imaging of the macula and mid periphery. Note the faint parafoveal hyperautofluorescent ring corresponding to the border between normal and dysfunctional photoreceptors. (**g, h**) Spectral domain optical coherent tomography (OCT) of the macula. Cystoid macular edema is present in both eyes (left greater than right). Diffuse paramacular outer retinal atrophy with photoreceptor and inner segment ellipsoid loss is noted

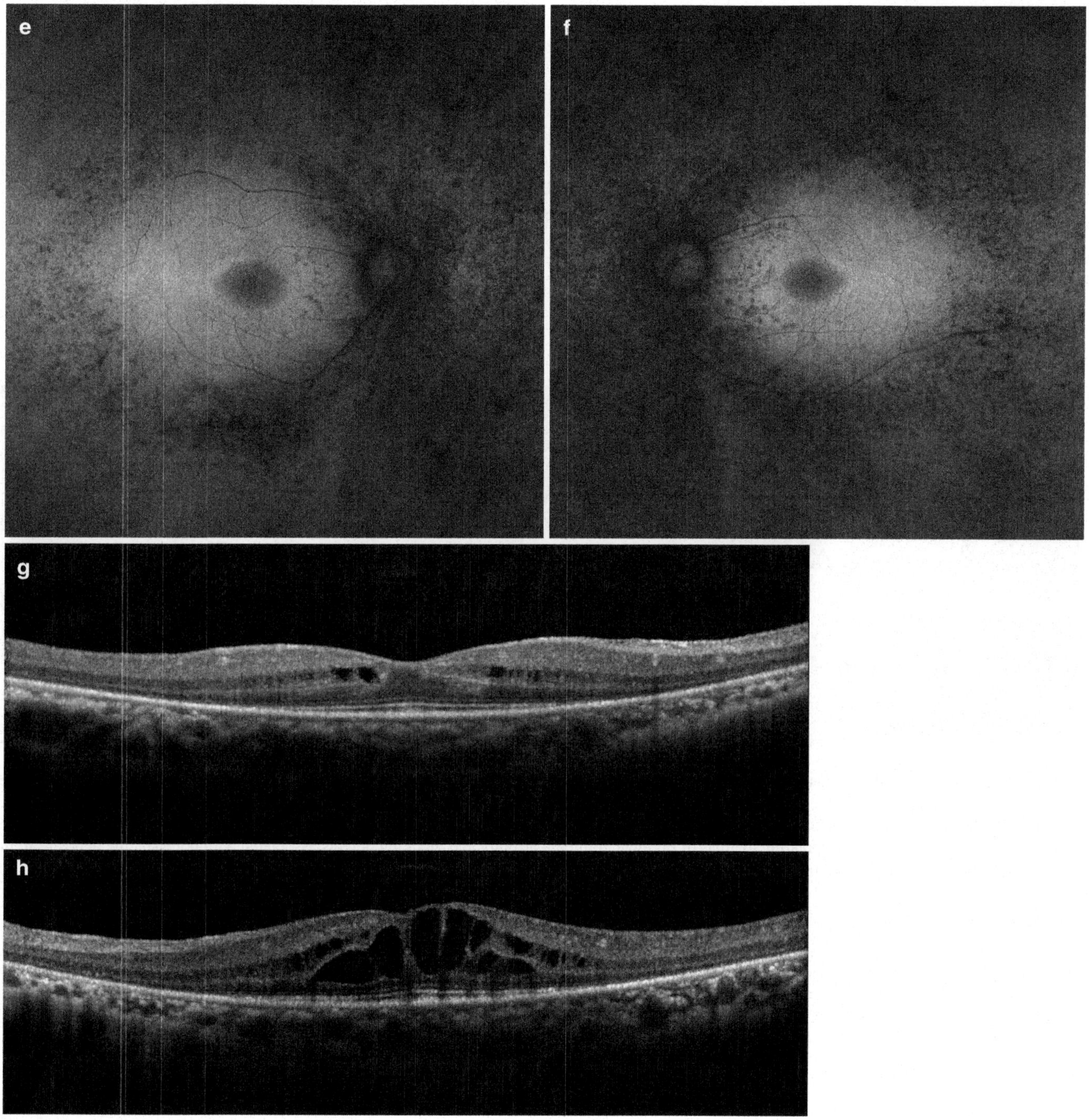

Fig. 1 (continued)

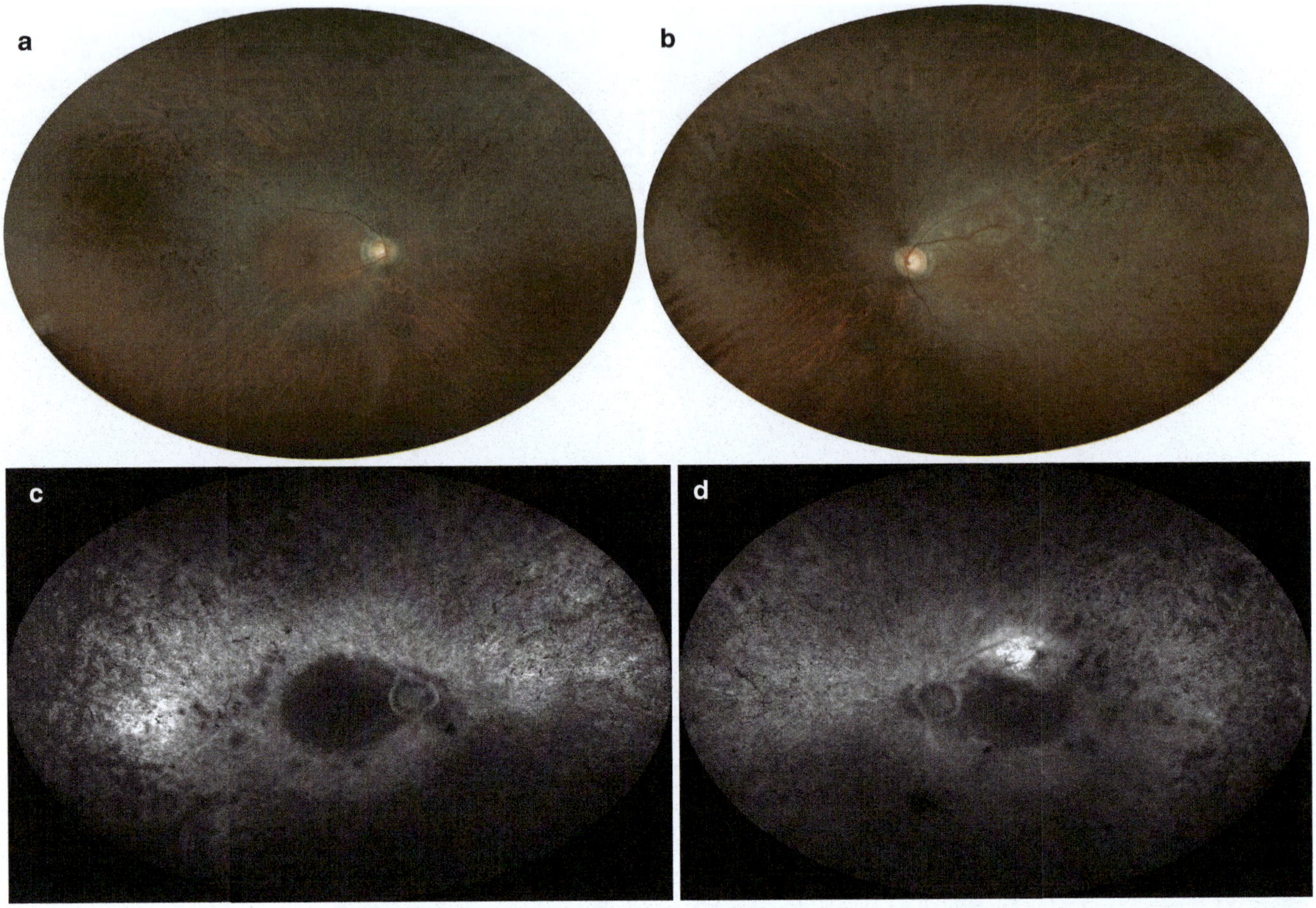

Fig. 2 Wide-field imaging of RP associated with a vasoproliferative tumor. (**a**, **b**) Wide-field color fundus photography. There is atrophy of the pigment epithelium concentric to the vascular arcades with associated peripheral bone spicule deposition. In the left eye, there is a vasoproliferative tumor along the superotemporal arcade with associated telangiectatic vessels and hard exudates. (**c**, **d**) Wide-field fluorescein angiography. There are bilateral window defects corresponding to areas of pigment epithelial atrophy and blocking defects associated with bone spicule deposition. In the left eye, there is late angiographic leakage overlying the vasoproliferative tumor and associated petalloid angiographic edema in the macula

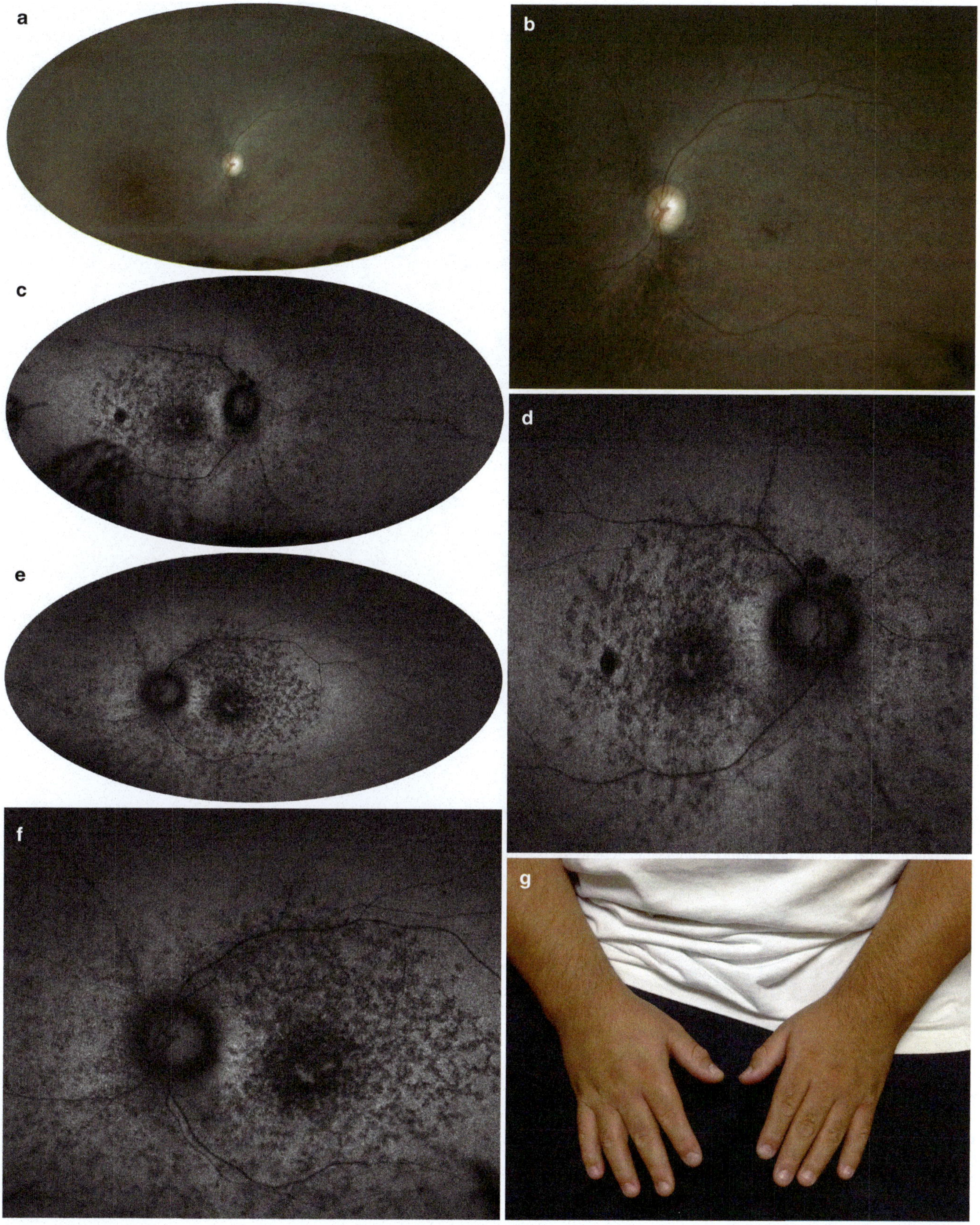

Fig. 3 Multimodal wide field imaging of Bardet-Biedl syndrome. (**a**, **b**) Wide-field color fundus photography of the left eye with perifoveal RPE mottling and an evolving bull's-eye maculopathy. (**c–f**) Wide-field fundus autofluorescence. A punctate pattern of hypoautofluorescence is present in the macula of both eyes. A paravenous pattern of hypoautofluorescence can be seen in the nasal periphery of both eyes. (**g**) This patient with Bardet-Biedl has short, thick digits. Polydactyly of the hands and toes may be seen in association with Bardet-Biedl

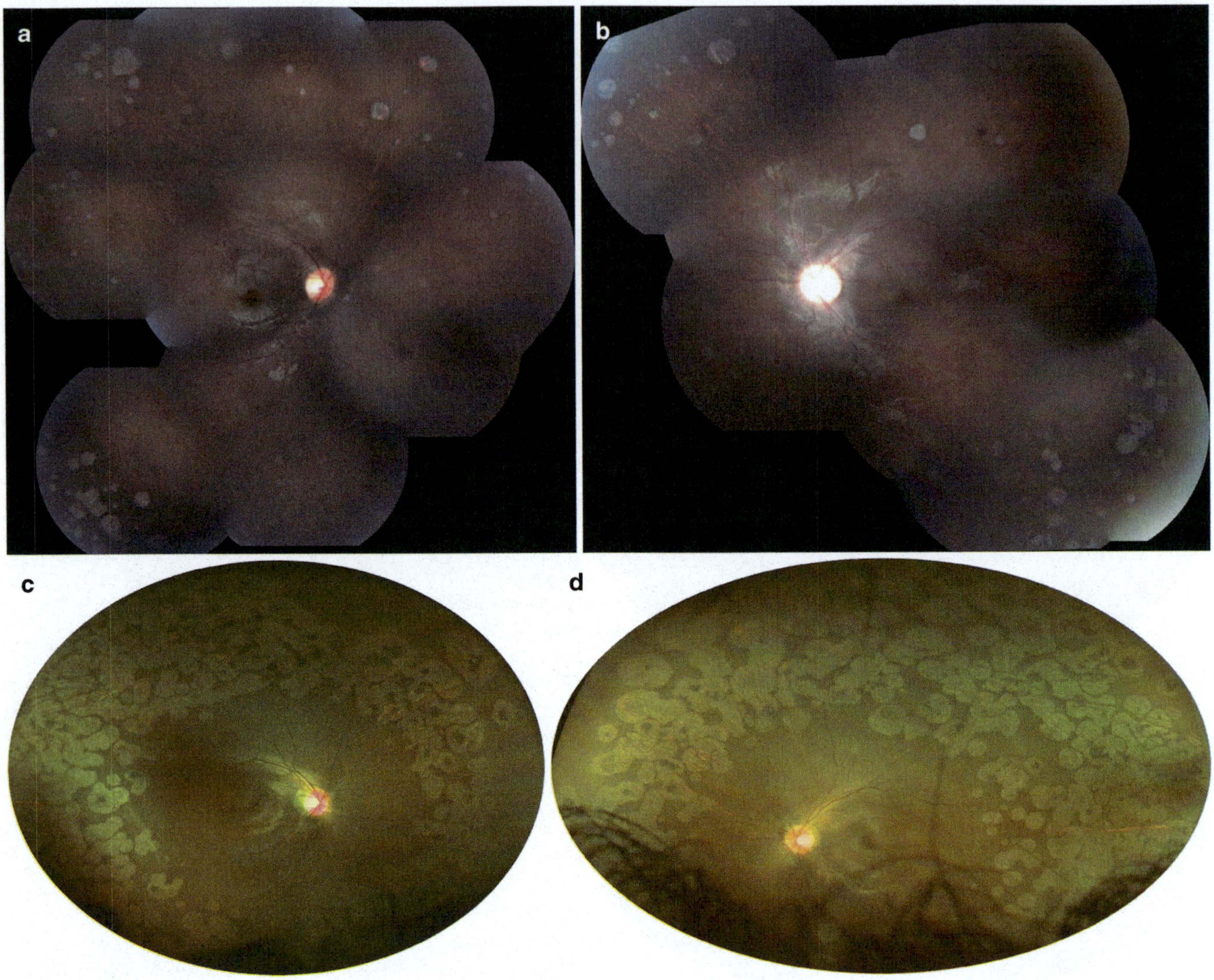

Fig. 4 Wide-field multimodal imaging of gyrate atrophy. (**a**, **b**) Color fundus photo montage of a patient with early gyrate atrophy. Note the patchy peripheral zones of chorioretinal atrophy. (**c**, **d**) Wide-field color fundus photography, 5 years later, shows progression and coalescence of peripheral chorioretinal atrophy in a sharply scalloped pattern (**a**–**d**) (Courtesy of Jesse Smith, Antonio Ciardella, Guillermo Salcedo-Villanueva, and Hugo Quiroz-Mercado)

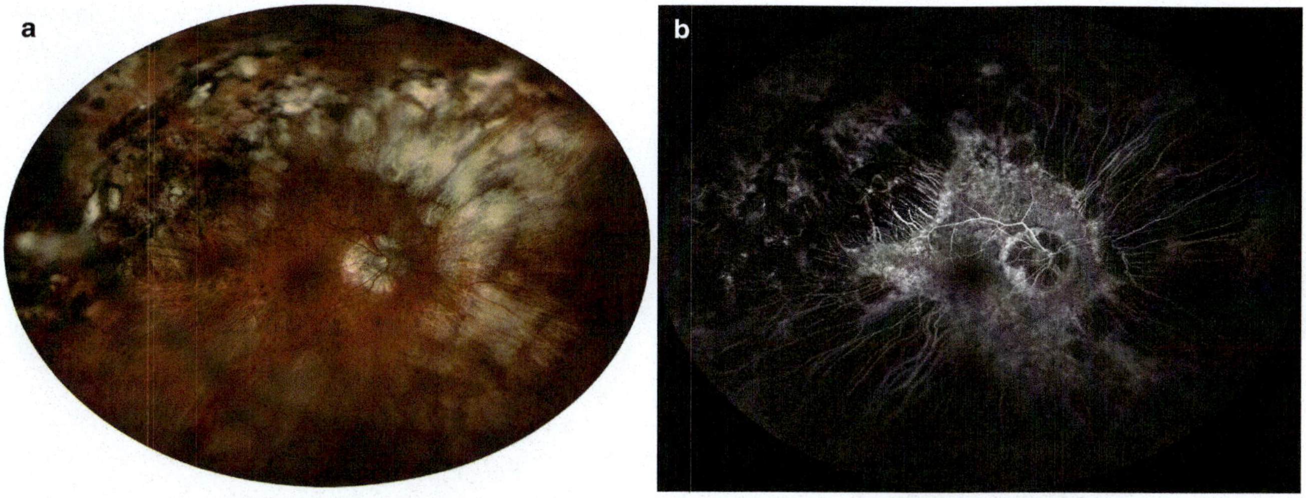

Fig. 5 Wide-field imaging of choroideremia. (**a**) Wide-field fundus photography demonstrates patchy areas of peripheral RPE atrophy and pigment deposition. (**b**) Wide-field fluorescein angiography demonstrates stellate preservation of the posterior pole with widespread peripheral pigment epithelial loss and attenuation of the choriocapillaris (**a** and **b**, Courtesy of Michael Gorin)

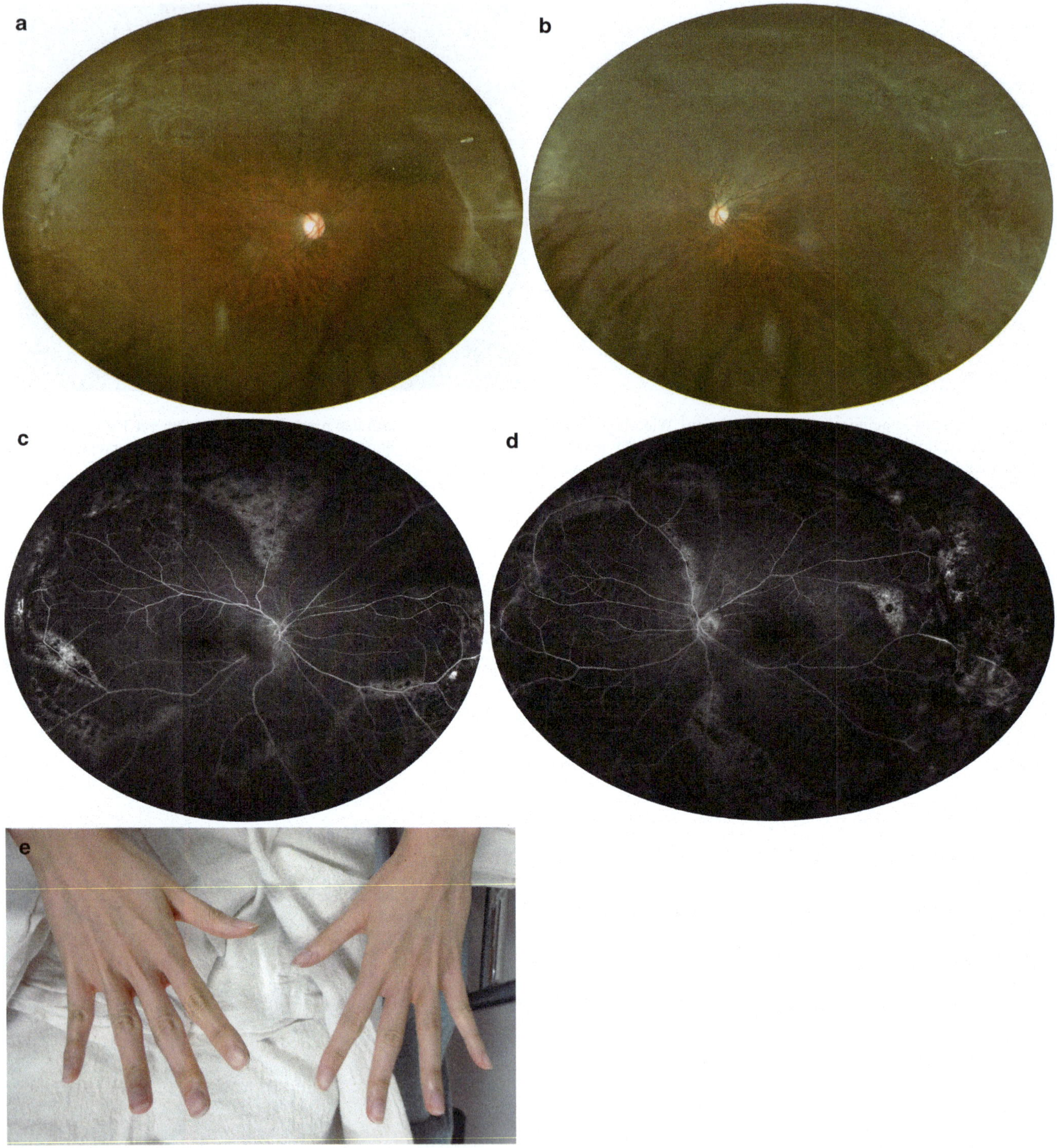

Fig. 6 Multimodal imaging of Stickler syndrome. (**a**, **b**) Wide-field color fundus photography demonstrates peripheral retinal pigment clumping, radial perivascular pigmentary degeneration, and peripheral vascular sclerosis in association with lattice degeneration. Prophylactic photocoagulation scars are present in the superotemporal periphery of the right eye corresponding to barricade treatment of a prior retinal tear. (**c**, **d**) Wide-field fluorescein angiogram of the same case of Stickler syndrome. Areas of blocking and window defect along the peripheral retinal vessels correspond to radial perivascular pigmentary alteration and lattice degeneration. (**e**) Arachnodactyly is one of many skeletal abnormalities associated with Stickler syndrome

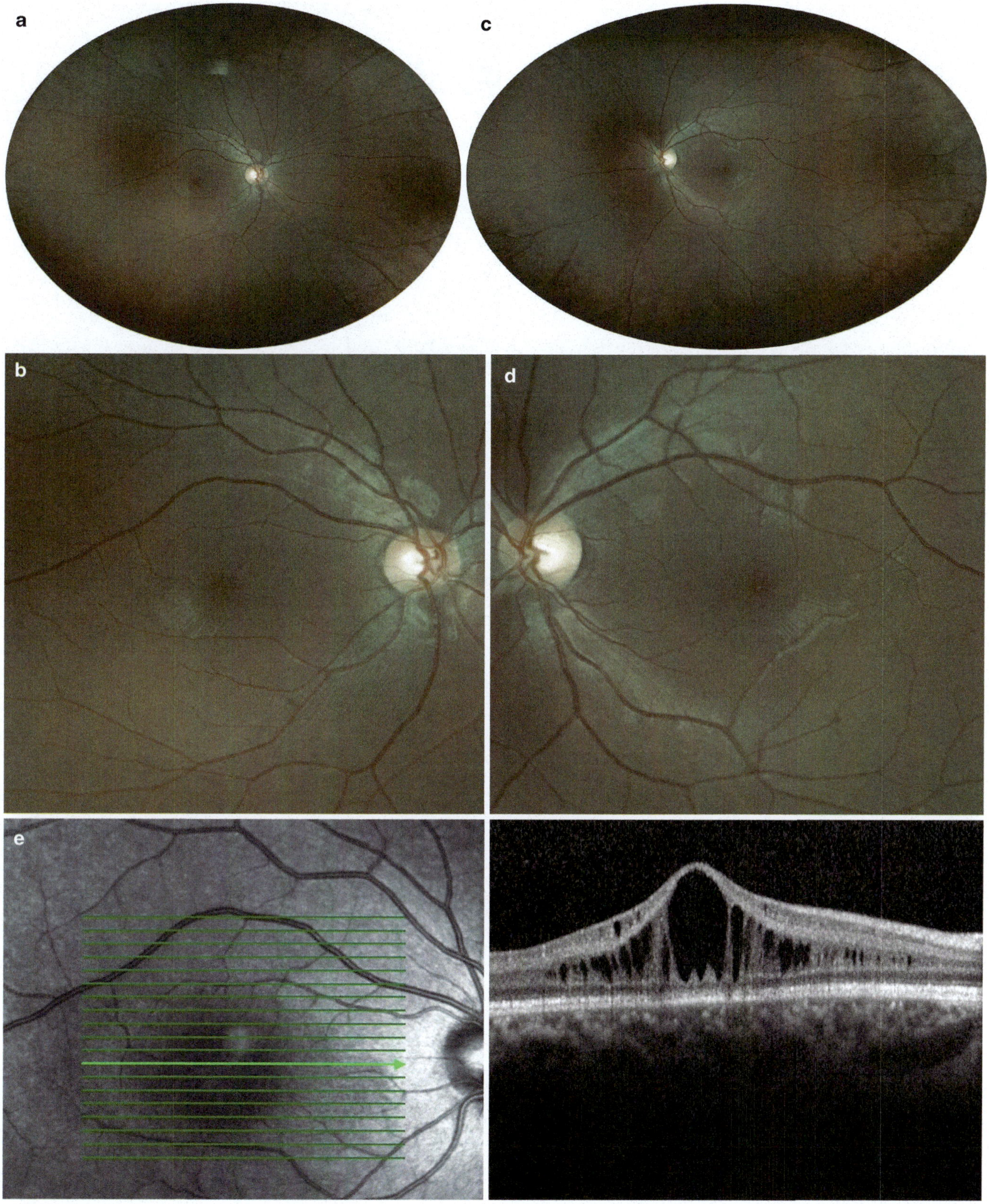

Fig. 7 Multimodal imaging of juvenile X-linked retinoschisis. (**a–d**) Wide-field color fundus photography with high-magnification view of the macula demonstrates radial, spokelike perifoveal changes consistent with macular schisis. (**e–f**) Spectral domain OCT demonstrates bilateral macular schisis

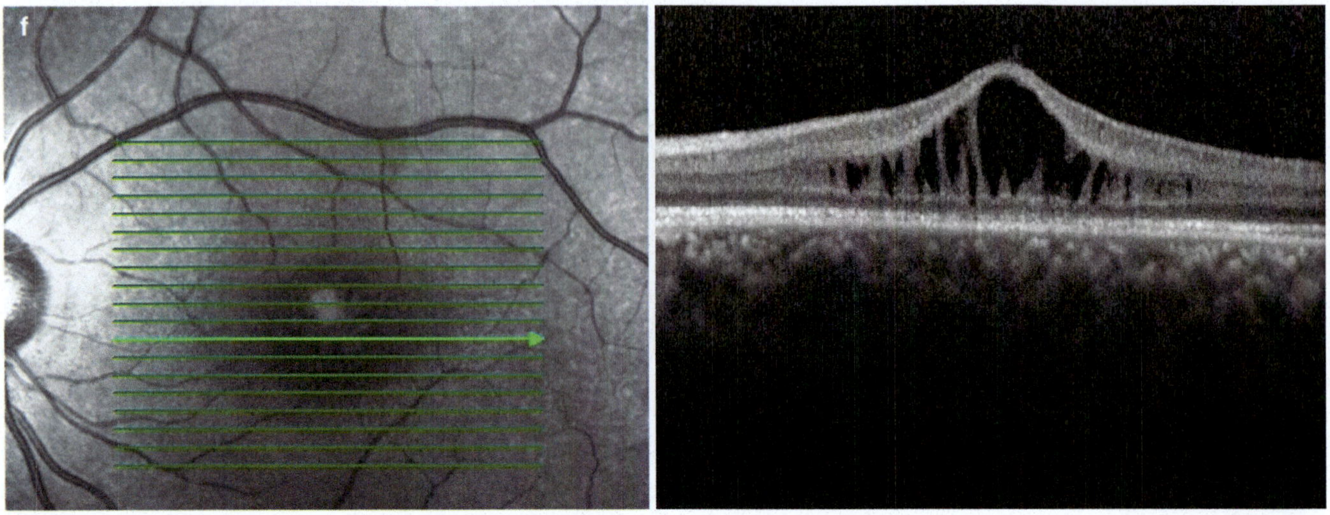

Fig. 7 (continued)

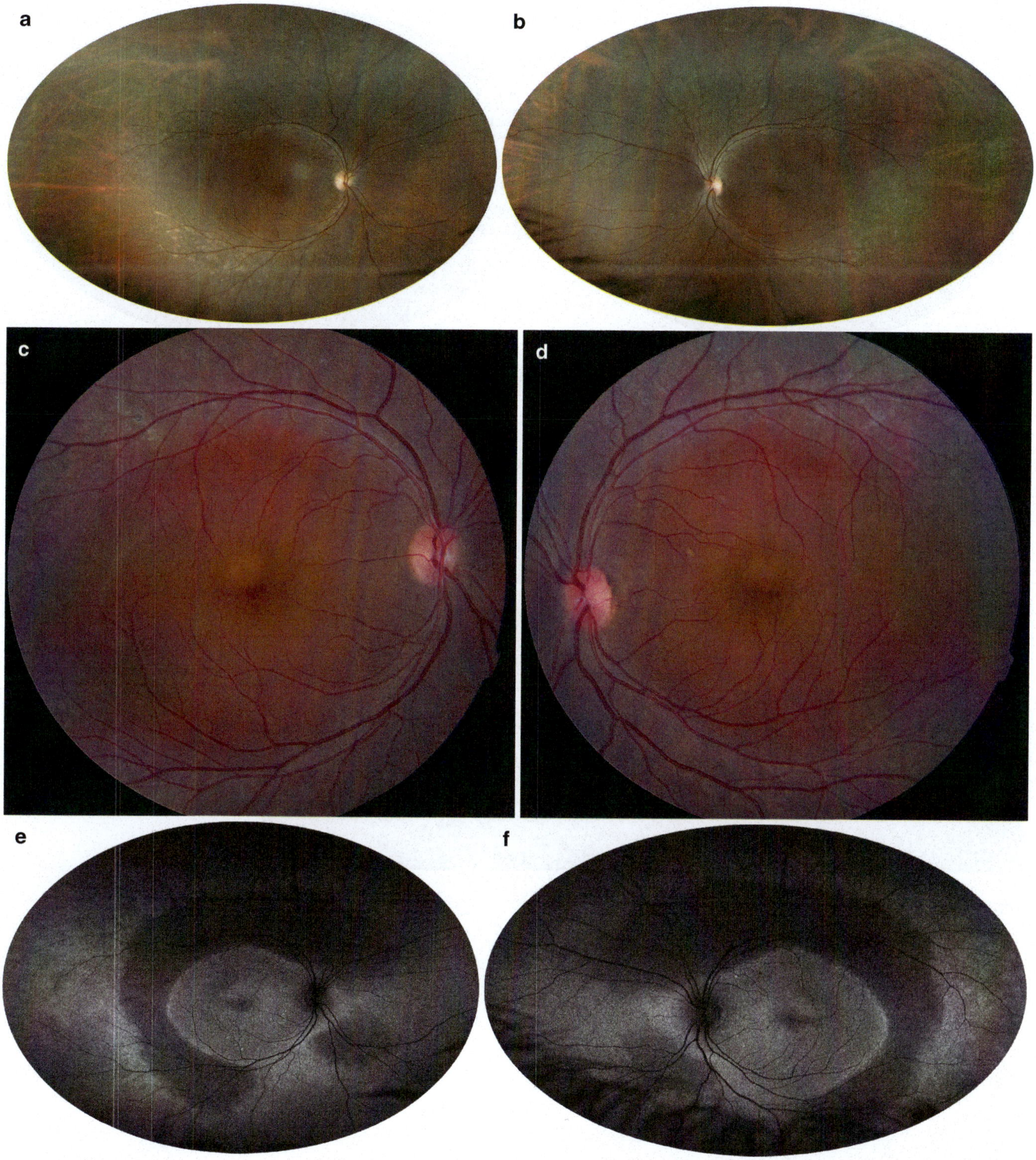

Fig. 8 Wide-field imaging of enhanced S-cone syndrome. (**a**, **b**) Wide-field color fundus photography of a case of enhanced s-cone syndrome shows concentric mid-peripheral RPE mottling. (**c**, **d**) Color fundus photography of the same patient demonstrates RPE mottling concentric to the vascular arcades. (**e**, **f**) Wide-field fundus autofluorescence demonstrates a mid-peripheral very symmetrical and tightly concentric band of hypo-autofluorescence in each eye. (**g**, **h**) Wide-field fluorescein angiography of the same case of enhanced S-cone syndrome. Areas of concentric mid-peripheral hyperfluorescence reflect window defects corresponding to RPE atrophy. (**i**, **j**) Spectral-domain OCT of the same case demonstrates macular schisis in both eyes

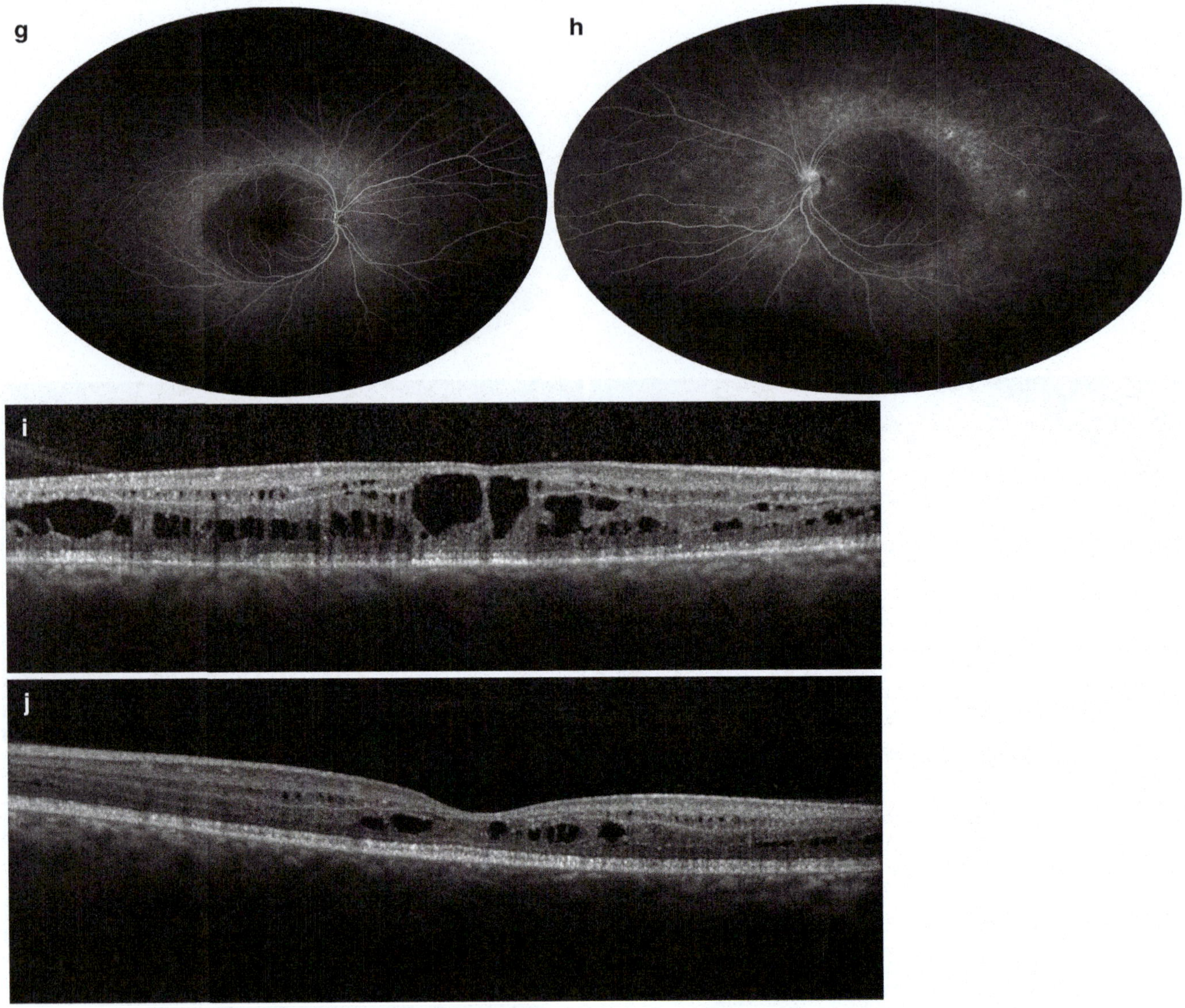

Fig. 8 (continued)

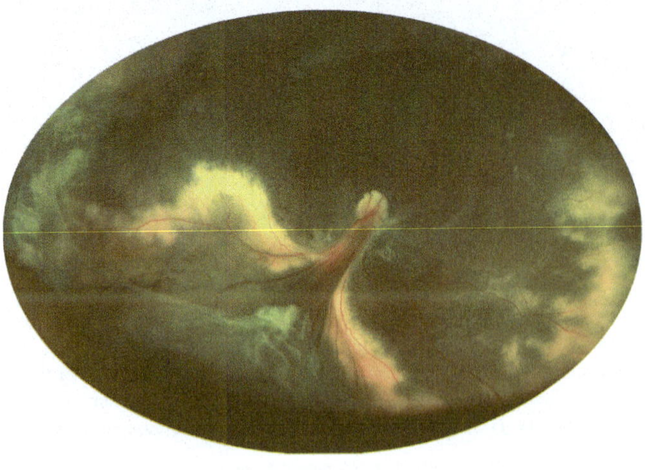

Fig. 9 Wide-field imaging of familial exudative vitreoretinopathy. Wide-field fundus photography of the right eye demonstrates dragging of the macula to the inferotemporal periphery. There is associated exudation and subretinal lipid accumulation

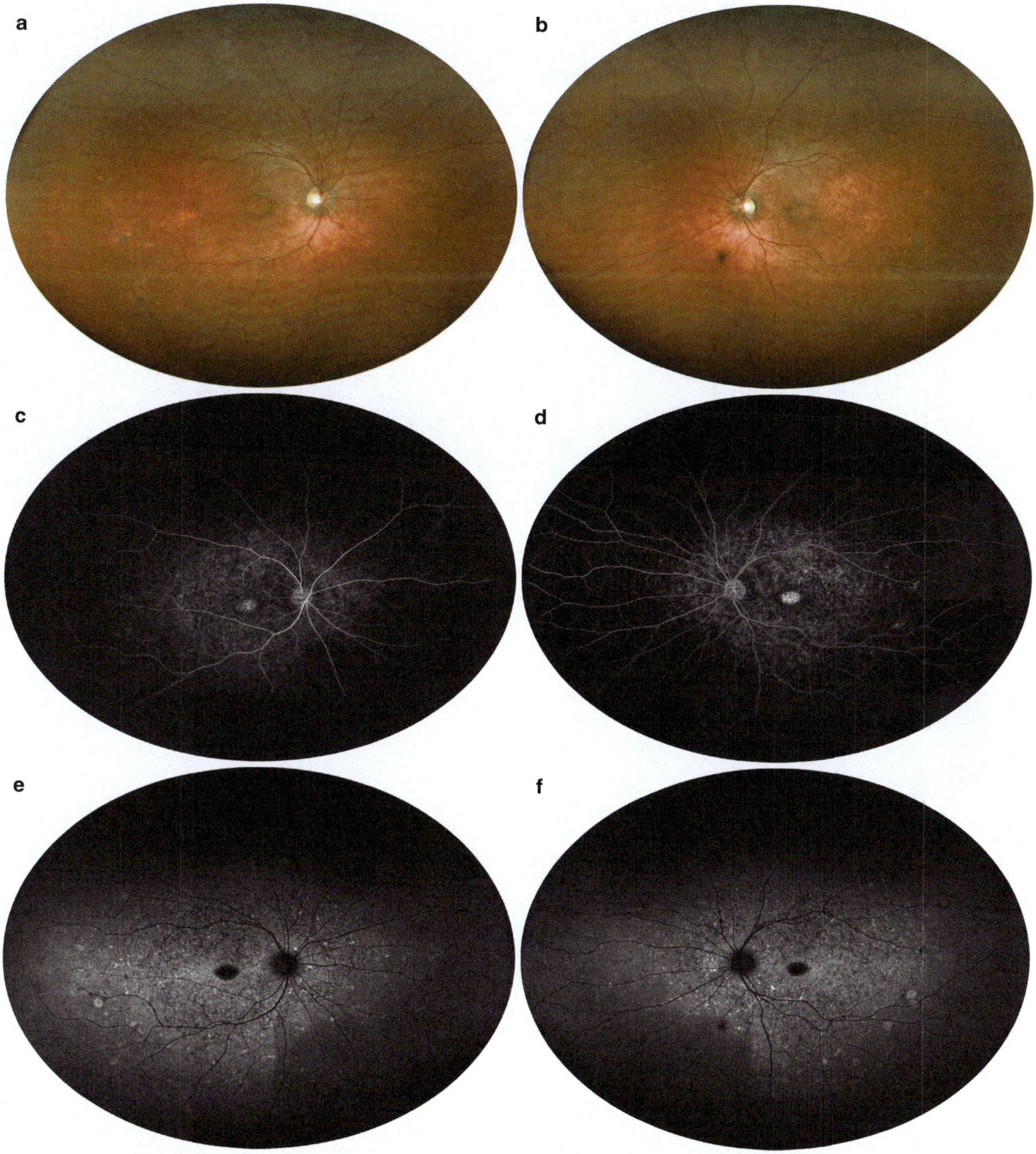

Fig. 10 Multimodal wide-field imaging of Stargardt disease. (**a**, **b**) Wide-field color fundus photography demonstrates a beaten-bronze sheen to the macula, numerous pisciform or triradiate flecks in the macula and perimacular area, and central RPE atrophy. (**c**, **d**) Wide-field fluorescein angiogram of the same case of Stargardt. Blocking defects correspond to areas of excess lipofuscin accumulation and contribute to the angiographic appearance of a "dark choroid." Window defects corresponding to RPE atrophy and staining of pisciform flecks can be seen in the macula. (**e**, **f**) Wide-field fundus autofluorescence. Hypoautofluorescence in the macula corresponds to areas of RPE atrophy. Abnormal lipofuscin accumulation with peripapillary sparing results in perimacular and peripheral hyperautofluorescence. New hyperautofluorescent and older hypoautofluorescent flecks can be seen. (**g**, **h**) Spectral domain OCT. Significant RPE and outer retinal atrophy of the macula can be appreciated

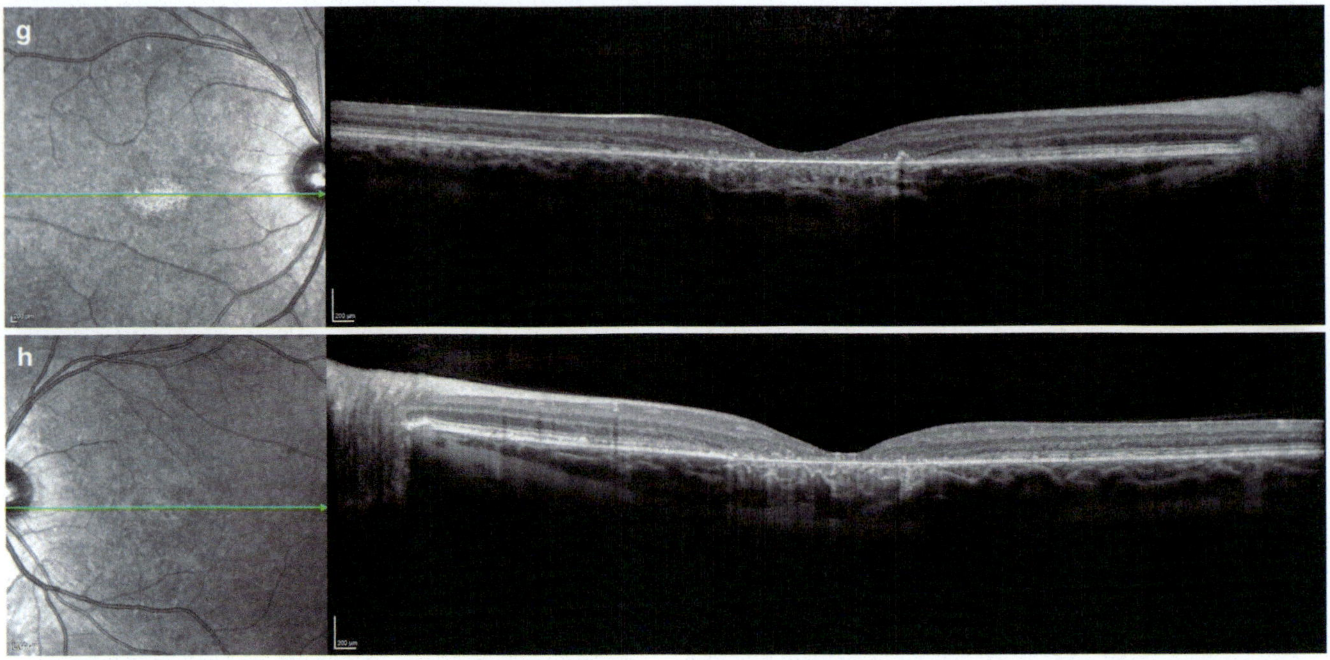

Fig. 10 (continued)

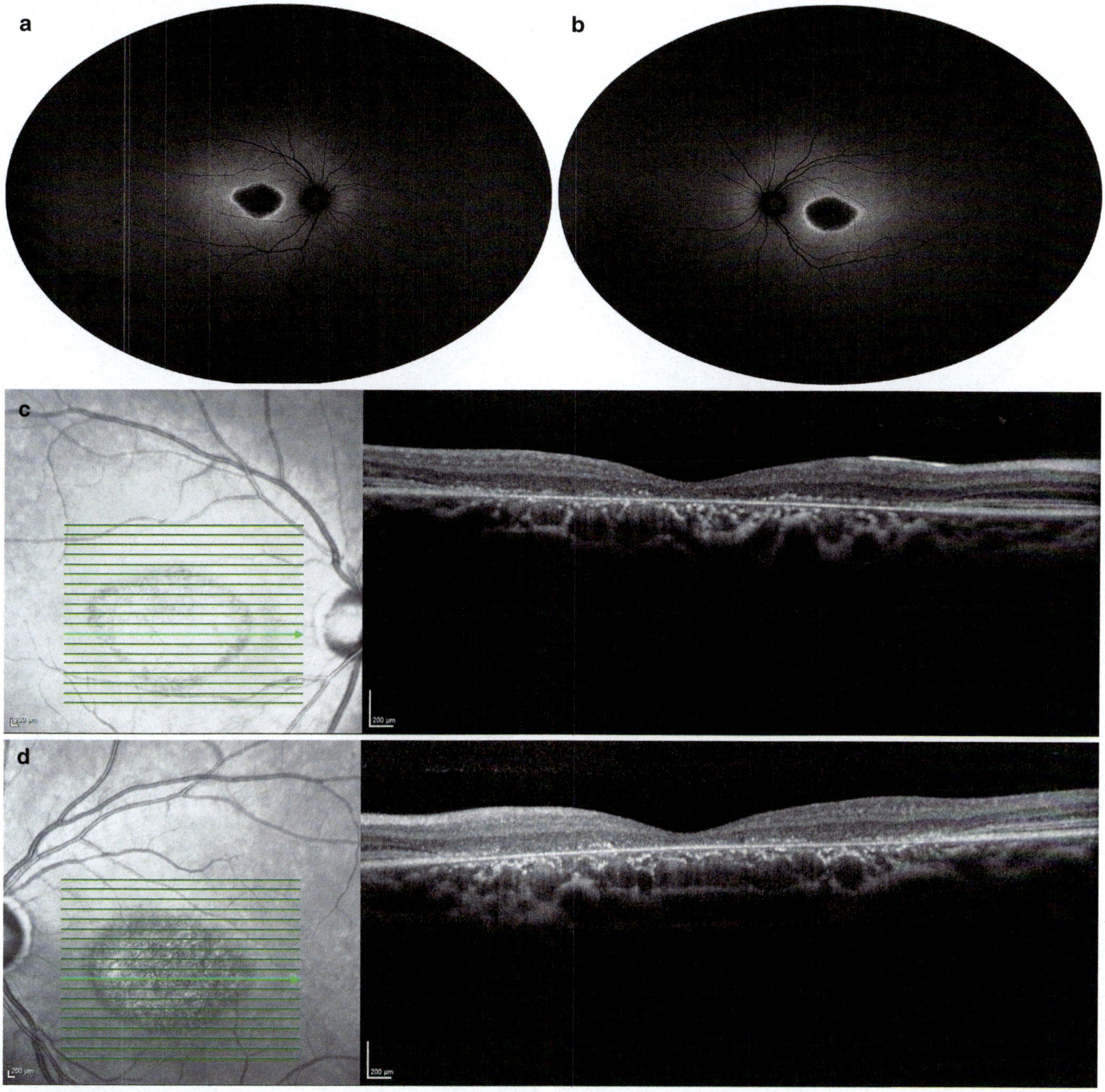

Fig. 11 Multimodal imaging of Stargardt disease. (**a**, **b**) Wide-field fundus autofluorescence demonstrates hypoautofluorescence with a rim of hyperautofluorescence consistent with geographic macular atrophy and minimal fleck deposition. (**c**, **d**) Spectral-domain OCT. Foveal and parafoveal outer retinal atrophy associated with an accumulation of punctate hyper-reflective flecklike material in the outer retina

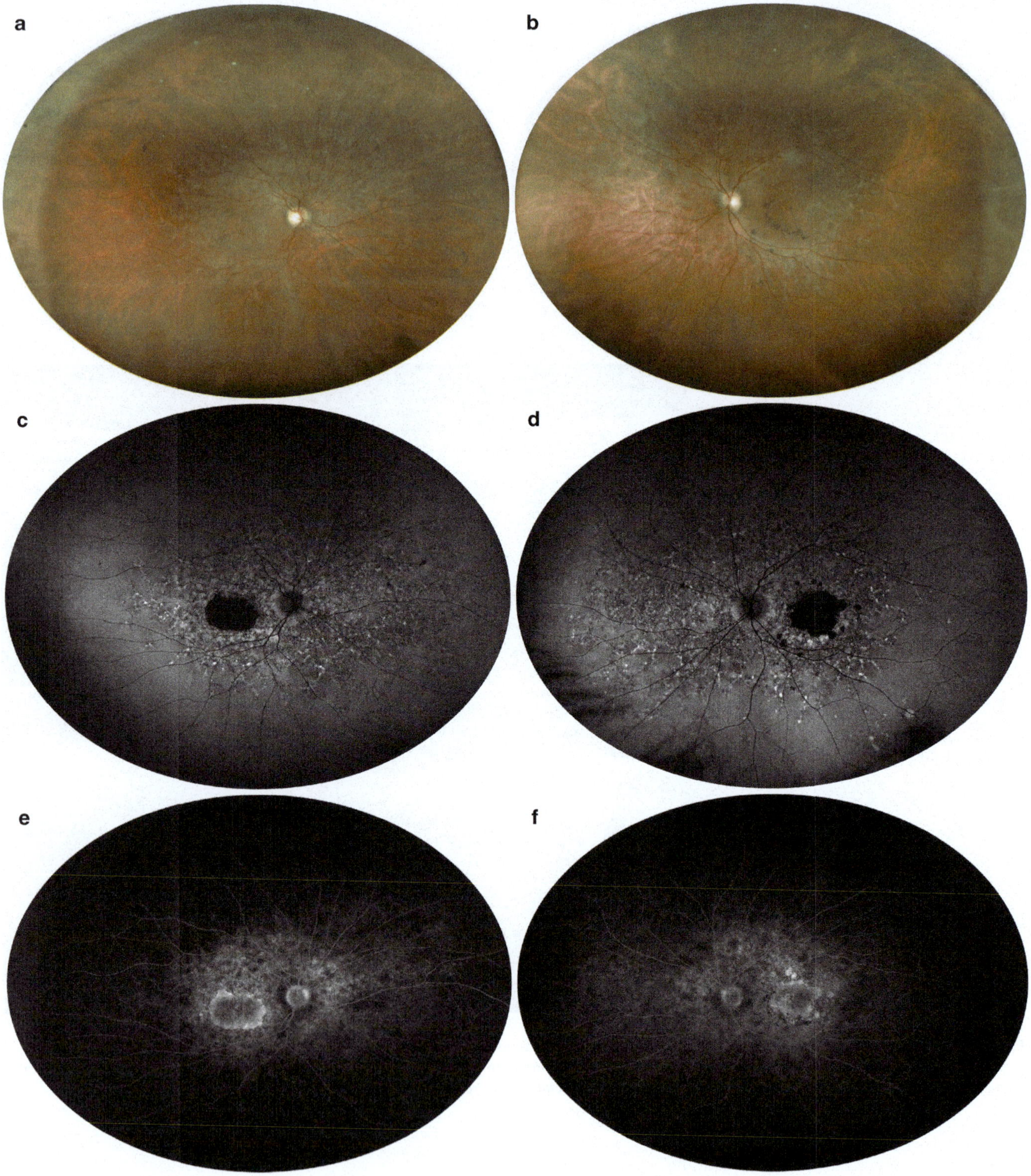

Fig. 12 Stargardt disease associated with a reticular pattern of fleck deposition and a large area of central RPE atrophy. (**a**, **b**) Wide-field color fundus photography shows peripheral fleck deposition. (**c**, **d**) Wide-field fundus autofluorescence demonstrates hyperfluorescence of the fleck deposits. (**e** and **f**), Wide-field fluorescein angiography shows macular window defects and late staining of the fleck depositions

Suggested Reading

Andreoli MT, Lim JI. Optical coherence tomography retinal thickness and volume measurements in X-linked retinoschisis. Am J Ophthalmol. 2014;158:567–73.

Chen Y, Roorda A, Duncan JL. Advances in imaging of Stargardt disease. Adv Exp Med Biol. 2010;664:333–40.

Edwards AO. Clinical features of the congenital vitreoretinopathies. Eye (Lond). 2008;22:1233–42.

Ferrara DC, Costa RA, Tsang S, Calucci D, Jorge R, Freund KB. Multimodal fundus imaging in best vitelliform macular dystrophy. Graefes Arch Clin Exp Ophthalmol. 2010;248:1377–86.

Gilmour DF. Familial exudative vitreoretinopathy and related retinopathies. Eye (Lond). 2015;29:1–14.

Gregori NZ, Lam BL, Gregori G, Ranganathan S, Stone EM, Morante A, et al. Wide-field spectral-domain optical coherence tomography in patients and carriers of X-linked retinoschisis. Ophthalmology. 2013;120:169–74.

Hayasaka S, Shoji K, Kanno C, Oura F, Mizuno K. Differential diagnosis of diffuse choroidal atrophies. Diffuse choriocapillaris atrophy, choroideremia, and gyrate atrophy of the choroid and retina. Retina. 1985;5:30–7.

Heussen F, Tan CS, Sadda SR. Prevalence of peripheral abnormalities on ultra-widefield greenlight (532 nm) autofluorescence imaging at a tertiary care center. Invest Ophthalmol Vis Sci. 2012;53(10):6525–31.

Jayasundera T, Rhoades W, Branham K, Musch DC, Heckenlively JR. Peripapillary dark choroid ring as a helpful diagnostic sign in advanced stargardt disease. Am J Ophthalmol. 2010;149:656–60.

Kang KB, Wessel MM, Tong J, D'Amico DJ, Chan RV. Ultra-widefield imaging for the management of pediatric retinal diseases. J Pediatr Ophthalmol Strabismus. 2013;50:282–8.

Krill AE, Archer D, Newell FW. Fluorescein angiography in retinitis pigmentosa. Am J Ophthalmol. 1970;69:826–35.

Lois N, Halfyard AS, Bird AC, Holder GE, Fitzke FW. Fundus autofluorescence in Stargardt macular dystrophy-fundus flavimaculatus. Am J Ophthalmol. 2004;138:55–63.

Manivannan A, Plskova J, Farrow A, Mckay S, Sharp PF, Forrester JV. Ultra-wide-field fluorescein angiography of the ocular fundus. Am J Ophthalmol. 2005;140:525–7.

Mitamura Y, Mitamura-Aizawa S, Nagasawa T, Katome T, Eguchi H, Naito T. Diagnostic imaging in patients with retinitis pigmentosa. J Med Invest. 2012;59:1–11.

Molday RS, Kellner U, Weber BH. X-linked juvenile retinoschisis: clinical diagnosis, genetic analysis, and molecular mechanisms. Prog Retin Eye Res. 2012;31:195–212.

Ogura S, Yasukawa T, Kato A, Usui H, Hirano Y, Yoshida M, et al. Wide-field fundus autofluorescence imaging to evaluate retinal function in patients with retinitis pigmentosa. Am J Ophthalmol. 2014;158:1093–8.

Oishi M, Oishi A, Ogino K, Makiyama Y, Gotoh N, Kurimoto M, et al. Wide-field fundus autofluorescence abnormalities and visual function in patients with cone and cone-rod dystrophies. Invest Ophthalmol Vis Sci. 2014;55:3572–7.

Oliveira TL, Andrade RE, Muccioli C, Sallum J, Belfort Jr R. Cystoid macular edema in gyrate atrophy of the choroid and retina: a fluorescein angiography and optical coherence tomography evaluation. Am J Ophthalmol. 2005;140:147–9.

Querques G, Regenbogen M, Quijano C, Delphin N, Soubrane G, Souied EH. High-definition optical coherence tomography features in vitelliform macular dystrophy. Am J Ophthalmol. 2008;146:501–7.

Renner AB, Kellner U, Cropp E, Preising MN, MacDonald IM, van den Hurk JA, et al. Choroideremia: variability of clinical and electrophysiological characteristics and first report of a negative electroretinogram. Ophthalmology. 2006;2066(113):e1–10.

Yuan A, Kaines A, Jain A, Reddy S, Schwartz SD, Sarraf D. Ultra-wide-field and autofluorescence imaging of choroidal dystrophies. Ophthalmic Surg Lasers Imaging. 2010;41:e1–5.

Yzer S, Barbazetto I, Allikmets R, van Schooneveld MJ, Bergen A, Tsang SH, et al. Expanded clinical spectrum of enhanced S-cone syndrome. JAMA Ophthalmol. 2013;131:1324–30.

10 Wide-Field Retinal Imaging of Peripheral Retinal Degenerations

Igor Kozak, J. Fernando Arevalo, Byung Ro Lee, and The KKESH Collaborative Retina Study Group*

Because many retinal diseases manifest with peripheral abnormality, there has been an ever-increasing pressure to better image the retinal periphery. Ultra-wide-field fluorescein angiography (UWFA), first described in 2004 by Friberg and Forrester for the Optos Imaging system, not only captures a wide field of retina at once, allowing visualization of many different areas of the retina at the same timepoint during angiography and reducing the amount of patient cooperation and technical expertise required for photography, but also visualizes the peripheral retina that was previously not photographed [1, 2]. Several imaging systems have been developed that provide a wide-field view of the retina. These include the Pomerantzeff camera [3], the Retcam (Clarity Medical Systems, Inc, Pleasanton, CA), the Panoret-1000 camera (Medibell Medical Vision Technologies, Haifa, Israel), the Optos camera (Optos PLC, Dunfermline, UK), the Staurenghi lens (Ocular Staurenghi 230 SLO Retina Lens; Ocular Instruments Inc, Bellevue, WA), and other wide-angle contact lenses [4–7].

A lesion is defined as predominantly peripheral in a specific field if more than 50 % of the lesions are in the retinal periphery compared with modified ETDRS (Early Treatment Diabetic Retinopathy Study) fields taking into account the number and extent. A lesion is uniformly distributed in a specific field if the severity of lesion (taking into account the number and extent) is approximately equivalent both within and outside of the ETDRS field. Peripheral lesions are lesions located outside of the modified ETDRS 7-standard field and ultra-wide-field comprises the fundus photography field that is 100° or more [8].

Wide-field imaging of the vitreous and retina is now possible with the introduction of a biomicroscopic wide-angle retinal and vitreous observation system utilizing a 3-CCD video camera and a personal computer for image display by

I. Kozak, MD, PhD (✉)
Senior Academic Consultant, Vitreoretinal Division, King Khaled Eye Specialist Hospital, Riyadh, Kingdom of Saudi Arabia
e-mail: ikozak@kkesh.med.sa

J.F. Arevalo, MD, FACS
Edmund F. and Virginia B. Ball Professor of Ophthalmology, Chairman, Department of Ophthalmology, Johns Hopkins Bayview Medical Center, Retina Division, Wilmer Eye Institute, The Johns Hopkins University School of Medicine, Baltimore, MD, USA
e-mail: arevalojf@jhmi.edu

B.R. Lee, MD, PhD
Department of Ophthalmology, Hanyang University, Seoul, Korea

I. Kozak, J.F. Arevalo (eds.), *Atlas of Wide-Field Retinal Angiography and Imaging*, DOI 10.1007/978-3-319-17864-6_10

Lee and Chang (Fig. 1) [9]. With this technique, various types of fundus lenses can be used. This approach is helpful for wide-field dynamic observation and documentation of vitreous in vitreoretinal relationship.

In this chapter, we review the applications of UWFA imaging in peripheral retinal degenerations.

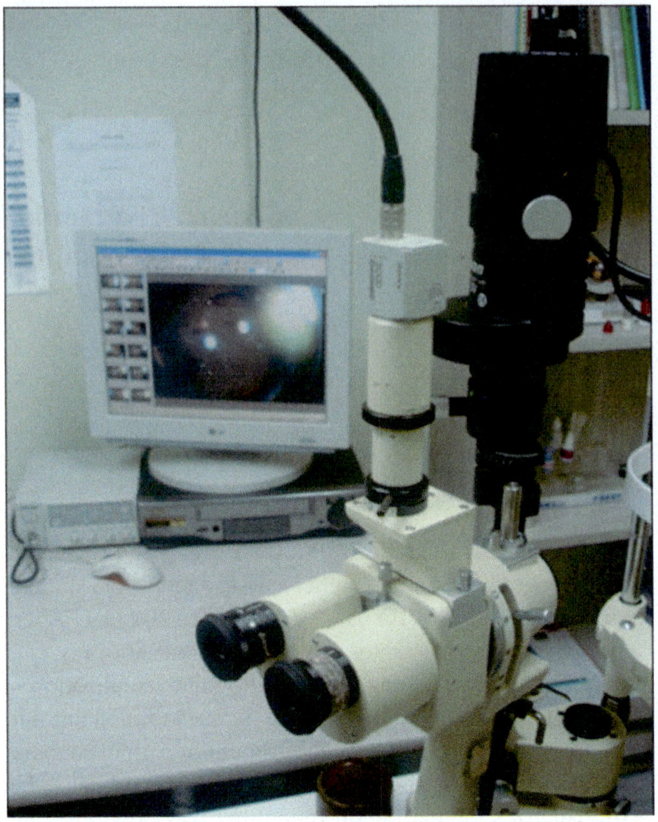

Fig. 1 The biomicroscopic observation system. It consists of a slit-lamp biomicroscope, a 3-CCD video camera, and a personal computer with an image capture and archiving software (Courtesy of Prof. B. Lee)

Peripheral Retinal Degenerations and UWFA Imaging

UWFA imaging may be useful to detect reticular cystoid degeneration, degenerative retinoschisis, paving-stone degeneration, peripheral tapetochoroidal degeneration, retinal holes, lattice degeneration, and retinal tears. Examining the peripheral retina and recording the findings require accurate and detailed knowledge of normal topography, anatomical relationships, common developmental variations, significant degenerations, and the manifestations of specific disease entities. UWFA imaging can significantly aid the clinician in documenting and preparing prophylactic management of these lesions when appropriate (Figs. 2, 3, 4, 5, 6, 7, 8, 9, 10, 11, 12, 13, 14, 15, 16, 17, 18, and 19).

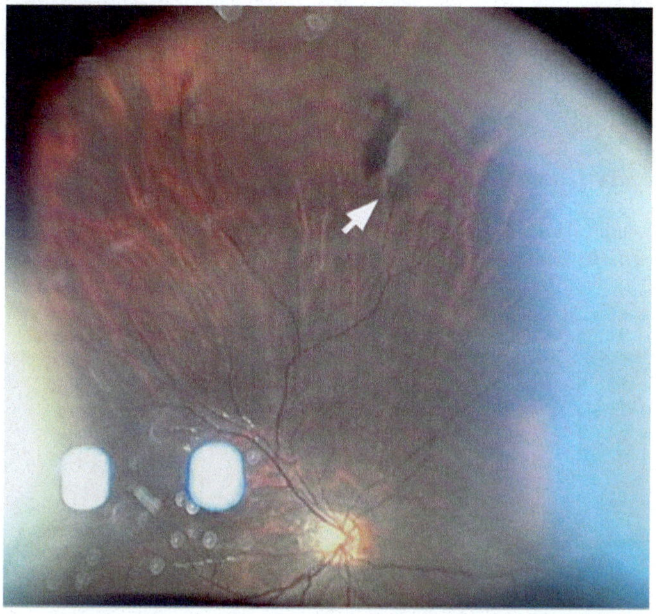

Fig. 2 Horseshoe tear. Wide-field biomicroscopic image of a horseshoe tear (*white arrow*) in the retinal periphery. Adjacent retina is attached

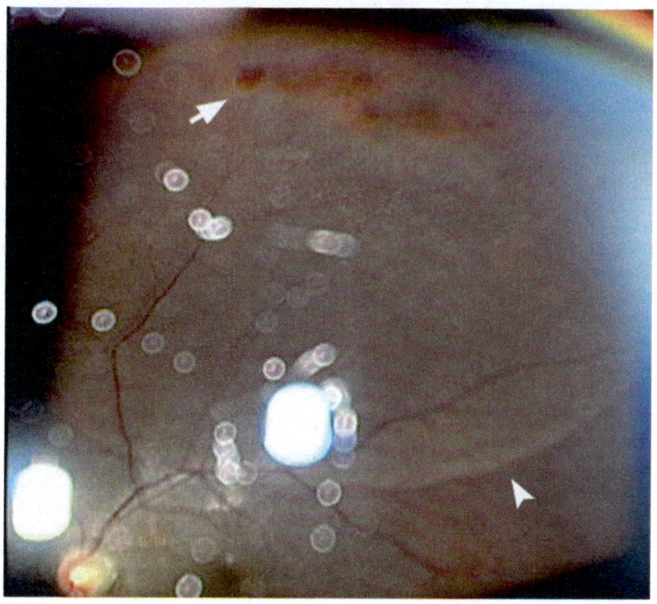

Fig. 3 Lattice degeneration with retinal hole. Wide-field biomicroscopic image of a peripheral retinal degeneration shows superotemporal lattice degeneration with atrophic hole (*white arrow*) leading to superotemporal retinal detachment (*arrowhead*)

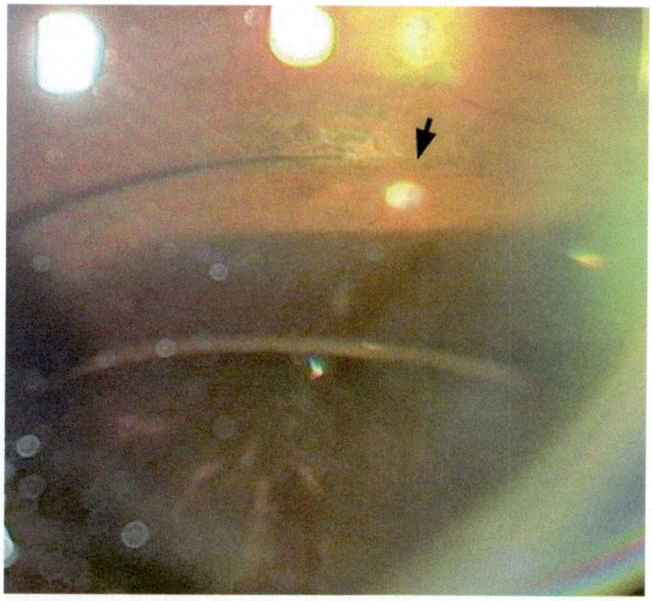

Fig. 4 Intravitreal gas. Wide-field biomicroscopic image of an eye after retinal detachment repair with intraocular gas. The image taken with a slit-lamp wide-field camera system is inverted. (*Black arrow*) points to the optic nerve head and the edge of intraocular gas bubble. Retina is attached

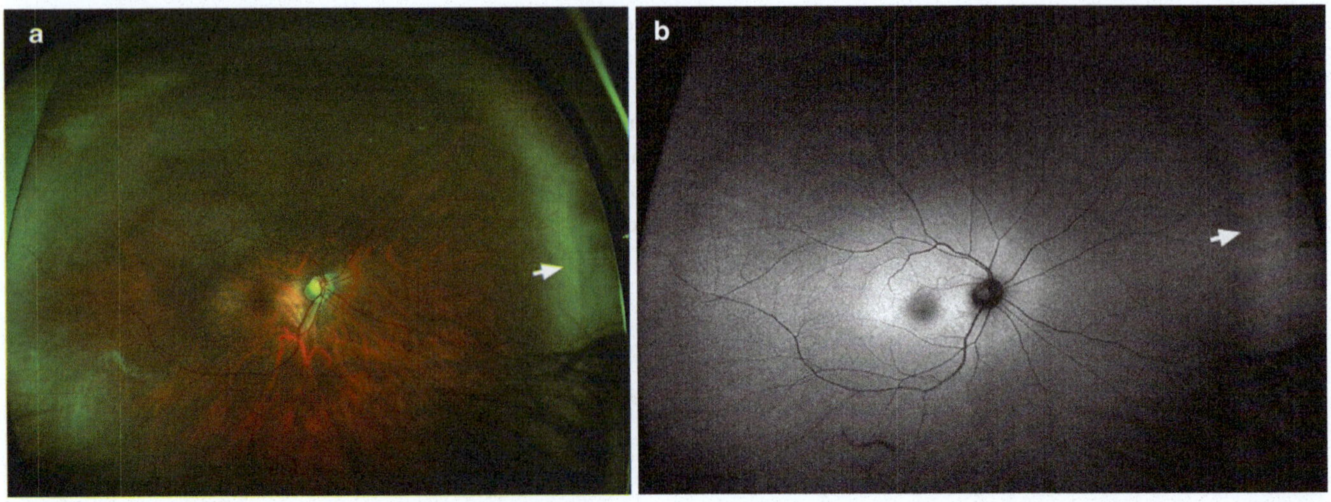

Fig. 5 (**a**) White without pressure. A 59-year-old man showed white without pressure on clinical examination. Wide-field retinal camera fundus image of the right eye shows peripheral white without pressure (*white arrow*). (**b**) White without pressure. Wide-field fundus autofluorescence of the same eye shows peripheral white without pressure (*white arrow*)

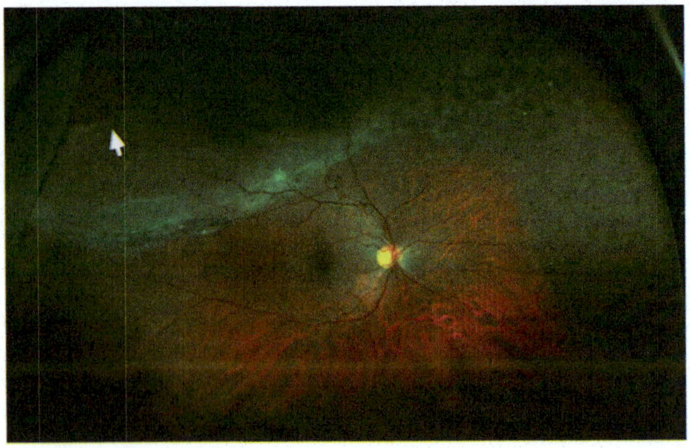

Fig. 6 Peripheral retinal break. Wide-field fundus color image of a 46-year-old diabetic man 9 years after barrier laser for peripheral retinal break (*white arrow*), which was an incidental finding at that time. Patient reports no complaints

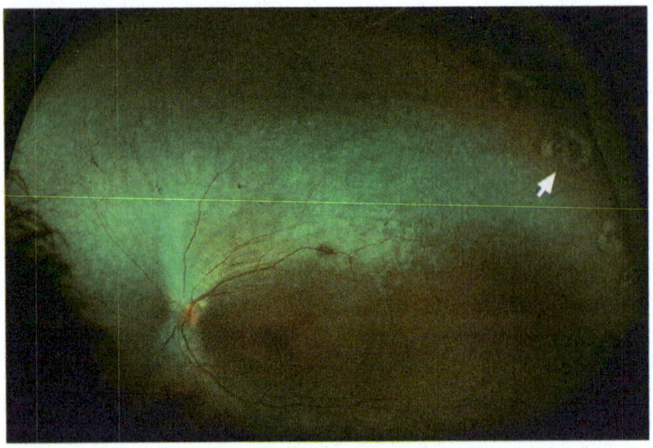

Fig. 7 Peripheral retinal degeneration. Wide-field fundus color image of the left eye of a patient with widespread atrophy of the retinal pigment epithelium demonstrates peripheral hyperpigmented lesions surrounded by hypopigmented circular rings (*white arrow*)

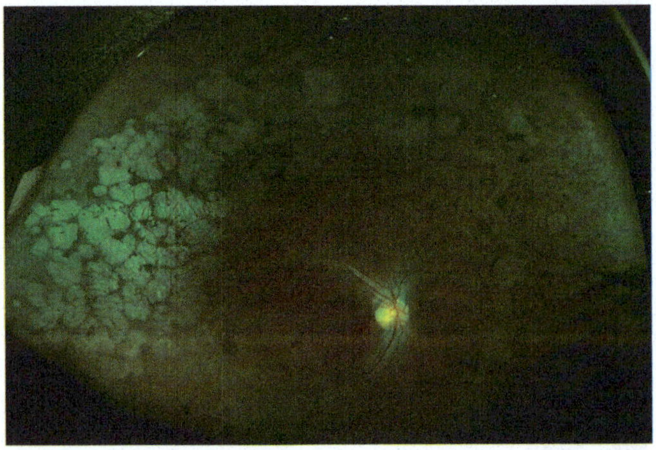

Fig. 8 Paving-stone (cobblestone) degeneration. Wide-field fundus color image of the right eye of a 45-year-old woman with no metabolic abnormalities or family history of similar lesions. Scalloped circular atrophic lesions are present in the retinal periphery and postequatorial area with hyperpigmented borders and visible choroidal vessels

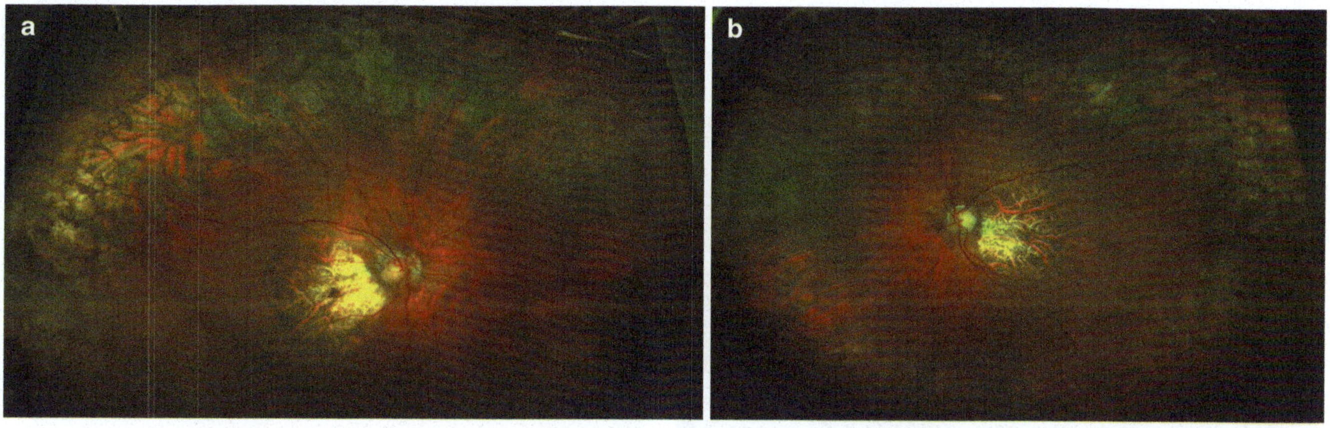

Fig. 9 (**a**) Paving-stone (cobblestone) degeneration in myopia. Wide-field fundus color image of the right eye of a 74-year-old woman with normal ornithine blood levels demonstrates central chorioretinal atrophy and scalloped circular atrophic lesions in the retinal periphery and postequatorial area with hyperpigmented borders. (**b**) Paving-stone (cobblestone) degeneration in myopia. Wide-field fundus color image of the left eye of the same patient shows an almost identical clinical picture

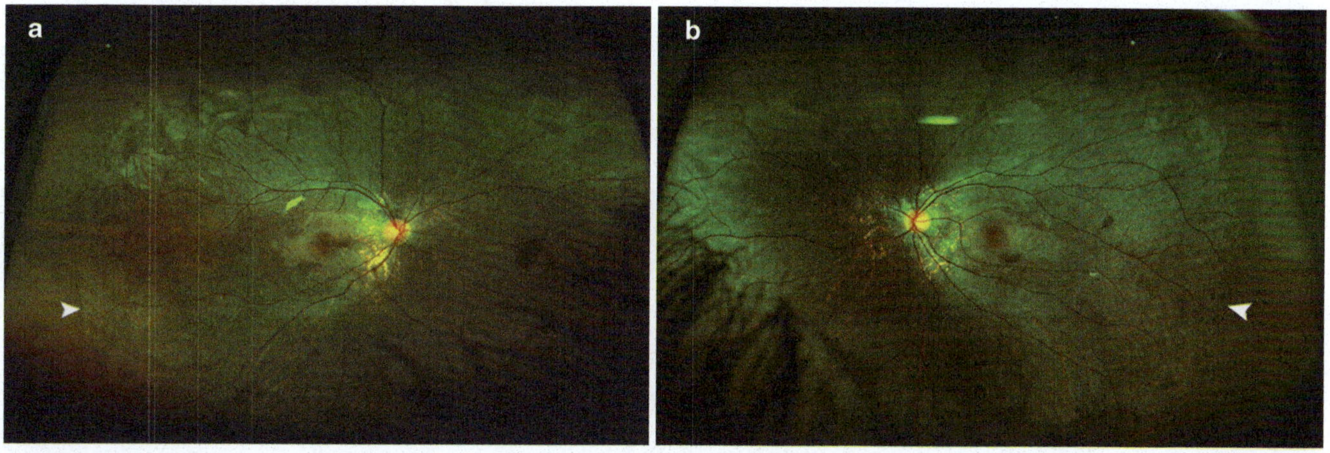

Fig. 10 (**a**) Gyrate atrophy. Wide-field fundus color image of the right eye of a 13-year-old boy with increased ornithine blood levels demonstrates widespread atrophy of the retinal pigment epithelium (*white arrowhead*) with scalloped circular atrophic lesions in the retinal periphery and postequatorial area with hyper-pigmented borders and central foveal sparing. (**b**) Gyrate atrophy. Wide-field fundus color image of the left eye of the same patient shows an almost identical clinical finding

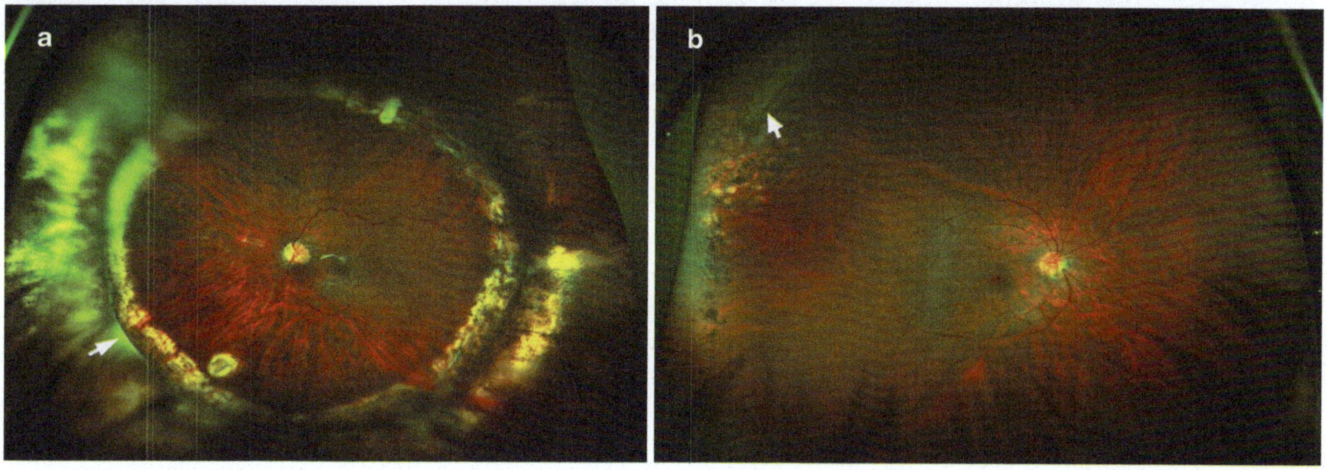

Fig. 11 (**a**) Status post retinal detachment repair. A 44-year-old man with a history of retinal detachment repair with combined scleral buckle and pars plana vitrectomy with gas tamponade in his left eye. Wide-field fundus color image shows flat retina, scleral buckle height (*white arrow*), and 360° laser at the edge of the buckle. (**b**) Prophylactic peripheral laser. Wide-field fundus color image of the right eye of the same patient shows prophylactic laser around the area of retinal degeneration with small break (*white arrow*). The finding has been stable for 5 years

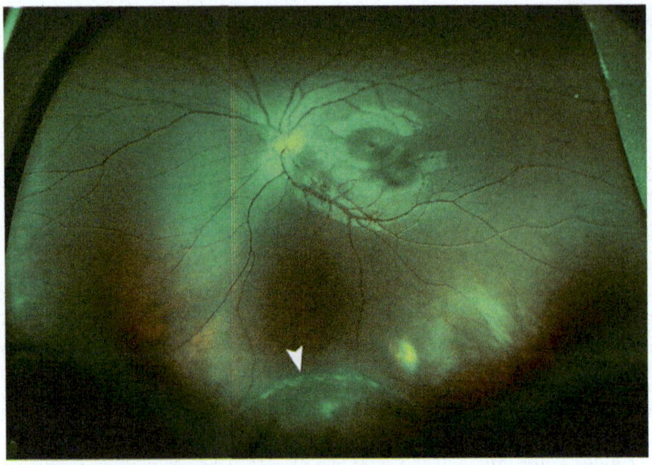

Fig. 12 Peripheral retinoschisis. Wide-field fundus color image of the left eye of a 22-year-old patient with no visual complaints shows peripheral retinoschisis in the inferior retina (*white arrowhead*) as an incidental finding

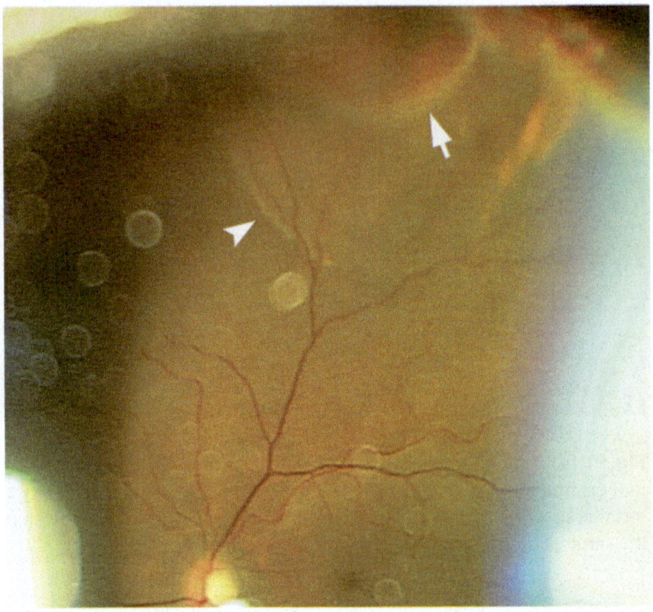

Fig. 13 Peripheral retinal cyst. Wide-field biomicroscopic image shows inferior (inverted image) retinal cyst (*white arrow*) with adjacent detachment (*white arrowhead*)

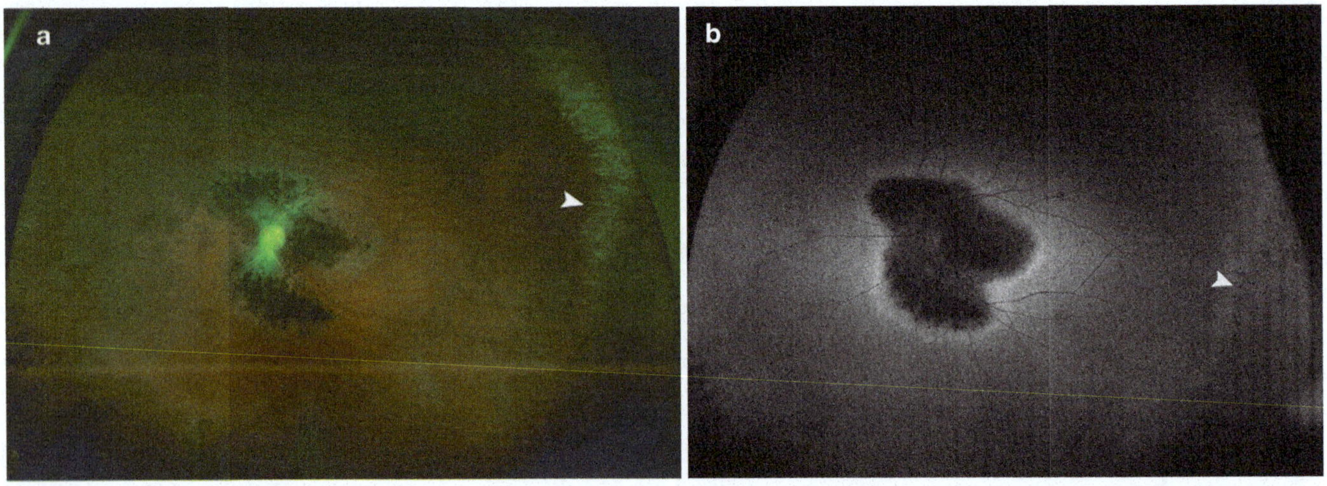

Fig. 14 (**a**) Peripheral thinning in retinal dystrophy. Wide-field fundus color image of the left eye of a 30-year-old man demonstrates extensive peripapillary hyperpigmentation and thinning of the peripheral retina (*white arrowhead*). (**b**) Peripheral thinning in retinal dystrophy. Wide-field fundus autofluorescence image of the same eye demonstrates central hyperautofluorescence with surrounding ring of hyperautofluorescence and peripheral pigmentary disturbances (*white arrowhead*)

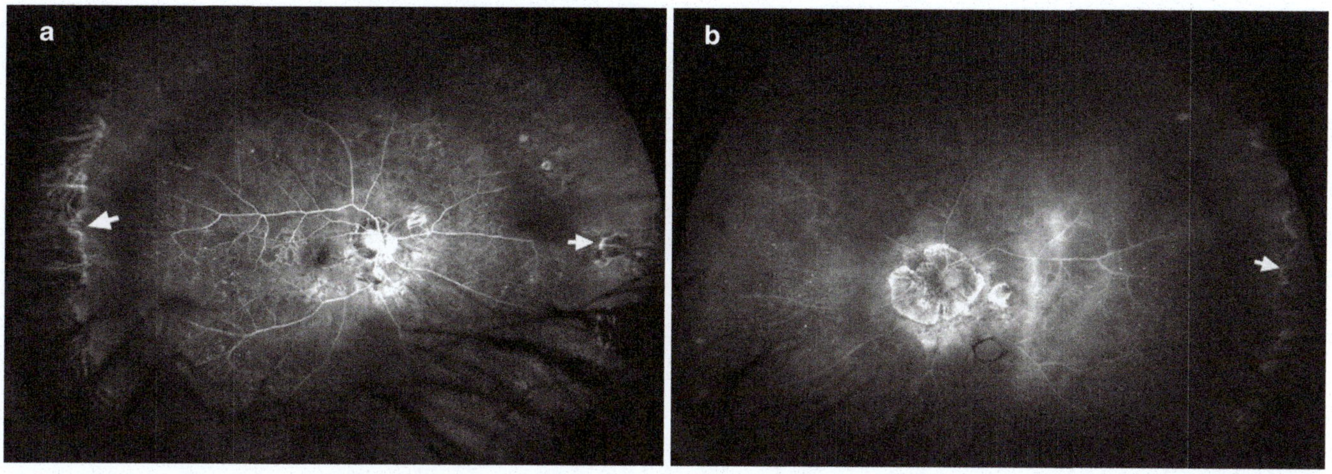

Fig. 15 (**a**) Peripheral retinal degeneration in myopia. Wide-field fundus fluorescein angiogram of the right eye of a 72-year-old myopic man demonstrates peripapillary atrophy and areas of atrophy in the retinal periphery (*white arrows*). (**b**) Peripheral retinal degeneration in myopia. Wide-field fundus fluorescein angiogram of the left eye of the same patient shows extensive peripapillary atrophy and peripheral retinal atrophy (*white arrow*)

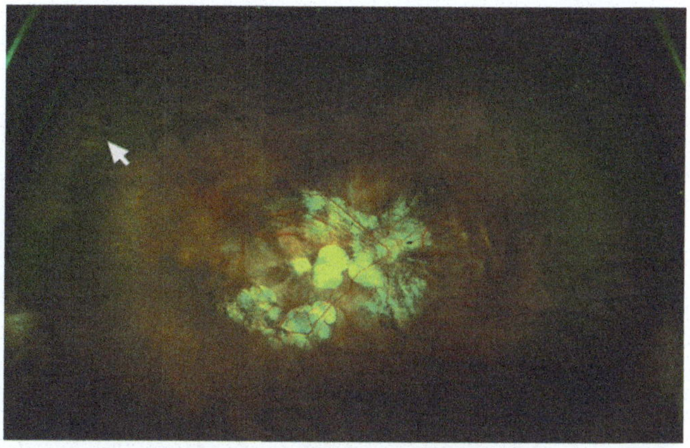

Fig. 16 Peripheral retinal degeneration in myopia. Wide-field fundus color image of the right eye of a 66-year-old myopic woman demonstrates extensive peripapillary atrophy and adjacent areas of geographic atrophy. Clinical examination with scleral indentation revealed areas of retinal thinning with hyperpigmentation (*white arrow*)

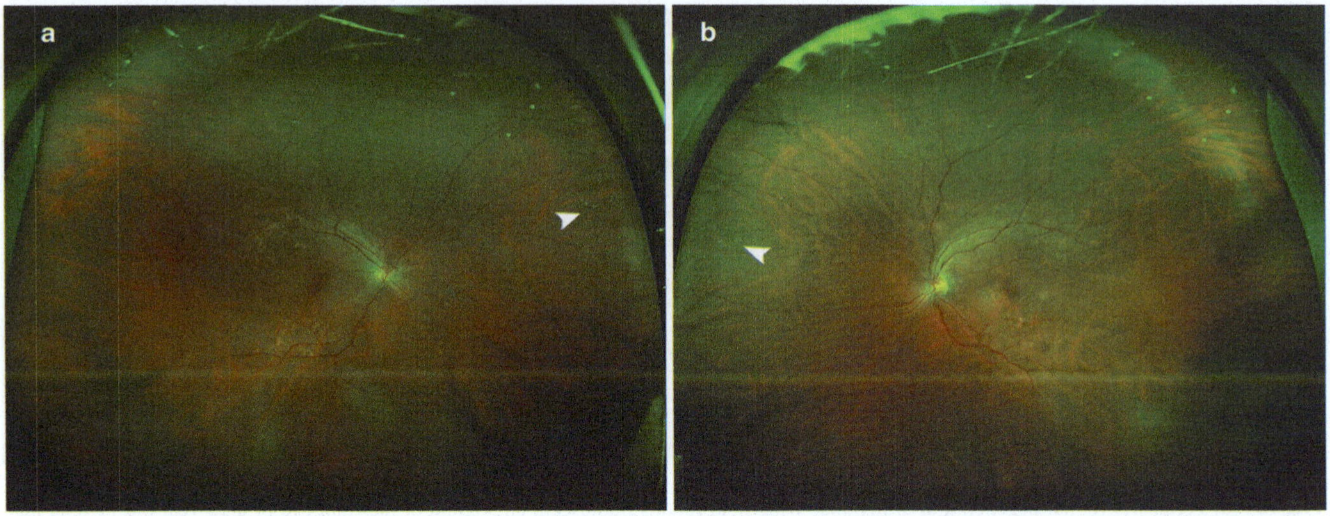

Fig. 17 (**a**) Peripheral drusen. Wide-field fundus color image of the right eye of a 72-year-old woman demonstrates drusen scattered around the posterior pole and in the nasal periphery (*white arrowhead*). (**b**) Peripheral drusen. Wide-field fundus color image of the left eye of the same patient demonstrates drusen scattered around the optic disc and posterior pole and in the nasal periphery (*white arrowhead*)

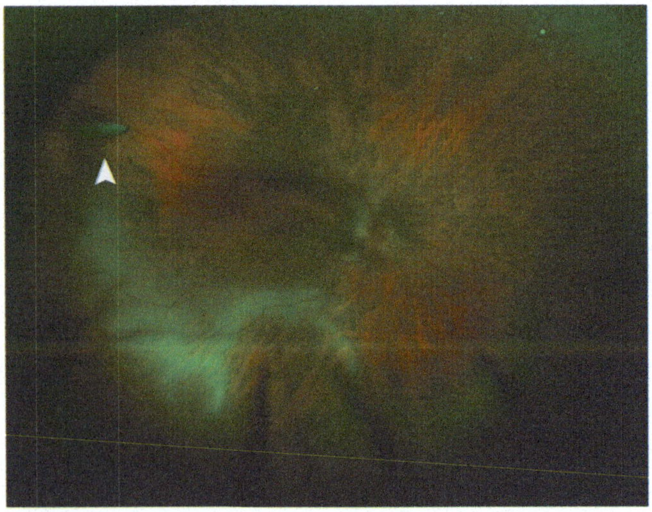

Fig. 18 Peripheral operculum. A 55-year-old man was seen in the emergency room with a complaint of floaters in the right eye. Wide-field fundus color image shows operculated tissue in the superotemporal retinal periphery (*white arrowhead*) with mild vitreous hemorrhage

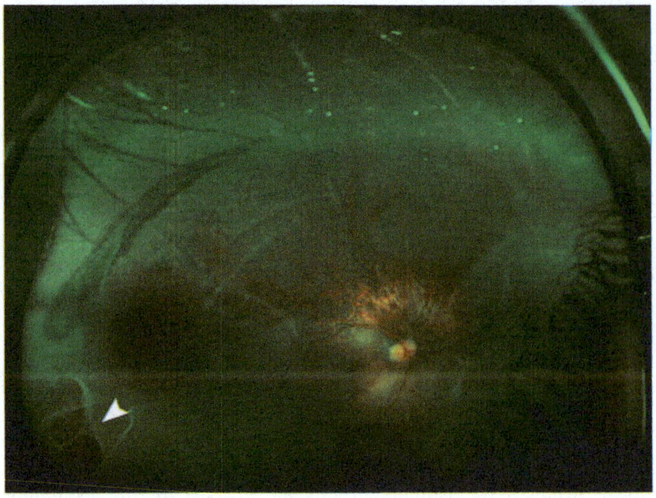

Fig. 19 Peripheral retinal holes with detachment. A 13-year-old boy presented with decreased vision in his right eye. Wide-field fundus color image shows numerous large holes in the temporal retina with subtotal retinal detachment (arrowhead)

UWFA Imaging and Age-Related Macular Degeneration

A good example for new insight provided by wide-field imaging is given by a recent study that showed clearly that even in dry age-related macular degeneration (AMD), which was primarily seen as a disease of the macula region and the posterior pole, typical peripheral retinal changes commonly occur, allowing the conclusion that AMD must now be better understood as primarily "panretinal" disease [10]. As a consequence, the peripheral retina may provide additional diagnostic information, allowing a better understanding of the disease.

UWFA imaging possesses great potential for the diagnosis and management of peripheral retinal degenerations. Because UWFA imaging has expanded our ability to evaluate the far periphery of the retina, we are identifying abnormality more frequently and earlier than we previously did. This is, in turn, changing our conception of the disease processes and how best to diagnose, follow, and treat them. With these gains, however, also comes the challenge of how to apply the findings toward clinical practice. Because we increasingly turn to UWFA imaging to diagnose and manage the retinal conditions, we will likewise have to increasingly reconcile the practice guidelines based on the older studies with the arsenal of new information now available through UWFA and imaging. Further clinical trials will be necessary to incorporate UWFA and imaging into evidence-based practice guidelines for the diagnosis and management of retinal disease.

Acknowledgment *The following investigators belong to The King Khaled Eye Specialist Hospital (KKESH) Collaborative Retina Study Group: J. Fernando Arevalo, MD, FACS (PI), Saba Al Rashaed, MD, Eman Al Kahtani, MD, Sawsan Nowilaty, MD, Hassan A. Al-Dhibi, MD, Yahya A. Al-Zahrani, MD, Igor Kozak, MD, PhD, Sulaiman Al-Sulaiman, MD, Patrik Schatz, MD, Abdulelah Al-Abdullah, MD, Khalid Al Rubaie, MD, Yousef Al Dhafiri, MD, Badr Al Ahmadi, MD, Abdulaziz Al Hadlaq, MD, Majed Al Harbi, MD, Abdulaziz Al Oreany, MD, Adel Al-Akeely, MD, Mohammad Hazzazi, MD, Mohammed Talea, MD, Ghazai Al-Thobaiti, MD.

References

1. Friberg TR, Forrester JV. Ultrawide angle (200+) fluorescein angiography using a modified Optos Panoramic 200TM imaging system. Invest Ophthalmol Vis Sci. 2004;45. ARVO E-Abstract 3001.
2. Friberg TR, Gupta A, Yu J, Huang L, Suner I, Puliafito CA, et al. Ultrawide angle fluorescein angiographic imaging: a comparison to conventional digital acquisition systems. Ophthalmic Surg Lasers Imaging. 2008;39:304–11.
3. Pomerantzeff O. Equator-plus camera. Invest Ophthalmol. 1975;14:401–6.
4. Staurenghi G, Viola F, Mainster MA, Graham RD, Harrington PG. Scanning laser ophthalmoscopy and angiography with a wide-field contact lens system. Arch Ophthalmol. 2005;123:244–52.
5. Noyori KS, Chino K, Deguchi T. Wide field fluorescein angiography by use of contact lens. Retina. 1983;3:131–4.
6. Spaide RF, Orlock DA, Herrmann-Delemazure B, Ciardella AP, Yannuzzi LA, Freund KB, et al. Wide-angle indocyanine green angiography. Retina. 1998;18:44–9.
7. Takahashi K, Muraoka K, Kishi S, Shimizu K. Watershed zone in the human peripheral choroid. Ophthalmology. 1996;103:336–42.
8. Diabetic Retinopathy Clinical Research Network website http://drcrnet.jaeb.org. Accessed 13 Feb 2015.
9. Lee BR, Chang HR. Biomicroscopic vitreous observation using a 3 CCD video camera and a personal computer for image capture and archiving. Korean J Ophthalmol. 2000;14:74–9.
10. Reznicek L, Wasfy T, Stumpf C, Kampik A, Ulbig M, Neubauer AS, et al. Peripheral fundus autofluorescence is increased in age-related macular degeneration. Invest Ophthalmol Vis Sci. 2012;53:2193–8.

Wide-Field Imaging of the Pediatric Retina

11

Mrinali Patel Gupta, Yoshihiro Yonekawa, Karyn E. Jonas, Anton Orlin, and R.V. Paul Chan

Traditionally, children posed a unique challenge to imaging in the clinical setting because significant compliance from the patient was required, especially if the pathology was peripheral and required direction of the patient's gaze into the necessary positions. As such, wide-field imaging of children was typically performed under anesthesia using handheld photography tools such as the RetCam (Clarity Medical Systems, Pleasanton, CA), which provides approximately 130° of visualization. The advent of ultra-wide-field (UWF) imaging technology, for example, the Optos (Optos, Marlborough, MA), enabled capturing a wider retinal area (approximately 200°) with potentially requisite cooperation from the young patient. In recent retrospective case series, ultra-wide-field outpatient imaging has shown to exhibit utility in the diagnosis of a variety of retinal conditions, allowing wide-field imaging and fluorescein angiography (FA) in the clinic, without the use of anesthesia [1, 2]. Retrospective case series of pediatric patients undergoing ultra-wide-field angiography (UWFA) using Optos in the clinic found that imaging was useful for the evaluation of conditions including uveitis (pars planitis), Coats' disease, retinopathy of prematurity, schisis, Stargardt's disease, Best disease, history of intraocular foreign body, toxoplasmosis, melanoma, and familial exudative vitreoretinopathy in children as young as 5 years old [1, 2]. It was noted in one series of 16 patients under age 12 that imaging of earlier phases (i.e. the choroidal phase) was limited, likely due to the time required to console the patient after intravenous injection and to reposition the head [1]. UWFA may therefore be limited in cases where visualization of early phases is critical. Conditions in which later phase imaging is sufficient may therefore be particularly amenable to ultra-wide-field angiography in the office, allowing the patient to avoid a trip to the operating room for examination under anesthesia. This chapter presents wide-field and ultra-wide-field fundus photographs and angiograms from a spectrum of pediatric retinal conditions.

Retinal Dystrophies and Degenerations

Retinitis Pigmentosa

Retinitis pigmentosa (RP) is a clinically and genetically heterogeneous disease with early rod photoreceptor degeneration and subsequent cone degeneration. Inheritance can be sporadic, X-linked, autosomal dominant, or autosomal recessive. Classic clinical signs include bilateral involvement (except in extremely rare cases), vascular attenuation, waxy disc pallor, bone spicule pigmentary changes (Fig. 1) that progressively increase with time, and possibly cystoid macular edema. Electroretinography reveals reduced scotopic responses early in the disease, with photopic responses also being affected in more advanced disease. Mid-peripheral visual field defects such as a ring scotoma expand over time, ultimately leaving a small central island, which ultimately can get extinguished as well [3]. Retinitis pigmentosa may be associated with a wide range of systemic findings, for example in Bassen-Kornzweig syndrome, Bardet-Biedl syndrome, Usher syndrome, and Refsum syndrome. While no studies specifically report the utility of wide-field imaging for pediatric patients with this condition, studies have demonstrated the utility of wide-field imaging in RP and have correlated the extent of wide field fundus hypoautofluorescence abnormalities with visual field loss by Goldmann testing [4, 5].

M.P. Gupta, MD
Department of Ophthalmology, Weill Cornell Medical College, New York–Presbyterian Hospital, New York, NY, USA
e-mail: mrp9003@med.cornell.edu

Y. Yonekawa, MD
Associated Retinal Consultants, Royal Oak, MI, USA
e-mail: yonekawa@gmail.com

K.E. Jonas, BSN, RN • R.V.P. Chan, MD (✉)
Department of Ophthalmology and Visual Sciences, Illinois Eye and Ear Infirmary, University of Illinois at Chicago, Chicago, IL, USA
e-mail: kj919@uic.edu; rvpchan@uic.edu

A. Orlin's, MD
Department of Ophthalmology, Weill Cornell Medical College, New York, NY, USA
e-mail: ano9028@med.cornell.edu

I. Kozak, J.F. Arevalo (eds.), *Atlas of Wide-Field Retinal Angiography and Imaging*, DOI 10.1007/978-3-319-17864-6_11

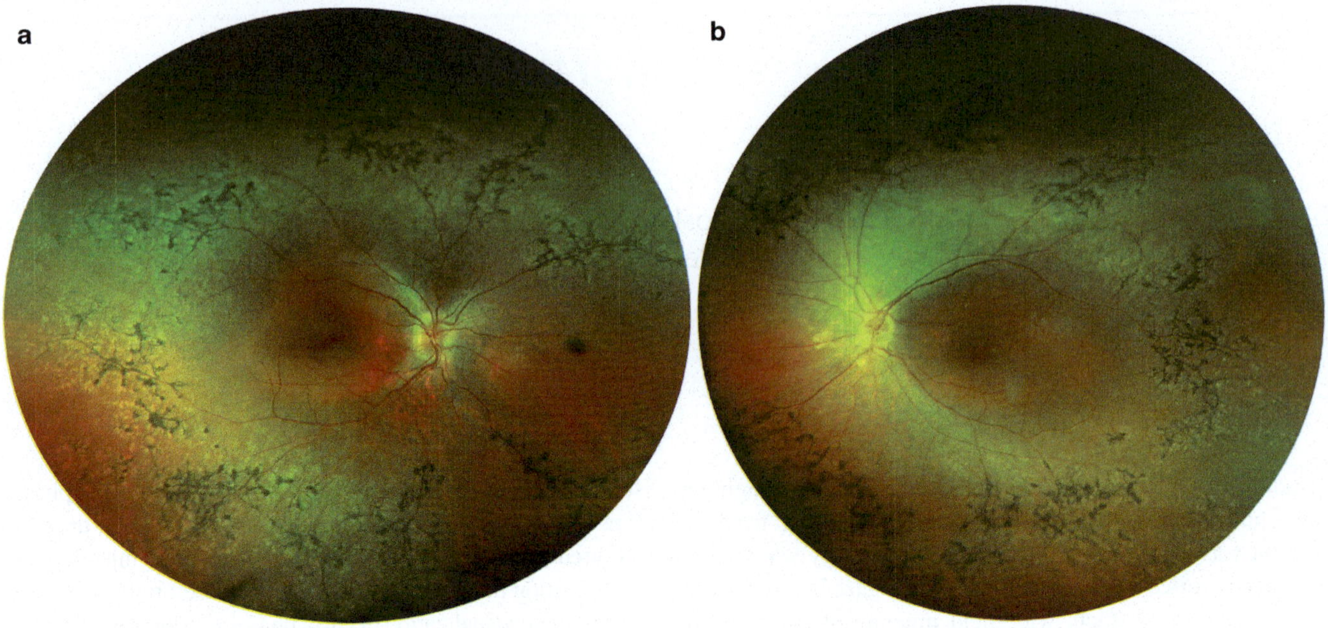

Fig. 1 UWF fundus photographs of a 9-year-old with autosomal recessive RP with attenuated vessels, granular fundus, and bone spicule pigmentary changes in each eye (OU). (**a**) Right eye (OD); (**b**) left eye (OS)

Albinism

Albinism represents a group of conditions involving a defect in one or more enzymes involved in melanin production in the hair, skin, and ocular structures. Oculocutaneous albinism is inherited in autosomal recessive fashion, whereas ocular albinism somewhat spares the skin and hair and is inherited in an X-linked recessive fashion. Findings include iris transillumination defects, foveal hypoplasia, and hypopigmentation of the fundus (Fig. 2), with poor vision and nystagmus. Visual evoked potentials show abnormal decussation of the optic nerve fibers. Associated systemic syndromes include Chediak-Higashi syndrome and Hermansky-Pudlak syndrome [6].

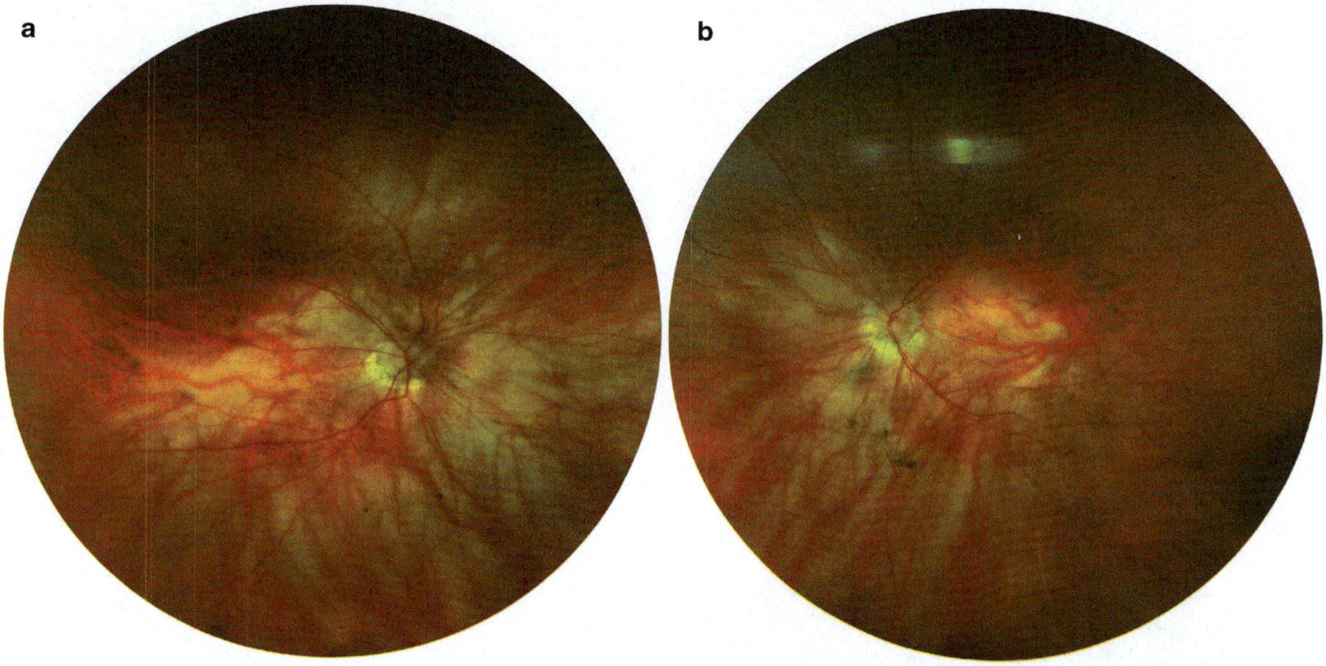

Fig. 2 UWF fundus photographs demonstrate hypopigmented fundus and foveal hypoplasia OU (**a** OD; **b** OS) in a female with ocular albinism

Doyne Honeycomb Dystrophy (Also Known as Malattia Leventinese, Familial Drusen, or Autosomal Dominant Radial Drusen)

Doyne honeycomb dystrophy is an autosomal dominant fashion condition owing to a mutation in the *EFEMP1* (epidermal growth factor–containing fibulin-like extracellular matrix protein-1) gene and is characterized by small perifoveal and peripapillary (especially nasal) drusen (Fig. 3) that progressively increase over time. Late in the disease, geographic atrophy, scarring, and rarely, choroidal neovascularization may develop [7].

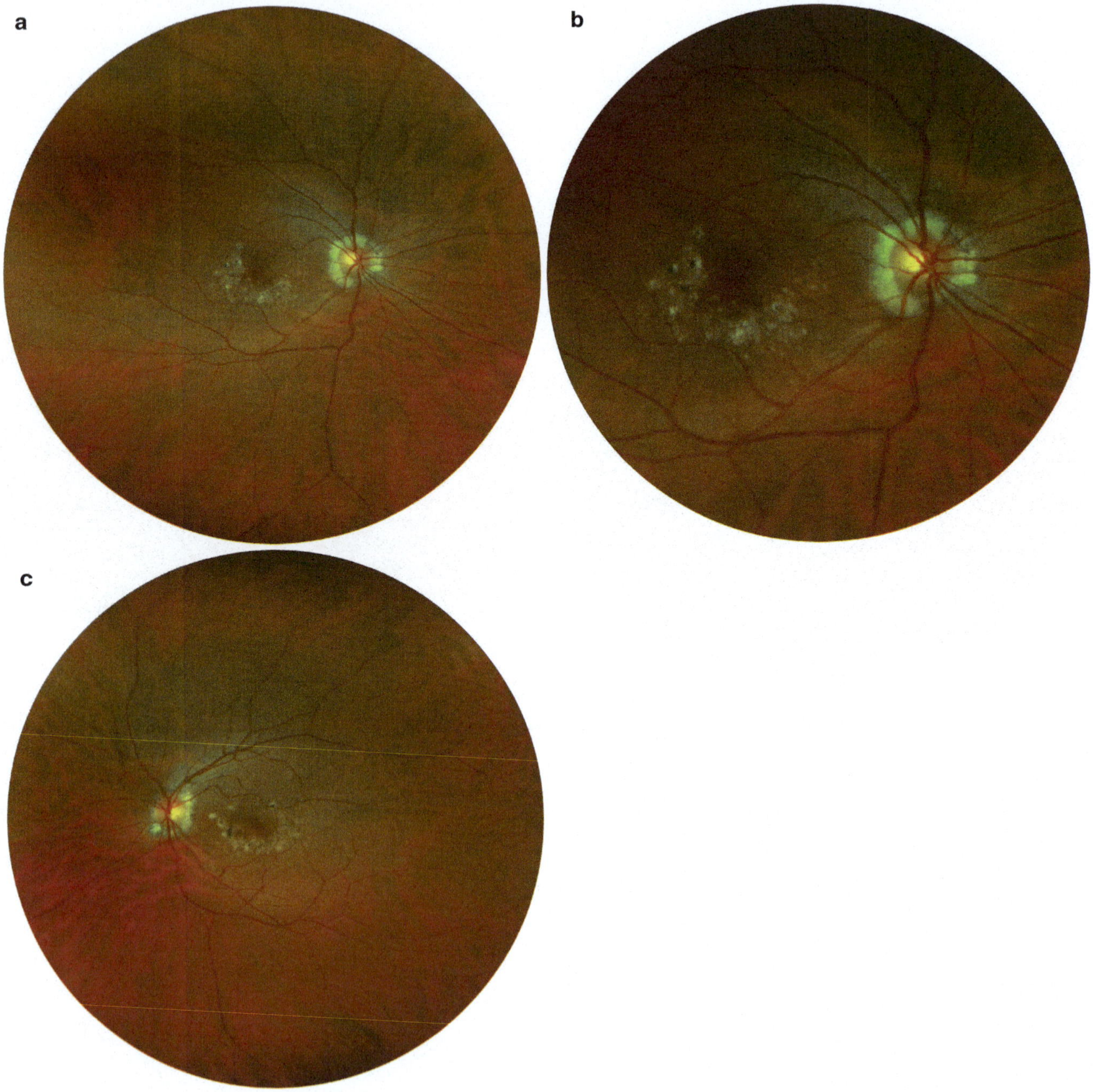

Fig. 3 UWF fundus photographs of a female with Doyne honeycomb dystrophy reveal a ring of perifoveal radiating drusen with scarring, as well as peripapillary large drusen OU (**a** OD; **b** magnified macular view OD; **c** OS)

Pediatric Retinal Vascular Disease

Coats' Disease

Coats' disease is an idiopathic, sporadic disease of retinal telangiectasia with intraretinal and subretinal exudation, sometimes with exudative retinal detachment (Figs. 4 and 5). The disease classically presents unilaterally, typically in boys, with an average age of presentation of 5 years. FA reveals hyperfluorescent telangiectatic bulbs with leakage and ischemia peripheral to the area of telangiectasias (Figs. 4 and 5). Several Coats' variants with bilateral involvement and systemic associations, including fascioscapulohumeral dystrophy and Coats plus disease, have been described [8]. UWF fundus photography and UWFA have been shown to be useful for the diagnosis of Coats' disease [1, 2], at times capturing peripheral vascular telangiectasias and areas of nonperfusion not visualized within the seven standard fields [2]. Wide-field imaging and angiography are critical for identification of peripheral nonperfusion and telangiectasias, as well as image-guided targeted panretinal photocoagulation to these areas [1, 2]. The presence of persistent areas of nonperfusion or leaking telangiectasias after treatment suggests need for repeat laser therapy.

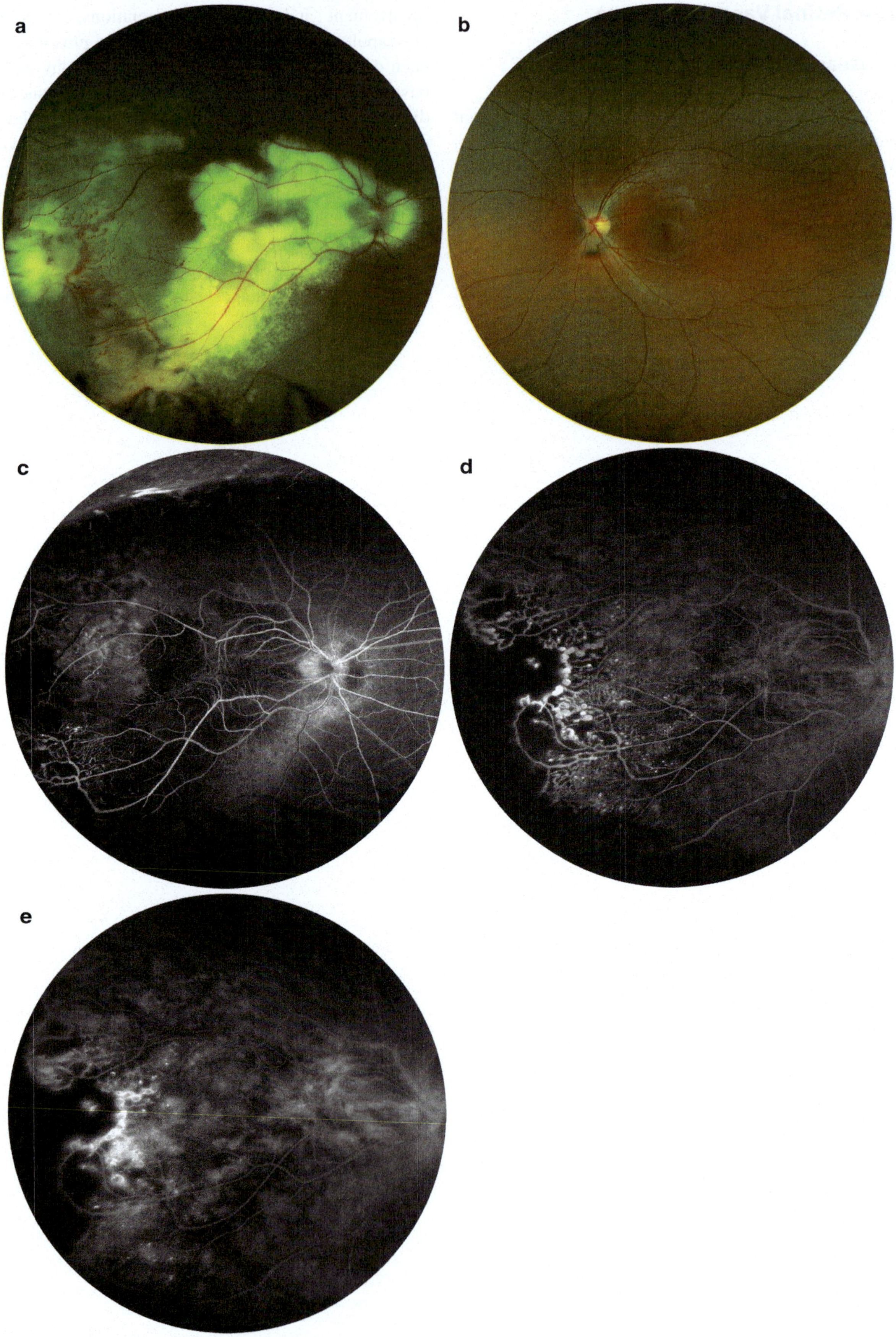

Fig. 4 UWF fundus photographs of a 10-year-old boy who presented with history of Coats disease status post laser elsewhere 1 year previously reveal temporal telangiectatic vessels with extensive retinal exudation OD (**a**) and normal fundus OS (**b**). UWFA reveals light bulb telangiectasias with leakage and ischemia (**c** 15 s; **d** 49 s; **e** 3 min 44 s)

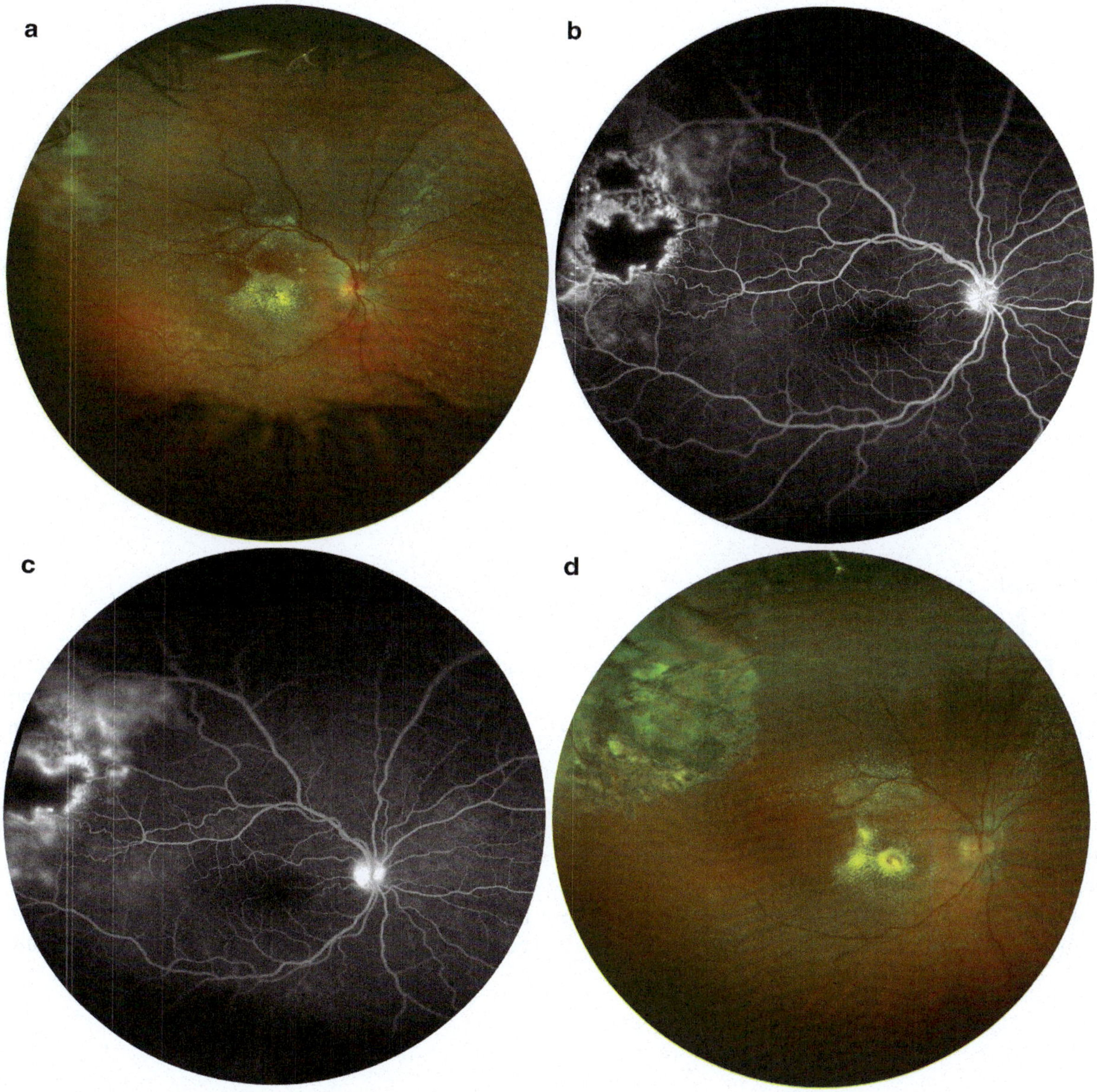

Fig. 5 UWF fundus photographs of a 9-year-old boy with Coats disease reveal macular and peripheral exudates with superotemporal retinal vascular telangiectasias OD (**a**), which leak on UWFA (**b** 1 min 48 s; **c** 5 min 40 s). The patient underwent targeted laser photocoagulation under anesthesia OD to areas of telangiectasia and nonperfusion on UWFA, with improved but persistent exudates at 3.5 months after laser (**d**). UWFA at that time showed no leaking telangiectasias (**e** 4 min 57 s). The patient was observed and gradual resolution of exudation was noted (**f** 16 months after laser). A small macular scar developed in the setting of chronic exudate (**f**)

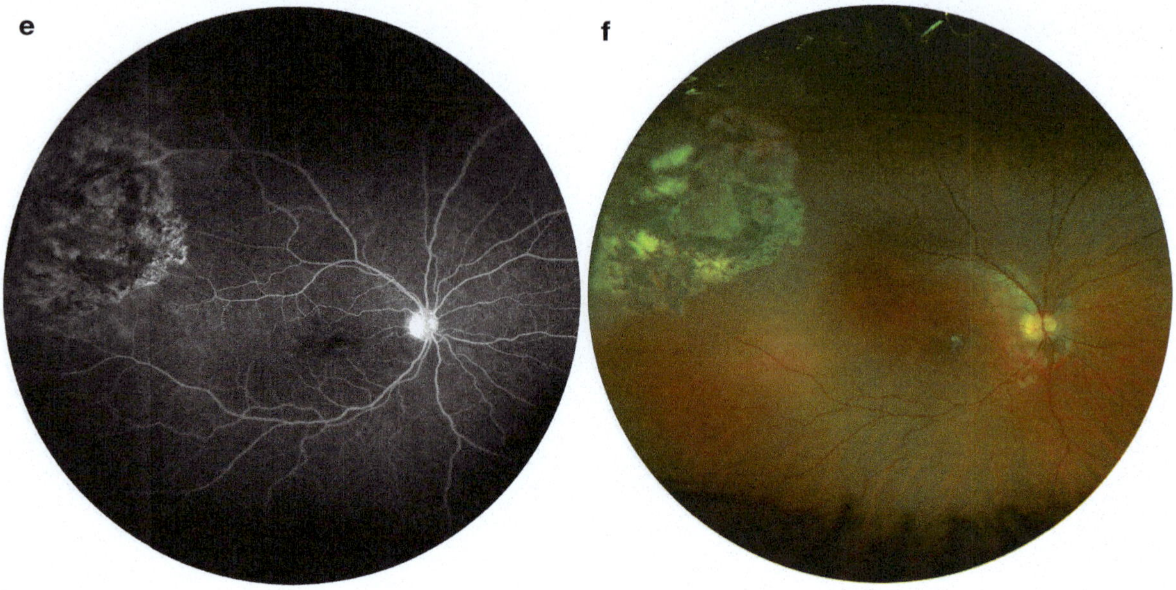

Fig. 5 (continued)

Familial Exudative Vitreoretinopathy

Familial exudative vitreoretinopathy (FEVR) is a condition of abnormal vascularization of the retinal periphery. Mutations in genes implicated in Wnt signaling have been associated with the disease. Clinical findings include avascular retinal periphery (Figs. 6 and 7) with vitreous degeneration and vitreoretinal interface changes, peripheral fibrovascular proliferation (Fig. 6c, e) with subsequent vitreous hemorrhage or retinal detachment (Fig. 7a), and vascular straightening (Figs. 6 and 7) and temporal dragging of the macula (Fig. 7a, b) [9]. UWF fundus photography and UWFA are useful for diagnosis, management, and monitoring of this condition given the characteristic peripheral nonperfusion and neovascularization. Recent studies have utilized UWFA to provide an update of the classification of FEVR and establish a more complete characterization of the early stages of FEVR [10]. Moreover, UWFA imaging can be used to guide targeted photocoagulation to areas of nonperfusion [2].

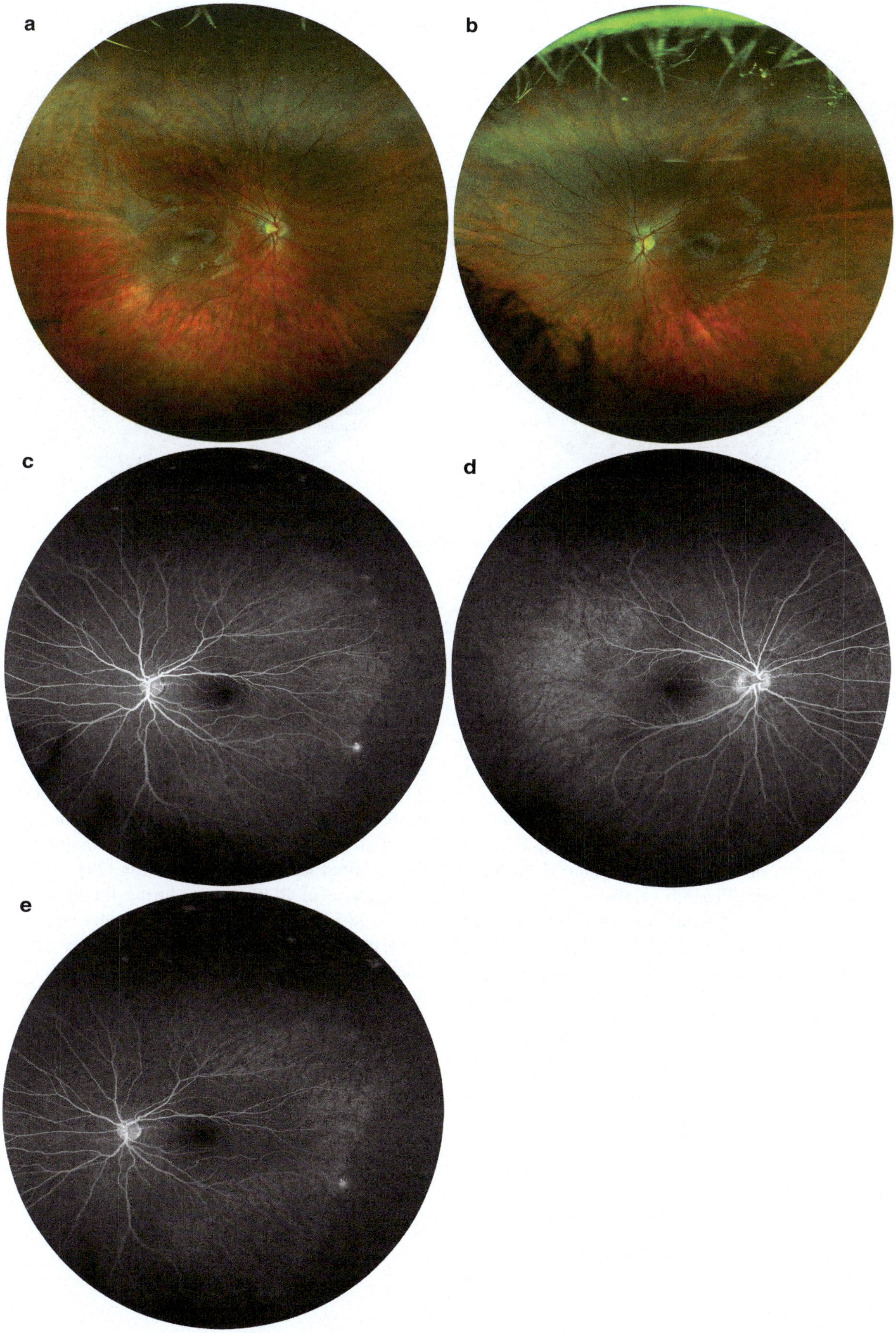

Fig. 6 UWF fundus photographs of an 11-year-old boy with FEVR reveal vascular straightening and pruning of the retinal vessels peripherally OU (**a**, **b**). UWFA demonstrates peripheral ischemia OU (**c** 1 min 24 s; **d** 3 min 22 s; **e** 5 min 22 s) and a tiny retinal neovascularization at the border of perfused and nonperfused retina OS (**c**, **e**)

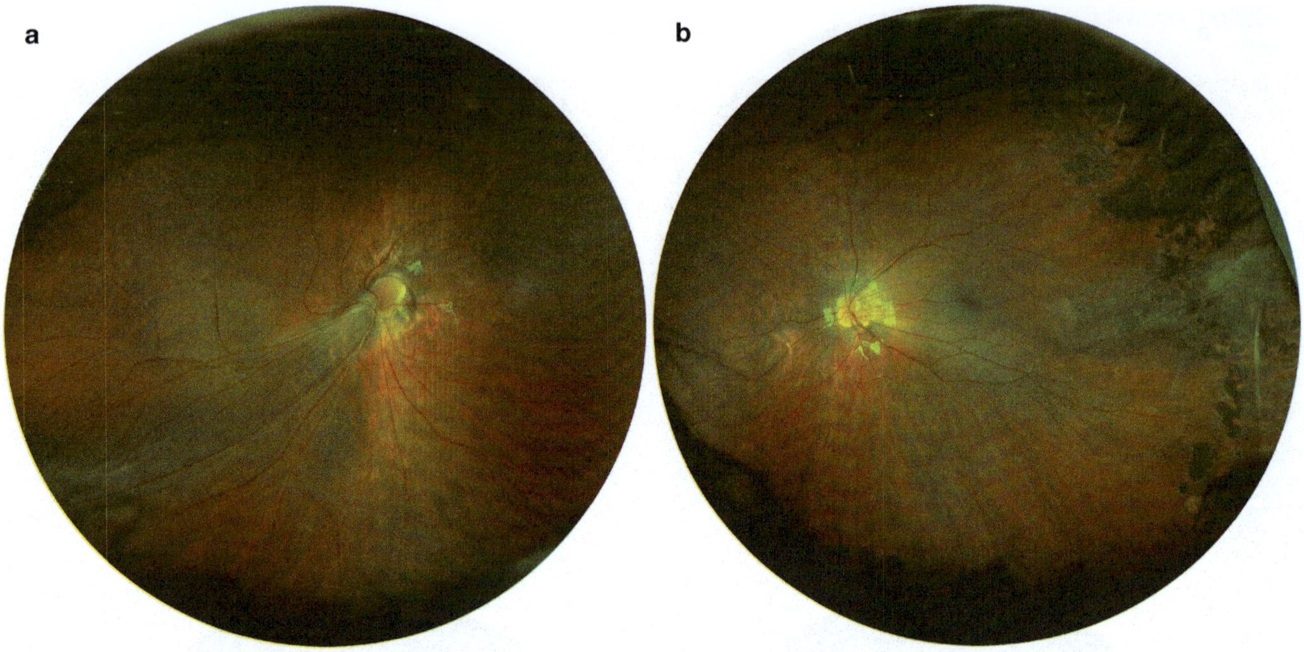

Fig. 7 UWF fundus photographs of a 5-year-old boy with FEVR reveal straightening of the retinal vessels and macular dragging OU (**a**, **b**), with an associated tractional retinal detachment OD (**a**). There are chorioretinal scars from peripheral laser OS (**b**)

Retinopathy of Prematurity

Retinopathy of prematurity (ROP) is a condition of the retinal vasculature that occurs in premature neonates. Risk factors include low birthweight and low gestational age at birth. ROP is characterized by the zone of involvement within the retina and stage of disease—stage 1: demarcation line (Fig. 8a); stage 2: elevated ridge (Fig. 8b); stage 3: extraretinal fibrovascular proliferation (Fig. 8c, d); stage 4: retinal detachment with (4B) or without (4A; Fig. 8e) foveal involvement; or stage 5: total retinal detachment (Fig. 8f), and presence (Fig. 8d) or absence (Fig. 8c) of plus disease. Cicatricial changes such as temporal vessel straightening and macular dragging (Figs. 9 and 10b), vitreoretinal interface changes (Fig. 10), retinal folds (Fig. 11), and tractional (Fig. 12) and rhegmatogenous detachments may occur [11].

Digital imaging and wide-field imaging for telemedicine-based screening of ROP has been gaining popularity, and studies suggest that the diagnosis of clinically relevant ROP through image based diagnosis may be accurate [12–22]. Wide-field imaging may also supplement clinical examination through objective documentation of clinical findings and improved ability to detect progression through comparison of serial photographs. One recent study suggests that compared to fundus photography alone, wide-field angiography may improve the sensitivity of ROP diagnosis, especially for stage 3 disease [23]. Use of RetCam imaging immediately after laser therapy for ROP can also identify skip areas of untreated ROP, potentially reducing the need for re-treatment due to inadequate initial laser photocoagulation [24]. Given that the active phase of ROP occurs during the neonatal period, wide-field imaging of ROP has generally been performed using the RetCam technology, either under anesthesia or after swaddling of the awake patient. UWF imaging with Optos technology has more often been performed in older children to document the late sequelae of ROP, though there are now reports of Optos imaging of neonates with ROP using the "flying baby" position, in which a technician or clinician holds the neonate upright in the Optos machine [25].

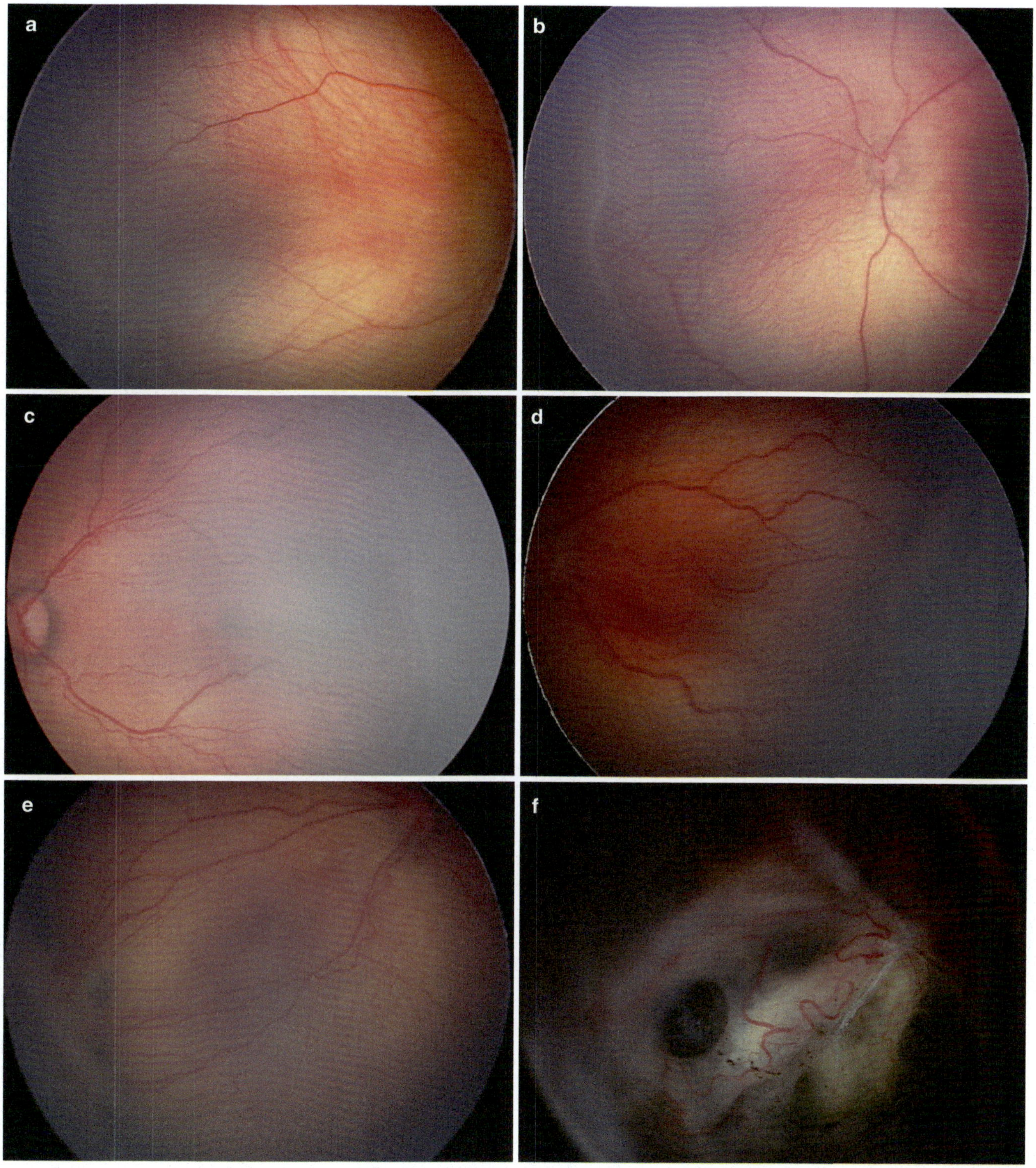

Fig. 8 Wide-field fundus photographs of ROP including stage 1 demarcation line (**a**), stage 2 elevated ridge (**b**), stage 3 neovascularization without plus disease (**c**), stage 3 neovascularization with plus disease (**d**), stage 4A retinal detachment not involving the fovea (**e**), and stage 5 total retinal detachment (**f**)

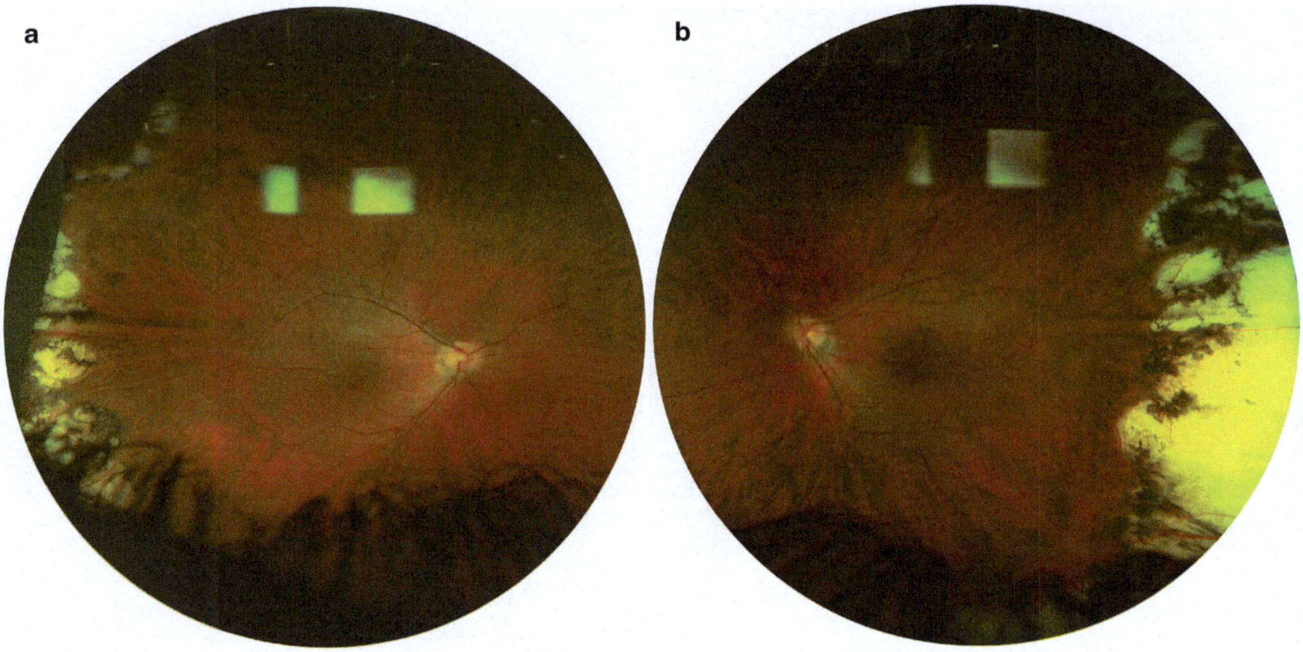

Fig. 9 UWF fundus photographs of a 16-year-old boy born at 23 weeks gestational age and with a history of ROP OU status post laser photocoagulation OU with mild temporal dragging of the retinal vasculature and peripheral chorioretinal scars from laser (**a** OD; **b** OS)

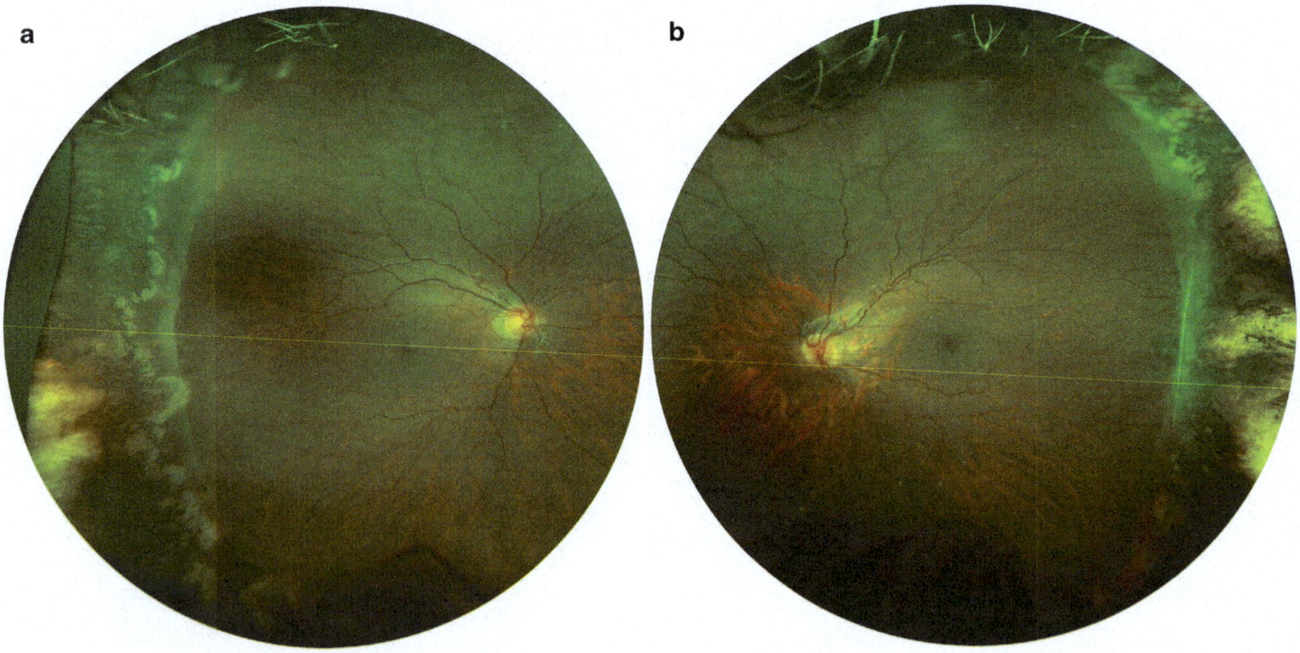

Fig. 10 UWF fundus photographs of a 12-year-old girl, born at 24 weeks gestational age, status post laser OU with peripheral laser scars and vitreoretinal interface changes OU (**a** OD; **b** OS) with some associated temporal dragging of the retinal vessels OS (**b**)

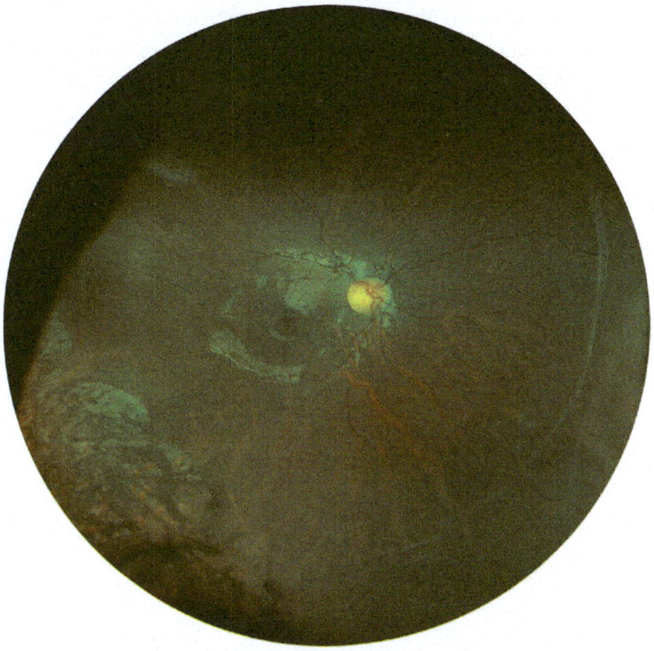

Fig. 11 UWF fundus photographs of a 9-year-old boy, born at 25 weeks gestational age and status post laser photocoagulation OU for ROP with stage 5 retinal detachment OS (not shown) and attached retina with temporal chorioretinal scars and nasal retinal fold OD

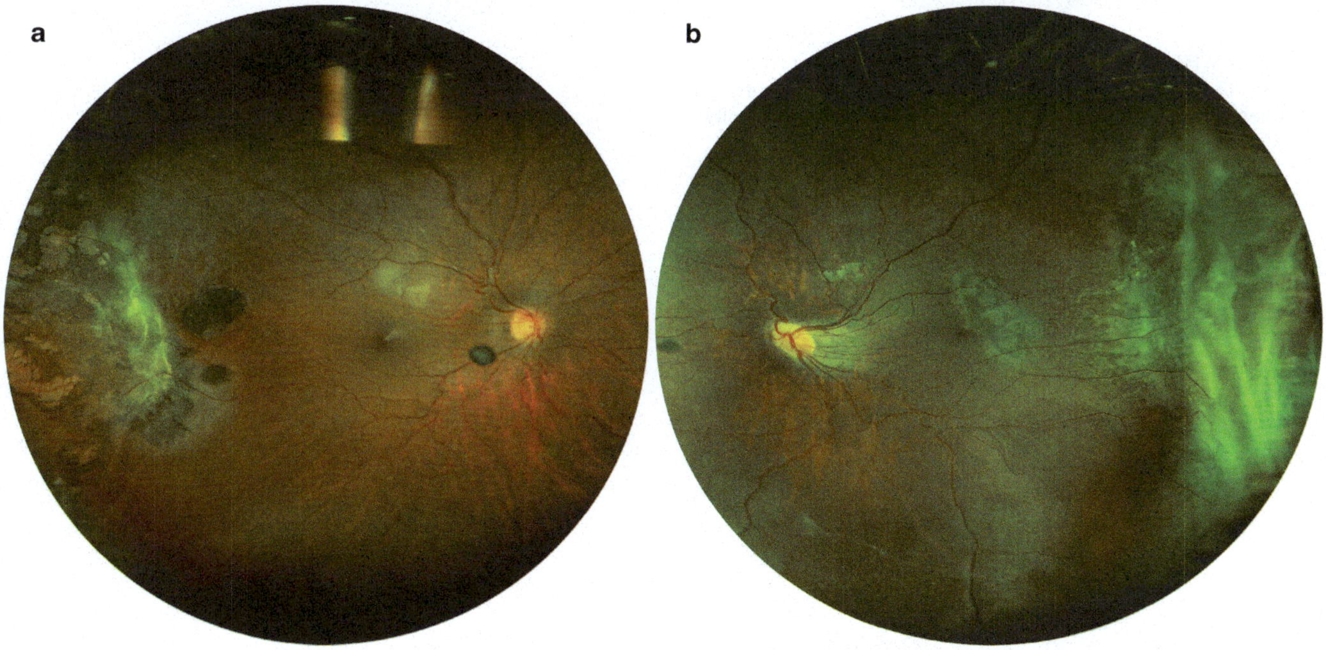

Fig. 12 UWF fundus photographs of an 11-year-old boy, born at 24 weeks gestation, weighing 850 g, status post laser OU with temporal dragging of the vessels and peripheral chorioretinal scars from laser OU (**a**, **b**) and tractional retinal detachment temporally, anterior to the laser scars, OS (**b**)

Persistent Fetal Vasculature

Persistent fetal vasculature (PVF) is a condition in which the fetal hyaloid artery fails to regress, resulting in ocular manifestations ranging from mild (prominent vessel remnants, Mittendorf dots on the lens, or Bergmeister papillae on the nerve) to severe (microophthalmia, dense cataract, thick persistent hyaloid artery (Fig. 13), elongated ciliary vessel, and even retinal dyspasia). Severe cases may develop angle-closure glaucoma, vitreous hemorrhage, or retinal detachment [26].

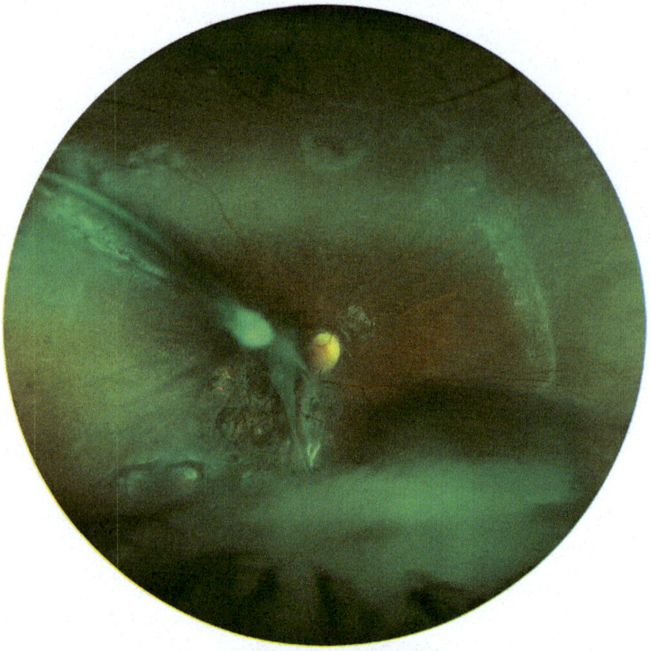

Fig. 13 UWF fundus photographs of a female with PFV reveal a rudimentary fibrovascular stalk coursing from the nerve anteriorly. The inferotemporal view is obscured by the associated lenticular opacity

Sickle Cell Retinopathy

Ocular manifestations of sickle cell disease include abnormal conjunctival vessels; iris atrophy; iris neovascularization; peripheral retinal arteriolar occlusions with avascularity; peripheral arteriovenous anastomoses (Fig. 14); neovascularization (sea fans) with subsequent hemorrhages or tractional detachments; retinal hemorrhages in the subretinal, intraretinal, or preretinal spaces include salmon patch hemorrhages; retinal pigment epithelial hyperplasia resulting in black sunburst lesions; and vascular occlusions [27, 28]. While wide-field imaging of sickle cell retinopathy has not been studied specifically in the pediatric population, studies in adult populations demonstrate a strong role for UWF imaging and UWFA for this condition, given the peripheral nature of the pathology. In one study of 12 eyes of 6 patients with sickle cell retinopathy, UWFA identified peripheral vascular findings not identified by the trainee or attending on clinical examination in 25 % of eyes. In all except one eye with macular ischemia, the pathology seen on UWFA was not visible on simulated seven standard fields [29, 30]. Thus, UWF imaging, and UWFA especially, are useful for monitoring the peripheral retina for active neovascularization, which should prompt laser photocoagulation if clinically significant or associated with hemorrhage or traction. For cases requiring laser therapy, UWFA may allow imaging-guided treatment specifically to areas of peripheral nonperfusion and neovascularization.

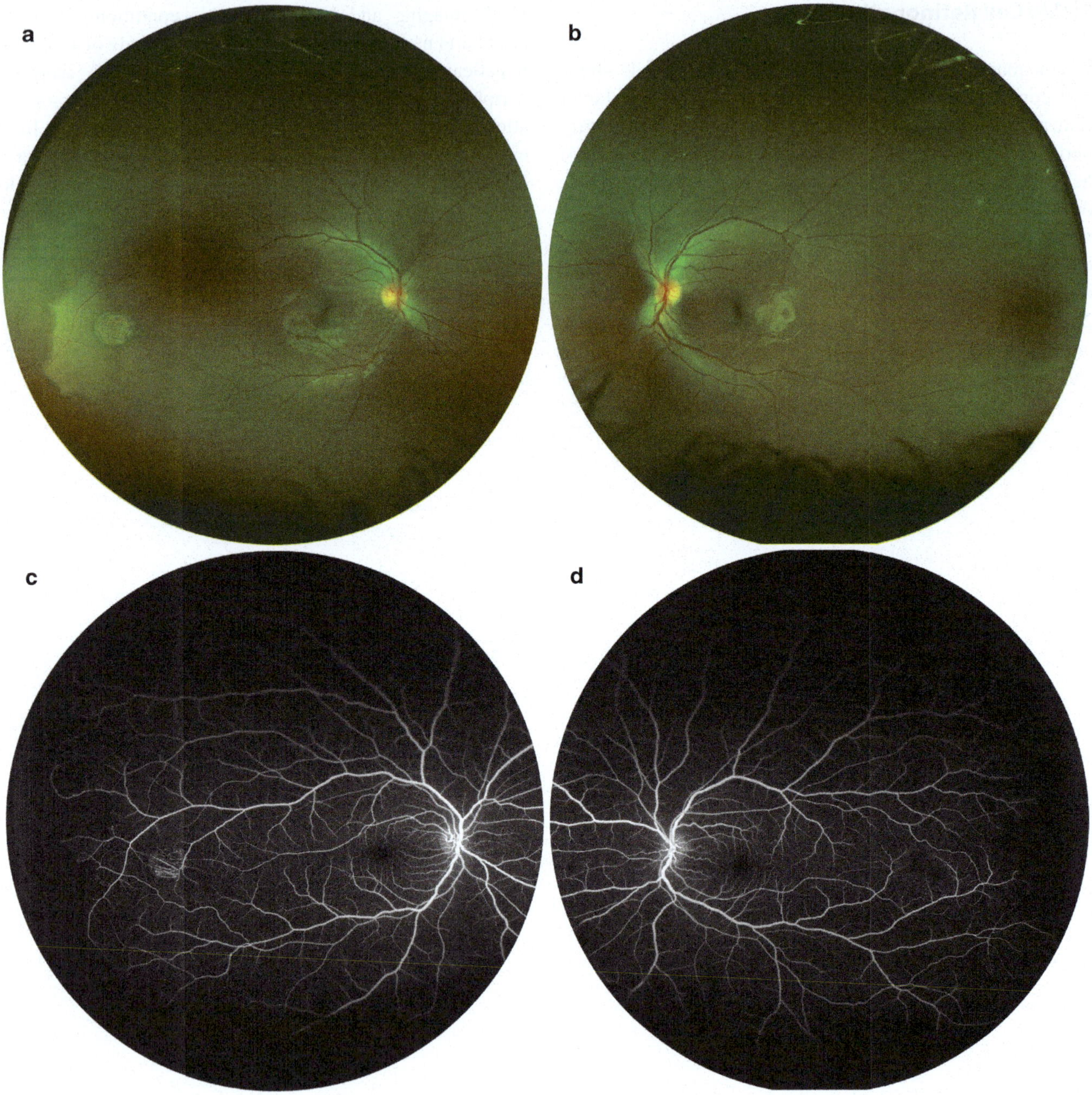

Fig. 14 UWF fundus photographs of a 12-year-old boy with sickle cell/betathalassemia with chorioretinal scar OD and peripheral retinal avascularity OU (**a**, **b**). UWFA shows peripheral avascularity and pruning of the retinal vessels without leakage suggestive of neovascularization (**c** 3 min 27 s; **d** 4 min 16 s)

Congenital Pediatric Retinal Conditions

X-Linked Retinoschisis

X-linked retinoschisis (XLRS) is a retinal degeneration due to a mutation in the *RS1* gene encoding retinoschisin that manifests with loss of vision, foveal schisis (Fig. 15a, b), an electronegative electroretinogram, and in 50 % of cases, peripheral schisis (Fig. 15c, d). Complications include vitreous hemorrhage from vessels within schisis cavities or schisis-associated retinal detachment (Fig. 15c) [29]. The use of UWFA to document both the macular and peripheral schisis cavities has been reported in the pediatric population [1], and may be useful for monitoring for progression or associated retinal detachments over time.

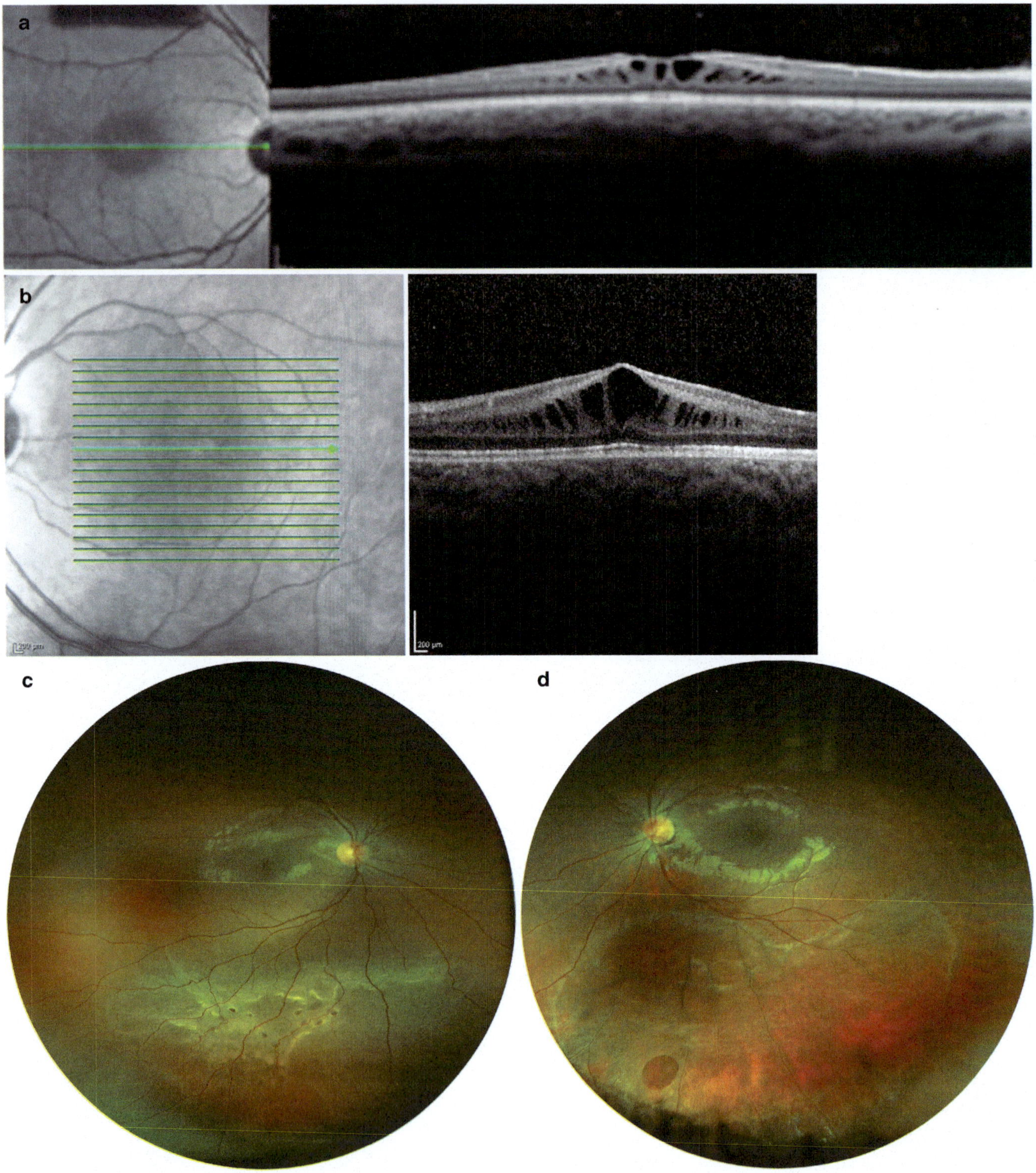

Fig. 15 Optical coherence tomography (OCT) images of a 6-year-old boy with XLRS reveal foveal schisis changes OU (**a**, **b**). The patient ultimately developed a retinoschisis-related retinal detachment with multiple holes OD (**c**), while the left eye revealed inferior retinoschisis with an inner retinal hole and no detachment (**d**) (With permission from Elsevier)

Retinal Coloboma/Optic Disc Coloboma/Optic Disc Pit

A coloboma refers to a localized area where there is a lack of tissue, often due to an incomplete closure of the embryonic fissure (Fig. 16). Complications include associated serous retinal detachment (Fig. 16b), rhegmatogenous retinal detachment, and choroidal neovascularization at the edge of the coloboma. Cases of bilateral coloboma or unilateral coloboma with associated systemic abnormality warrant genetic testing. Optic disc pit is a defect in the optic disc, often temporally, which is related to optic disc coloboma. It, too, may be associated with a serous retinal detachment (Fig. 17) [31, 32].

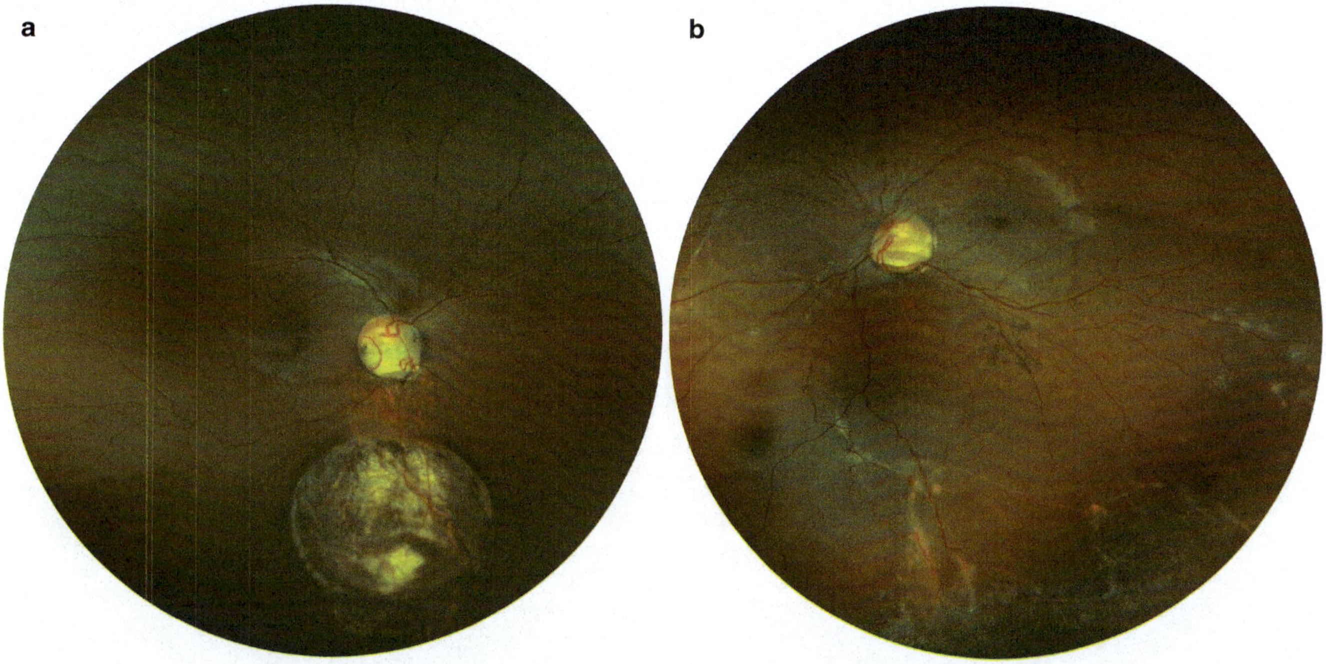

Fig. 16 UWF fundus photographs of a 16-year-old boy with a history of DiGeorge syndrome with retinal coloboma OD (**a**) and bilateral optic disc colobomas (**a, b**) with disc coloboma-associated retinal detachment with proliferative vitreoretinopathy OS (**b**)

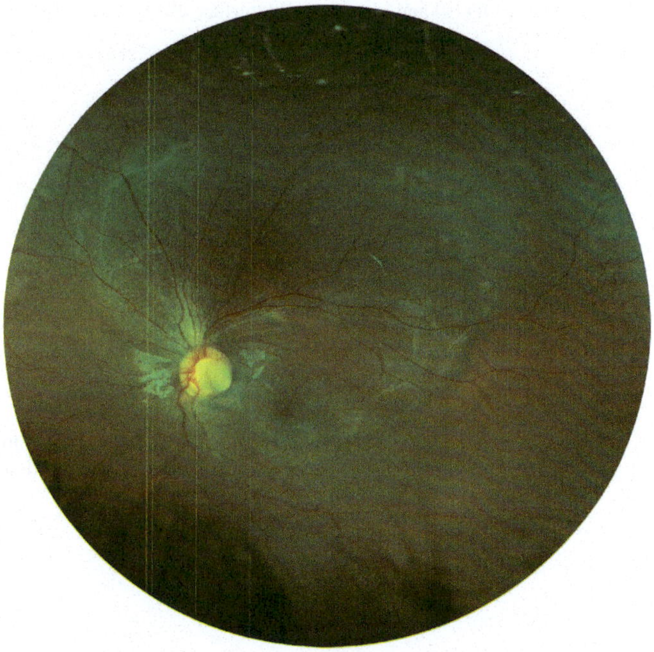

Fig. 17 UWF fundus photographs of a 10-year-old girl with optic disc pit with associated retinal detachment OS

Vitreoretinopathies and Retinal Detachments

Stickler Syndrome

Stickler syndrome is the most common vitreoretinopathy associated with retinal detachments in children. It is a hereditary arthro-ophthalmopathy due to defective collagen connective tissue. Stickler manifests with characteristic facial abnormalities (including Pierre Robin sequence), arthropathy, deafness, and/or ocular findings including optically empty vitreous, vitreoretinal interface changes (Fig. 18b), high myopia, and risk of retinal tear and detachment (Fig. 18) [33]. As described in section "Rhegmatogenous retinal detachment", there is a role for UWF fundus photography and autofluorescence in documentation of the presence and extent of retinal detachments such as those associated with Stickler syndrome.

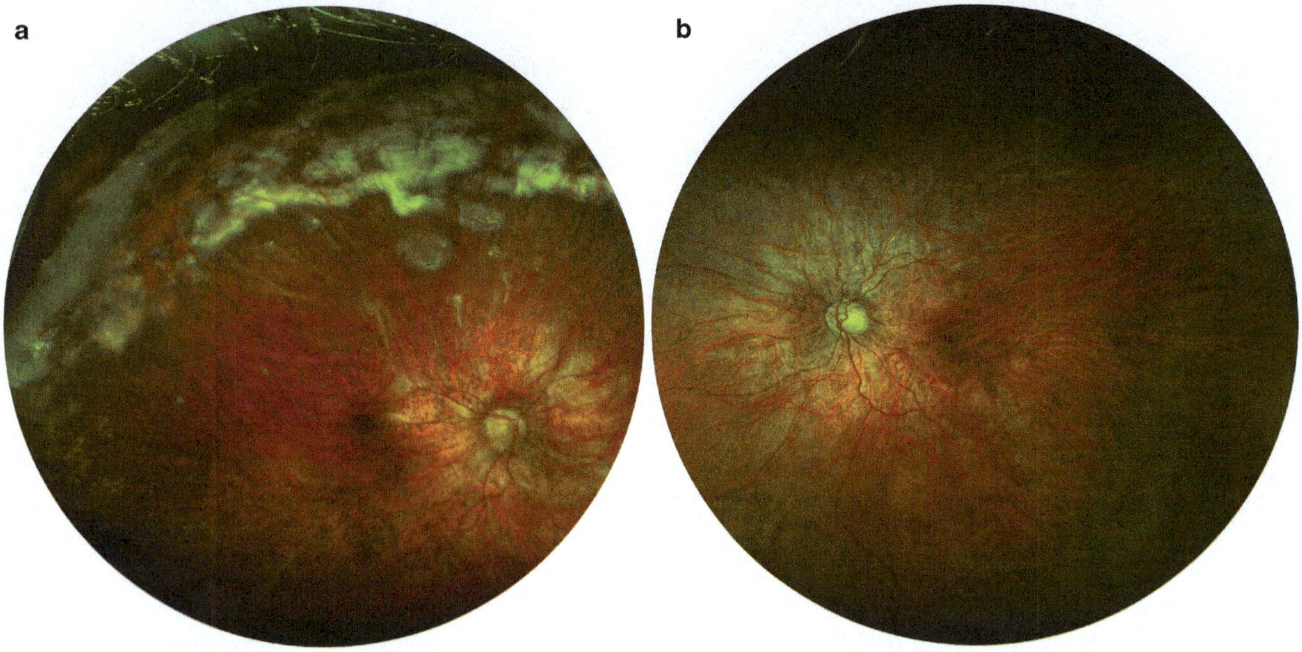

Fig. 18 An 8-year-old boy with a history of Stickler syndrome had developed a giant retinal tear retinal detachment OD and underwent scleral buckle and pars plana vitrectomy with silicon oil placement OD. UWF fundus photographs postoperatively reveal attached retina with giant retinal tear visualized over the buckle (**a**). There are also emulsified oil droplets inferotemporally OD (**a**) and vitreoretinal interface changes OS (**b**)

Rhegmatogenous Retinal Detachment

Rhegmatogenous retinal detachments (Fig. 19) are uncommon in the pediatric population but may be seen in the setting of trauma (with associated tear or dialysis), vitreoretinopathies (such as Stickler syndrome; see above and Fig. 18), retinal vascular diseases such as ROP or FEVR (see above and Fig. 7), prior intraocular surgery, or high myopia [34]. Studies report as high as a 33 % risk of peripheral retinal pathology in pediatric patients with high myopia [35], suggesting an important role for careful examination under anesthesia in this population. In the setting of rhegmatogenous detachment, the tight adherence of the hyaloid to the retina, the formed vitreous, and the phakic status of these patients inform the management strategy. UWF imaging seems to be a useful adjunct for documentation of rhegmatogenous retinal detachments, although studies suggest that the detection of causative breaks and tears is poor [36]. UWF autofluorescence may be used to accurately identify the edges of rhegmatogenous retinal detachment [37].

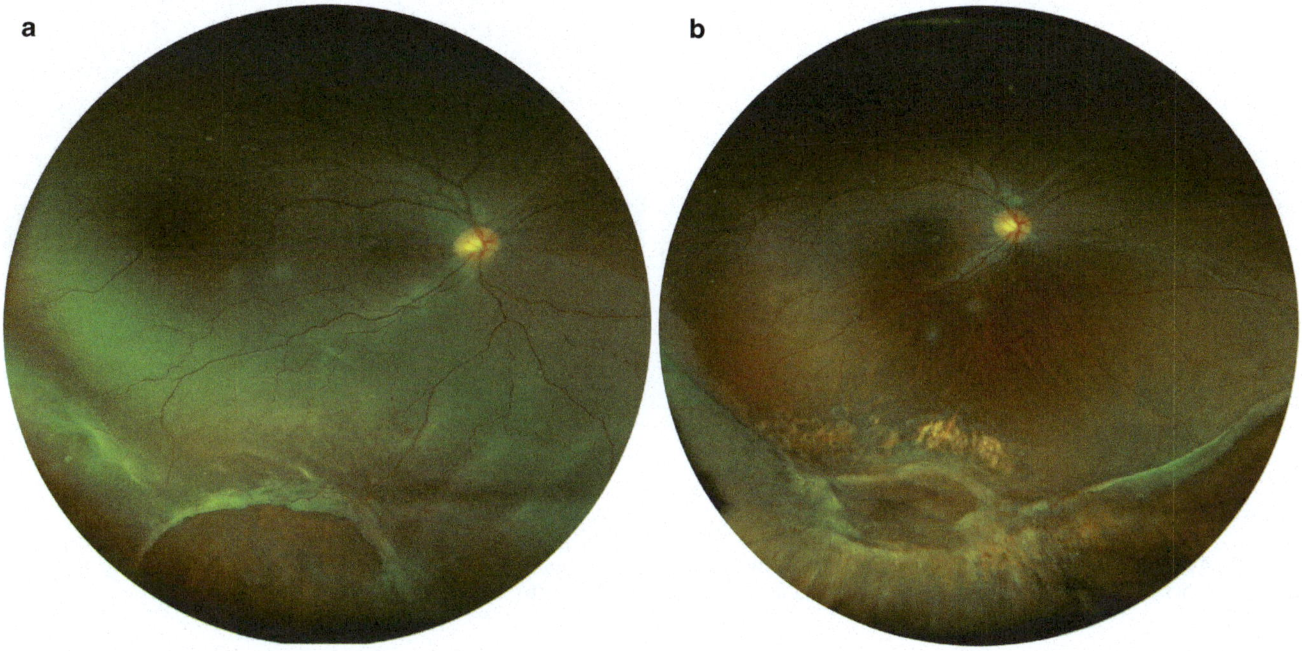

Fig. 19 UWF fundus photographs of a 10-year-old boy with failed vision screening diagnosed with macula-involving retinal detachment with large inferior retinal tear OD (**a**), who underwent cryotherapy and scleral buckle surgery (41 band), with subsequent supplemental laser photocoagulation of the retinal tear, with successful reattachment of the retina (**b**)

Phakomatoses

Tuberous Sclerosis

Tuberous sclerosis is inherited in an autosomal dominant fashion due to mutations on chromosome 9 or 16 and features a classic triad of seizures, mental retardation, and adenoma sebaceum. A variety of other skin findings including ash leaf spots, café-au-lait spots, Shagreen patches, and others may be noted, as well as intracranial paraventricular subependymal astrocytic hamartomas (tubers), renal angiomyolipomas, cardiac rhabdomyosarcomas, and pulmonary tumors. Retinal findings include astrocytomas (Fig. 20) [38].

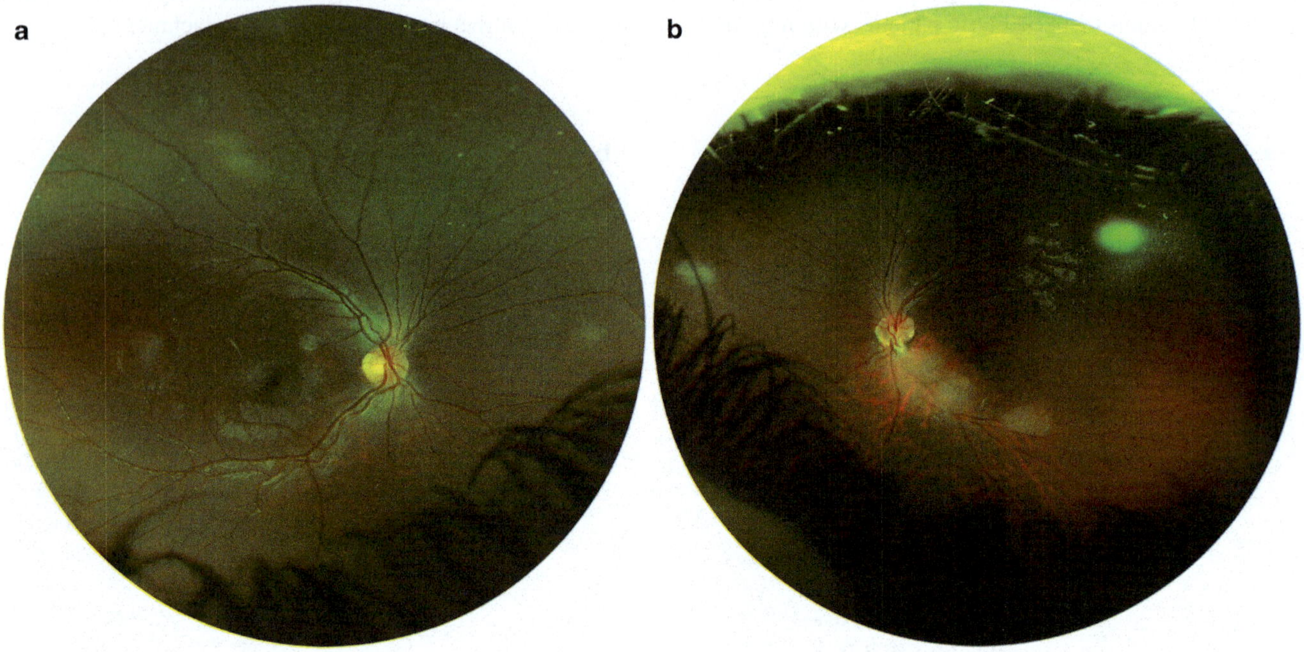

Fig. 20 UWF fundus photographs of a 10-year-old girl with tuberous sclerosis with retinal hamartomas (astrocytomas) superiorly, temporally, and nasally OD (**a**) and nasally, superotemporally, and along the inferior arcade OS (**b**)

Neurofibromatosis

Neurofibromatosis (NF) is an autosomal dominant condition due to a mutation in the *NF1* gene on chromosome 17 or the *NF2* gene on chromosome 22. NF1 manifests with café-au-lait spots, neurofibromas, axillary or inguinal freckling, optic nerve gliomas or meningiomas, iris hamartomas (Lisch spots), ectropion uvea, or sphenoid wing dysplasia. Retinal findings include increased frequency of choroidal nevi (which may be multifocal or bilateral; Fig. 21) or rarely, retinal astrocytomas (Fig. 20). NF2 manifests with bilateral acoustic neuromas, neurofibromas, meningioma, glioma, and schwannoma. Retinal findings may include combined hamartomas of the retinal pigment epithelium and retina [38].

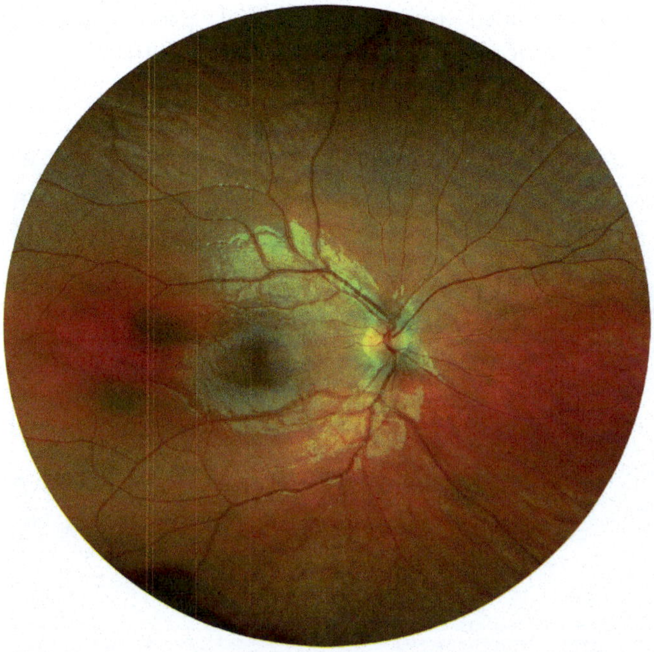

Fig. 21 UWF fundus photographs of a 4-year-old girl with NF1, with multiple small flat choroidal nevi near the nerve and within the macula OD

Incontinentia Pigmenti

Incontinentia pigmenti (IP), also known as Bloch-Sulzberger syndrome, is an X-linked dominant condition involving the eyes, skin, and central nervous system. Ocular findings are usually unilateral, although sometimes they may be asymmetrically bilateral. The spectrum of ocular findings includes strabismus, microophthalmos, ptoshisos, blue sclera, corneal changes, cataract, optic atrophy, and myopia. The most typical findings, however, are retinal and include peripheral retinal avascularity (Fig. 22), often with fibrovascular proliferation and detachment similar to that seen in ROP [39]. Systemic findings include microcephaly, seizures, spastic paralysis, and mental retardation. Given the relatively peripheral nature of nonperfusion and neovascularization in this condition, wide-field imaging and angiography are critical. Recently, the use of UWF imaging and angiography using the "flying baby" position in the office was reported for the diagnosis of this condition, as well as for UWF imaging-guided targeted panretinal photocoagulation treatment of a 3-month-old infant with IP [40].

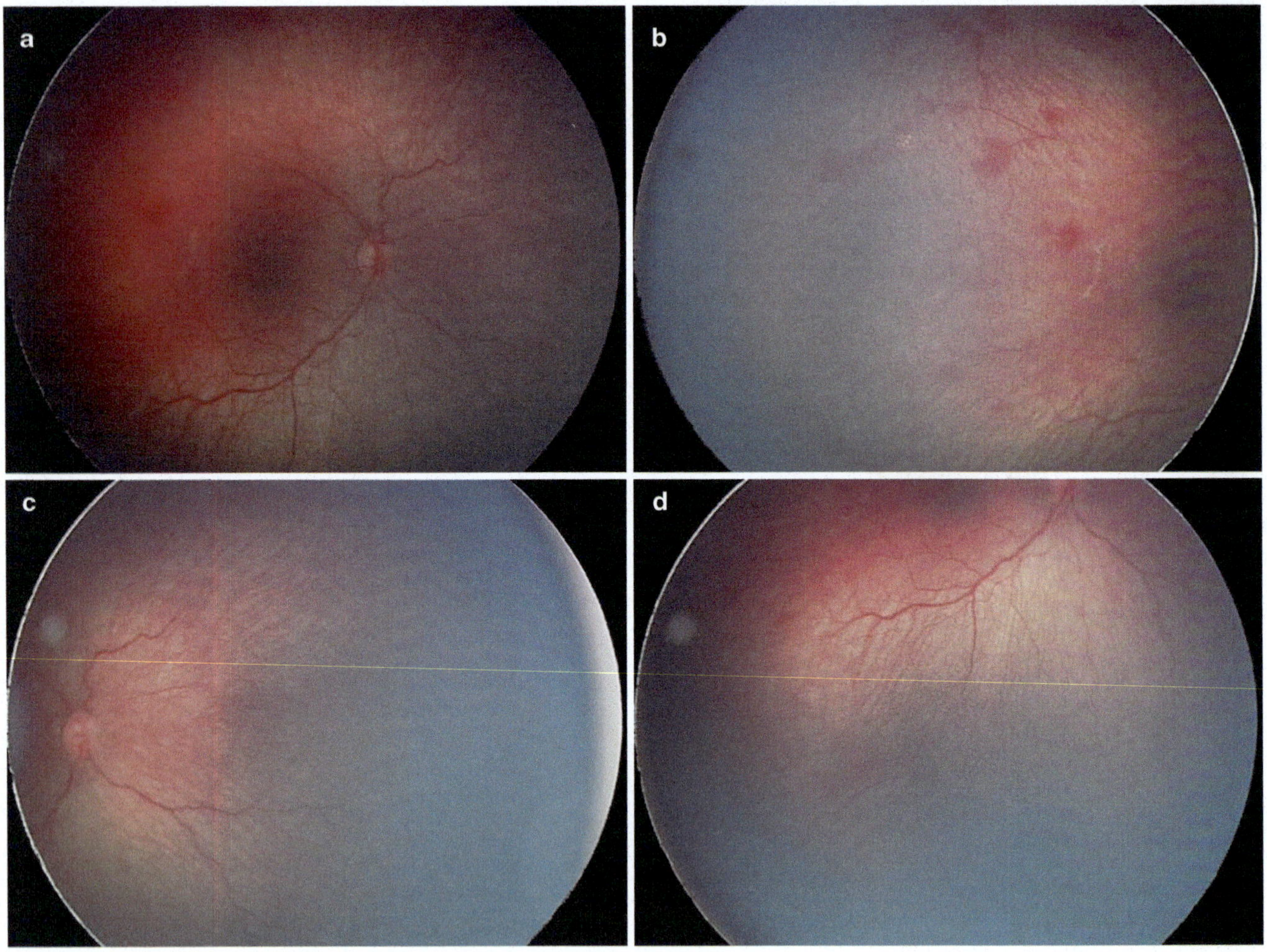

Fig. 22 Wide-field fundus photos of a 4-month-old girl admitted to the hospital for intracranial hemorrhage and seizures revealing peripheral retinal hemorrhages and avascularity OD (**a–e**) and normal fundus examination OS (**f**). Wide-field FA reveals peripheral avascularity OD (**g**) and normal OS (**h**). Laser photocoagulation was applied to areas of ischemia peripherally OD (**i**)

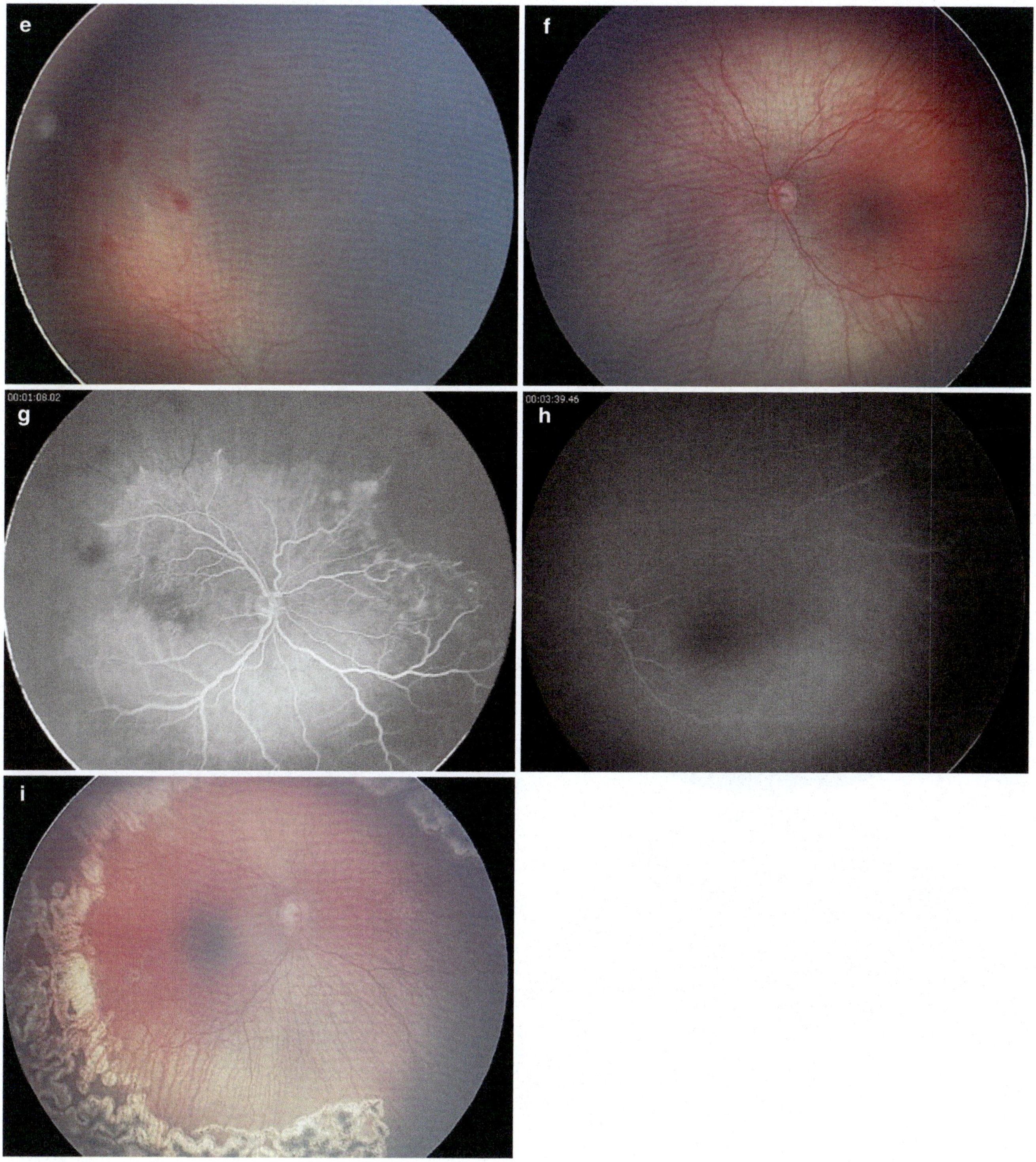

Fig. 22 (continued)

Manifestations of Systemic Disease

Leukemic Optic Neuropathy and Retinopathy

Retinal findings in leukemia include hemorrhages or white-centered hemorrhages in the setting of anemia and thrombocytopenia or leukemic infiltration of the optic nerve and/or retina itself (Fig. 23). Hyperviscosity may also predispose to retinal vascular occlusions.

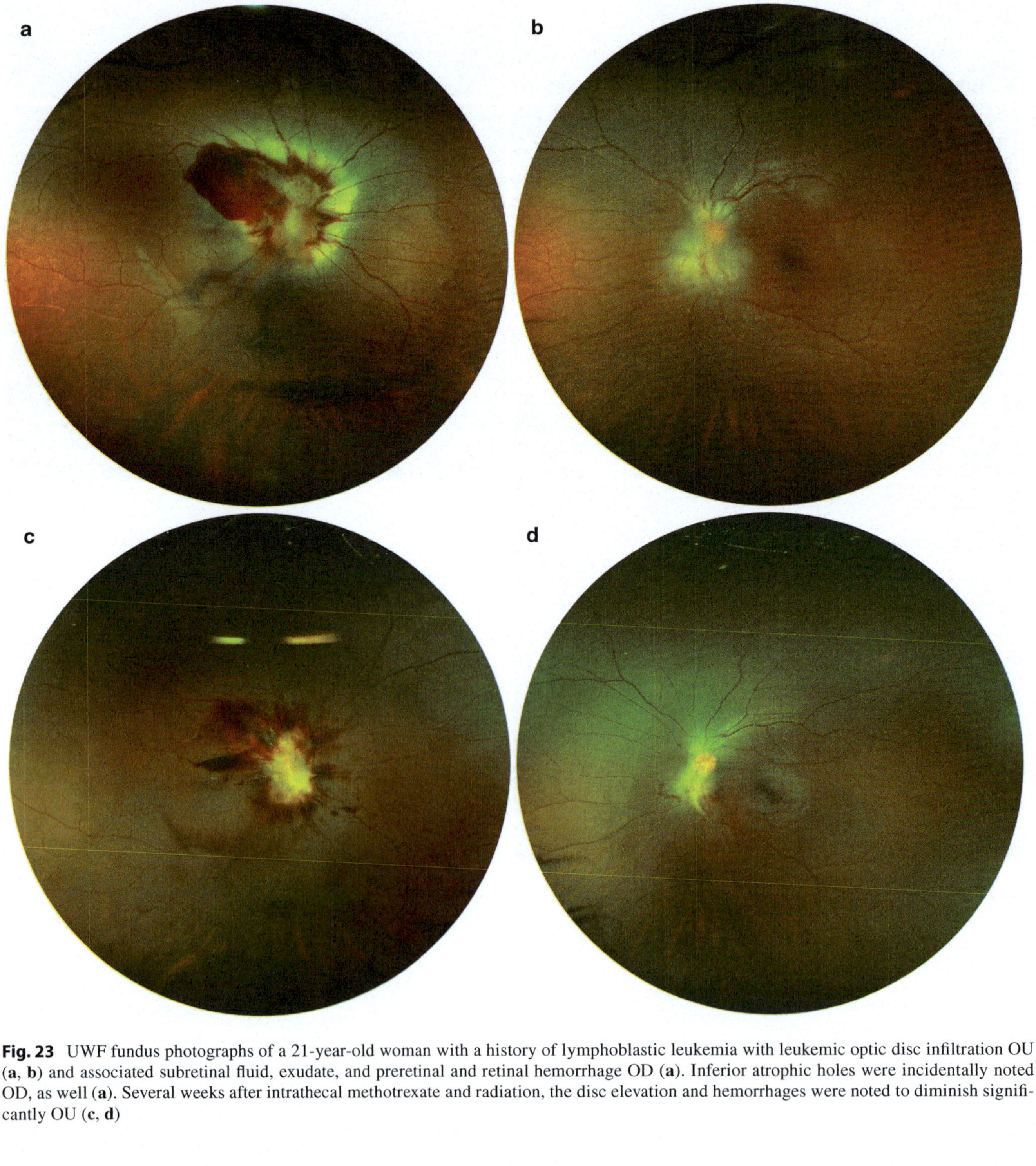

Fig. 23 UWF fundus photographs of a 21-year-old woman with a history of lymphoblastic leukemia with leukemic optic disc infiltration OU (**a**, **b**) and associated subretinal fluid, exudate, and preretinal and retinal hemorrhage OD (**a**). Inferior atrophic holes were incidentally noted OD, as well (**a**). Several weeks after intrathecal methotrexate and radiation, the disc elevation and hemorrhages were noted to diminish significantly OU (**c**, **d**)

Fungal Chorioretinitis

Fungal chorioretinitis manifests with fluffy white lesions that initially present in the choroidal and subretinal space and may migrate inward to the inner retina, ultimately breaking through into the vitreous (Fig. 24) with associated vitritis.

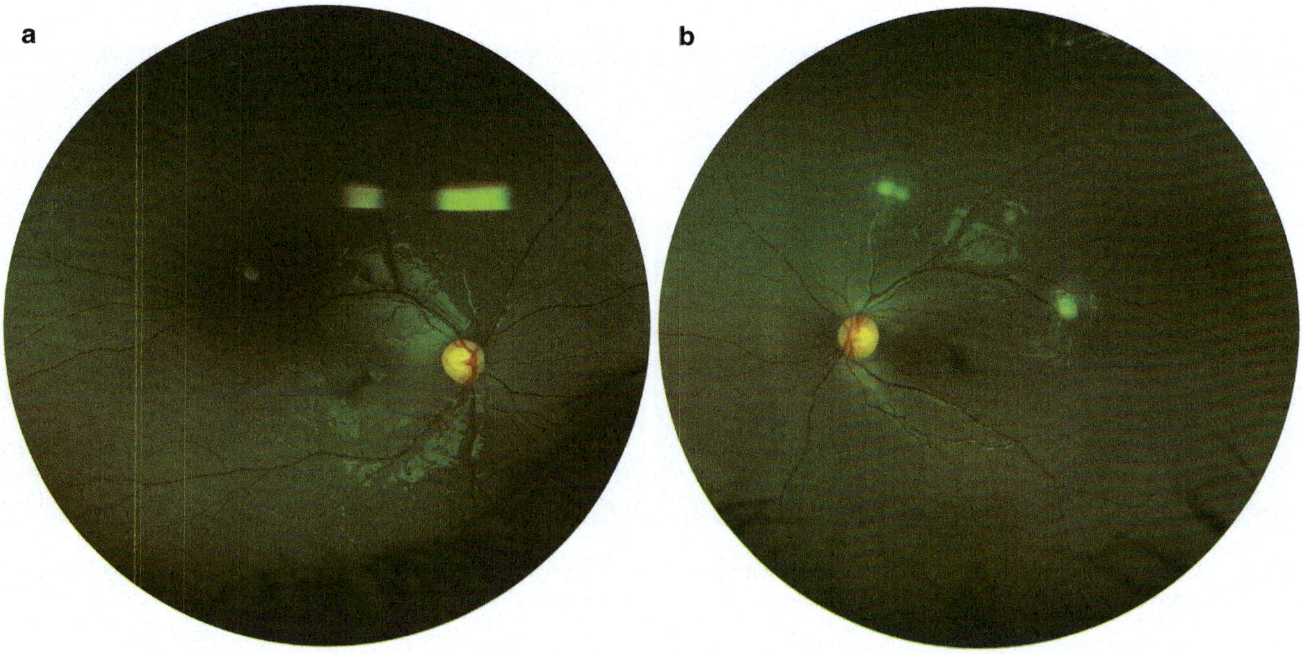

Fig. 24 UWF fundus photographs of a 5-year-old girl with fungemia and disseminated fungal infection with *Trichosporon asahii*, complicated by fungal chorioretinitis OU, status post intravenous antifungals and intravitreal injections of voriconazole OS. UWF fundus photos 3 months after diagnosis show consolidated fungal lesions OU (**a**, **b**)

Trauma

Nonaccidental Trauma (Abusive Head Trauma)

Retinal findings in nonaccidental trauma include retinal hemorrhages, often in multiple layers (preretinal, intraretinal, and/or subretinal), that are typically present in the posterior pole and can extend as far out as the ora serrata in some cases (Fig. 25) [41]. Perimacular folds and macular schisis may also occur, which are quite specific signs for repeated acceleration-deceleration injuries. Although the pathology is typically present posteriorly, wide-field imaging using the RetCam or Optos systems are useful for documentation of the pathology in this condition for clinical, social, and legal purposes.

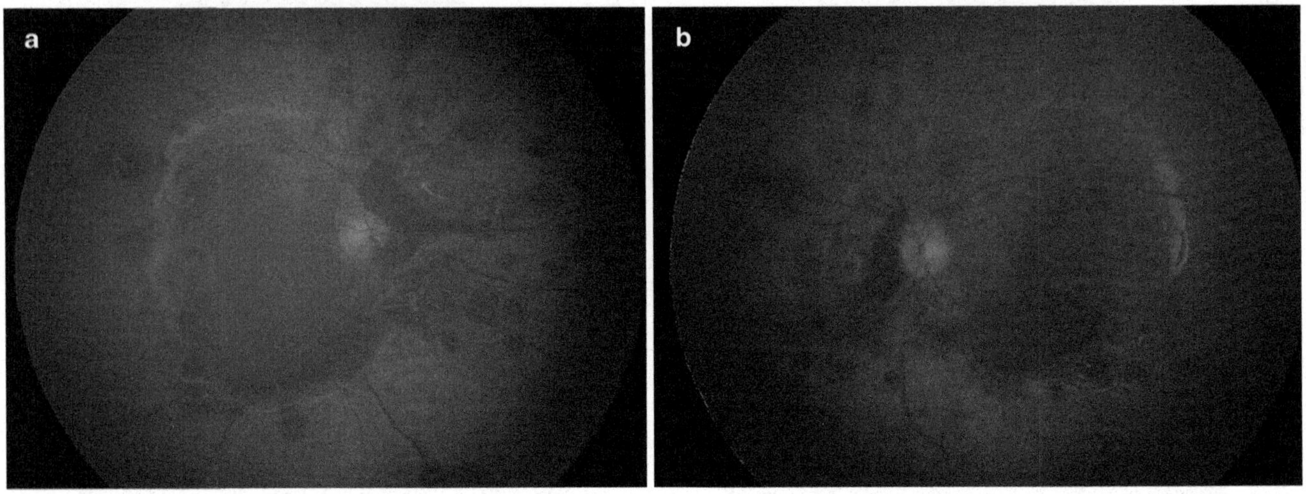

Fig. 25 Wide-field fundus photos of a baby who suffered nonaccidental trauma reveal numerous retinal hemorrhages in the posterior pole OU (**a**, **b**), including preretinal, intraretinal, and subretinal hemorrhages, as well as some white-centered hemorrhages

References

1. Tsui I, Franco-Cardenas V, Hubschman JP, Schwartz SD. Pediatric retinal conditions imaged by ultra wide field fluorescein angiography. Ophthalmic Surg Lasers Imaging Retina. 2013;44:59–67.
2. Kang KB, Wessel MM, Tong J, D'Amico DJ, Chan RV. Ultra-widefield imaging for the management of pediatric retinal diseases. J Pediatr Ophthalmol Strabismus. 2013;50:282–8.
3. Pagon RA. Retinitis pigmentosa. Surv Ophthalmol. 1988;33:137–77.
4. Oishi A, Ogino K, Makiyama Y, Nakagawa S, Kurimoto M, Yoshimura N. Wide-field fundus autofluorescence imaging of retinitis pigmentosa. Ophthalmology. 2013;120(9):1827–34.
5. Ogura S, Yasukawa T, Kato A, Usui H, Hirano Y, Yoshida M, Ogura Y. Wide-field fundus autofluorescence imaging to evaluate retinal function in patients with retinitis pigmentosa. Am J Ophthalmol. 2014;158(5):1093–8.
6. Oetting WS, Summers CG, King RA. Albinism and the associated ocular defects. Metab Pediatr Syst Ophthalmol. 1995;17:5–9.
7. Marmorstein L. Association of EFEMP1 with malattia leventinese and age-related macular degeneration: a mini-review. Ophthalmic Genet. 2004;25:219–26.
8. Sigler EJ, Randolph JC, Calzada JI, Wilson MW, Haik BG. Current management of Coats disease. Surv Ophthalmol. 2014;59:30–46.
9. Warden SM, Andreoli CM, Mukai S. The Wnt signaling pathway in familial exudative vitreoretinopathy and Norrie disease. Semin Ophthalmol. 2007;22:211–7.
10. Kashani AH, Brown KT, Chang E, Drenser KA, Capone A, Trese MT. Diversity of retinal vascular anomalies in patients with familial exudative vitreoretinopathy. Ophthalmology. 2014;121(11):2220–7.
11. Hellstrom A, Smith LEH, Dammann O. Retinopathy of prematurity. Lancet. 2013;382:1445–57.
12. Fierson WM, Capone Jr A, American Academy of Pediatrics Section on Ophthalmology, American Academy of Ophthalmology, American Association of Certified Orthoptists. Telemedicion for evaluation of retinopathy of prematurity. Pediatrics. 2015;135(1):e238–54.
13. Chiang MF, Melia M, Buffenn AN, Lambert SR, Recchia FM, Simpson JL, Yang MB. Detection of clinically significant retinopathy of prematurity using wide-angle digital retinal photography: a report by the American Academy of Ophthalmology. Ophthalmology. 2012;119(6):1272–80.
14. Ells AL, Holmes JM, Astle WF, Williams G, Leske DA, Fielden M, Uphill B, Jennet P, Hebert M. Telemedicine approach to screening for severe retinopathy of prematurity: a pilot study. Ophthalmology. 2003;110(11):2113–7.
15. Chiang MF, Keenan JD, Starren J, Du YE, Schiff WM, Barile GR, Li J, Johnson RA, Hess DJ, Flynn JT. Accuracy and reliability of remote retinopathy of prematurity diagnosis. Arch Ophthalmol. 2006;124(3):322–7.
16. Wu C, Petersen RA, VanderVeen DK. RetCam imaging for retinopathy of prematurity screening. J AAPOS. 2006;10(2):107–11.
17. Silva RA, Murakami Y, Jain A, Gandhi J, Lad EM, Moshfeghi DM. Stanford University Network for Diagnosis of Retinopathy of Prematurity (SUNDROP): 18-month experience with telemedicine screening. Graefes Arch Clin Exp Ophthalmol. 2009;247(1):129–36.
18. Photographic Screening for Retinopathy of Prematurity (Photo-ROP) Cooperative Group. The photographic screening for retinopathy of prematurity study (photo-ROP). Primary outcomes. Retina. 2008;28 Suppl 3:S47–54.
19. Quinn GE, Ying GS, Daniel E, Hildebrand PL, Ells A, Baumritter A, Kemper AR, Schron EB, Wade K, e-ROP Cooperative Group. Validity of a telemedicine system for the evaluation of acute-phase retinopathy of prematurity. JAMA Ophthalmol. 2014;132(10):1178–84.

20. Chiang MF, Wang L, Busuioc M, Du YE, Chan P, Kane SA, Lee TC, Weissgold DJ, Berrocal AM, Coki O, Flynn JT, Starren J. Telemedical retinopathy of prematurity diagnosis: accuracy, reliability, and image quality. Arch Ophthalmol. 2007;125(11):1531–8.
21. Scott KE, Kim DY, Wang L, Kane SA, Coki O, Starren J, Flynn JT, Chiang MF. Telemedical diagnosis of retinopathy of prematurity intraphysician agreement between ophthalmoscopic examination and image-based interpretation. Ophthalmology. 2008;115(7):1222.e3–28.e3.
22. Dhaliwal C, Wright E, Graham C, McIntosh N, Fleck BW. Wide-field digital retinal imaging versus binocular indirect ophthalmoscopy for retinopathy of prematurity screening: a two-observer prospective, randomised comparison. Br J Ophthalmol. 2009;93(3):355–9.
23. Klufas MA, Patel SN, Ryan MC, Gupta MP, Jonas KE, Ostmo S, Martinez-Castellanos MA, Berrocal AM, Chiang MF, Chan RV. Influence of fluorescein angiography on the diagnosis and management of retinopathy of prematurity. Ophthalmology. 2015;122(8):1601–8.
24. Kang KB, Orlin A, Lee TC, Chiang MF, Chan RV. The use of digital imaging in the identification of skip areas after laser treatment for retinopathy of prematurity and its implications for education and patient care. Retina. 2013;33(10):2162–9.
25. Patel CK, Fung TH, Mugit MM, Mordant DJ, Brett J, Smith L, Adams E. Non-contact ultra-widefield imaging of retinopathy of prematurity using the Optos dual wavelength scanning laser ophthalmoscope. Eye (Lond). 2013;27(5):589–96.
26. Shastry BS. Persistent hyperplastic primary vitreous; congenital malformation of the eye. Clin Experiment Ophthalmol. 2009;37:884–90.
27. Elagouz M, Jyothi S, Gupta B, Sivaprasad S. Sickle cell disease and the eye: old and new concepts. Surv Ophthalmol. 2010;55:359–77.
28. Rosenberg JB, Hutcheson KA. Pediatric sickle cell retinopathy: correlation with clinical factors. J AAPOS. 2011;15:49–53.
29. Molday S, Kellner U, Weber BHF. X-linked juvenile retinoschisis: clinical diagnosis, genetic analysis, and molecular mechanisms. Prog Retin Eye Res. 2012;31:195–212.
30. Cho M, Kiss S. Detection and monitoring of sickle cell retinopathy using ultra wide-field color photography and fluorescein angiography. Retina. 2011;31:738–47.
31. Taylor D. Developmental abnormalities of the optic nerve and chiasm. Eye (Lond). 2007;21:1271–84.
32. Pagon RA. Ocular coloboma. Surv Ophthalmol. 1981;25:223–36.
33. Edwards AO. Clinical features of the congenital vitreoretinopathies. Eye (Lond). 2008;22:1233–42.
34. Fivgas GD, Capone Jr A. Pediatric rhegmatogenous retinal detachment. Retina. 2001;21:101–6.
35. Bansal AS, Hubbard III GB. Peripheral retinal findings in highly myopic children < or = 10 years of age. Retina. 2010;3:S15–9.
36. Kornberg DL, Klufas MA, Yannuzzi NA, Orlin A, D'Amico DJ, Kiss S. Clinical utility of ultra-widefield imaging with the Optos Optomap compared with indirect ophthalmoscopy in the setting of non-traumatic rhegmatogenous retinal detachment. Semin Ophthalmol. 2014;17:1–8.
37. Witmer MT, Cho M, Favarone G, Chan RV, D'Amico DJ, Kiss S. Ultra-wide-field autofluorescence imaging in non-traumatic rhegmatogenous retinal detachment. Eye (Lond). 2012;26(9):1209–16.
38. Font RL, Ferry AP. The phakomatoses. Int Ophthalmol Clin. 1972;12:1–50.
39. O'Doherty M, McCreery K, Green AJ, Tuwir I, Brosnahan D. Incontinentia pigmenti—ophthalmological observation of a series of cases and review of the literature. Br J Ophthalmol. 2011;95:11–6.
40. Patel CK, Fung TH, Mugit MM, Mordant DJ, Geh V. Non-contact ultra-widefield retinal imaging and fundus fluorescein angiography of an infant with incontinentia pigmenti without sedation in an ophthalmic office setting. J AAPOS. 2013;17(3):309–11.
41. Forbes BJ, Rubin SE, Margolin E, Levin A. Evaluation and management of retinal hemorrhage sin infants with and without abusive head trauma. J AAPOS. 2010;14:267–73.

Wide-Field Retinal Imaging of Retinal and Choroidal Tumors

12

Carol L. Shields and Jerry A. Shields

Wide-field imaging is important in the field of ocular oncology. This technology allows a panretinal image that includes tumor margins and relationships to surrounding structures with imaging of associated features and, most importantly, allows for accurate planning of tumor therapy. Several tumors in the eye arise from the retina, retinal pigment epithelium (RPE), choroid, and optic disc. Some of these tumors are benign and others are malignant. Wide-field imaging, in conjunction with other diagnostic testing, has improved our understanding of ocular tumors and provided better documentation of tumor appearance and effects. In this chapter, we provide images of intraocular tumors with various wide-field cameras.

Tumors of the Retina

The neurosensory retina is composed of neural, glial, and vascular tissue, each of which can produce specific retinal tumors. Most retinal tumors are congenital or develop in childhood. Some are benign; others are malignant. These tumors include retinoblastoma, retinal astrocytic hamartoma, retinal vascular tumors (hemangioblastoma, cavernous hemangioma, racemose hemangioma, and vasoproliferative tumor), and lymphoid/leukemic infiltrations.

C.L. Shields, MD (✉) • J.A. Shields, MD
Ocular Oncology Service, Wills Eye Hospital,
Philadelphia, PA, USA
e-mail: carolshields@gmail.com; jerryashields@gmail.com

I. Kozak, J.F. Arevalo (eds.), *Atlas of Wide-Field Retinal Angiography and Imaging*, DOI 10.1007/978-3-319-17864-6_12

Retinoblastoma

Retinoblastoma is a highly malignant intraocular tumor of childhood [1–4]. Retinoblastoma accounts for approximately 11 % of cancers in children during the first year of life, and most cases are detected before 5 years old. Worldwide, it is estimated that there are approximately 7,000–8,000 new cases per year. The diagnosis of retinoblastoma is established by recognition of classic clinical and imaging features without the need for biopsy. Retinoblastoma can appear endophytic with tumor invasion into the vitreous or exophytic with tumor invasion under the retina. Management of retinoblastoma includes methods of chemotherapy, radiotherapy, laser photocoagulation, thermotherapy, cryotherapy, and enucleation (Figs. 1, 2 and 3).

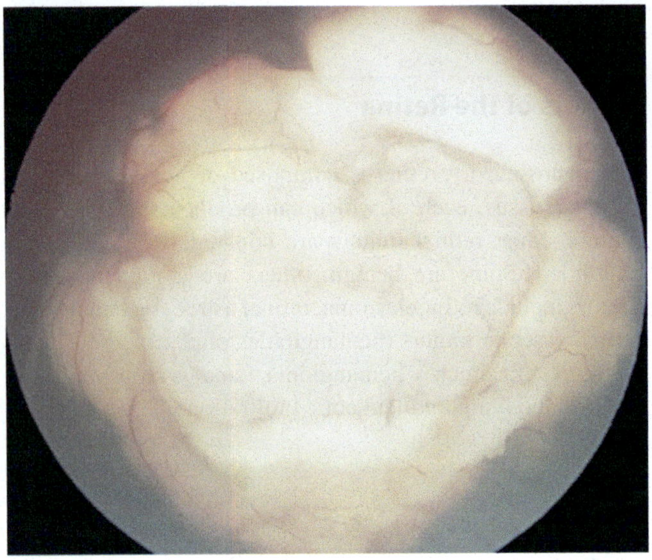

Fig. 1 Endophytic retinoblastoma

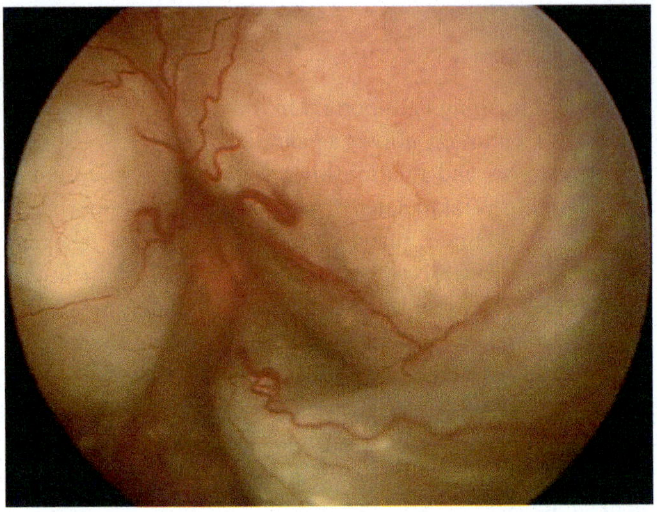

Fig. 2 Exophytic retinoblastoma

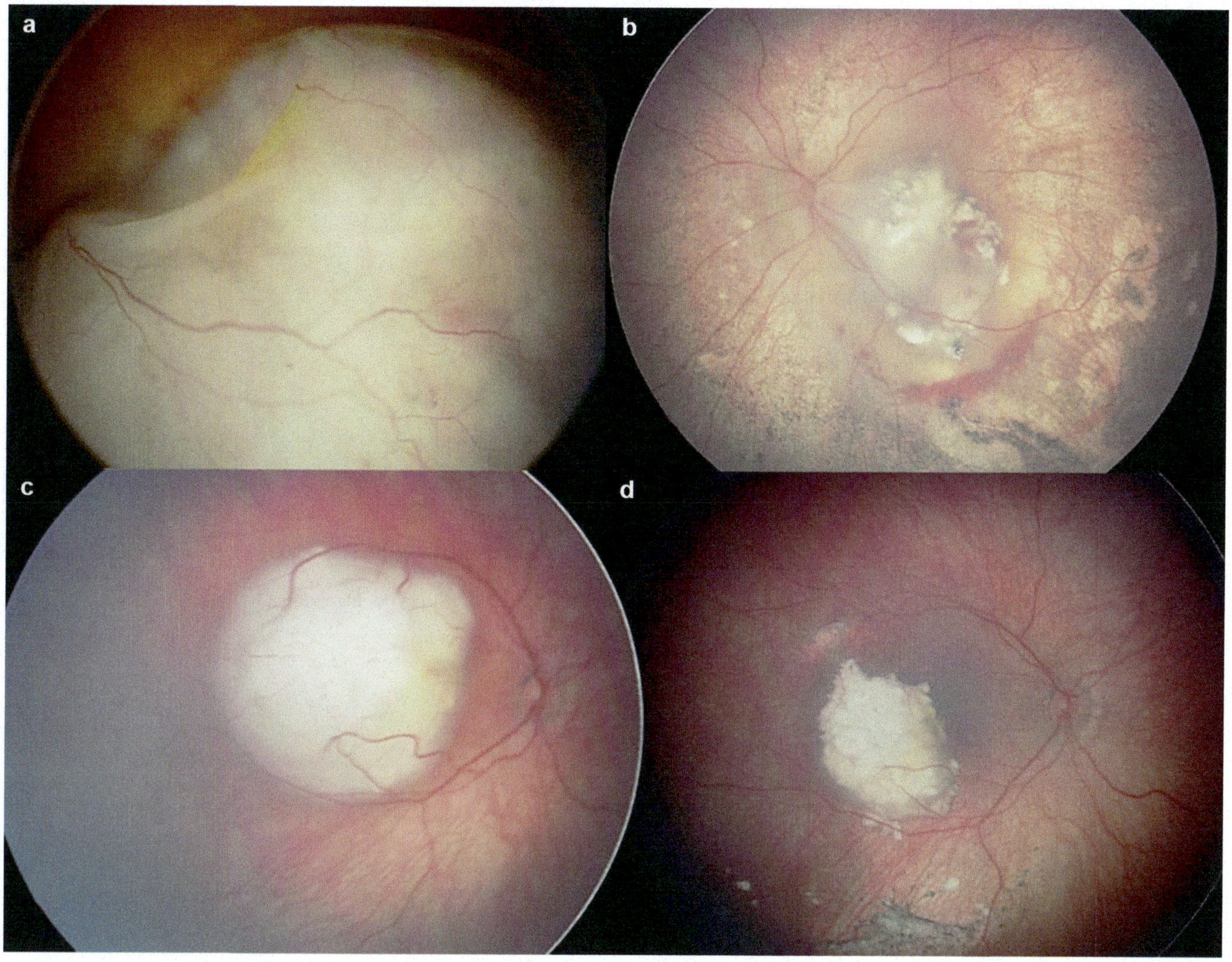

Fig. 3 Retinoblastoma treated with intra-arterial chemotherapy shows advanced retinoblastoma before (**a**) and after (**b**) treatment and less advanced retinoblastoma before (**c**) and after (**d**) treatment, leaving a calcified regressed tumor

Retinal Astrocytic Hamartoma

Retinal astrocytic hamartoma is a benign and classically stable retinal tumor found in patients with tuberous sclerosis complex or as a sporadic condition [5]. This retinal lesion is classified into three morphological groups: types 1, 2, and 3. Type 1 occurs in about 50 % of cases and is characterized by a circular or oval flat semitransparent solitary lesion in the retinal nerve fiber layer with an average size of 0.5 disc diameter [5]. Type 2 shows multiple calcified nodular areas of variable size with a mulberry-like appearance. Type 3 shows features of both type 1 and type 2 with a whitish-gray glistening central calcification and a peripheral semitranslucent, irregular rim. Occasionally, depigmented RPE "punched-out" lesions can be seen with this tumor as part of tuberous sclerosis complex (Fig. 4) [6].

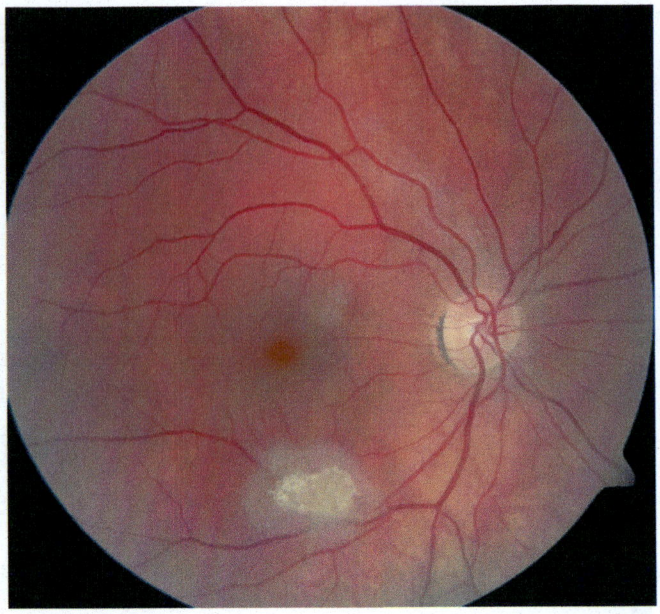

Fig. 4 Retinal astrocytic hamartoma with classic "mulberry-like" calcification

Retinal Hemangioblastoma

Retinal hemangioblastoma is a vascular hamartoma with a circumscribed orange-colored mass with dilated feeding vessels, often producing subretinal fluid and exudation (Fig. 5). This tumor can be a feature of von Hippel–Lindau syndrome [7]. Management includes laser photocoagulation, photodynamic therapy, cryotherapy, plaque radiotherapy, external beam radiotherapy, surgical resection, or anti–vascular endothelial growth factor (anti-VEGF) medications.

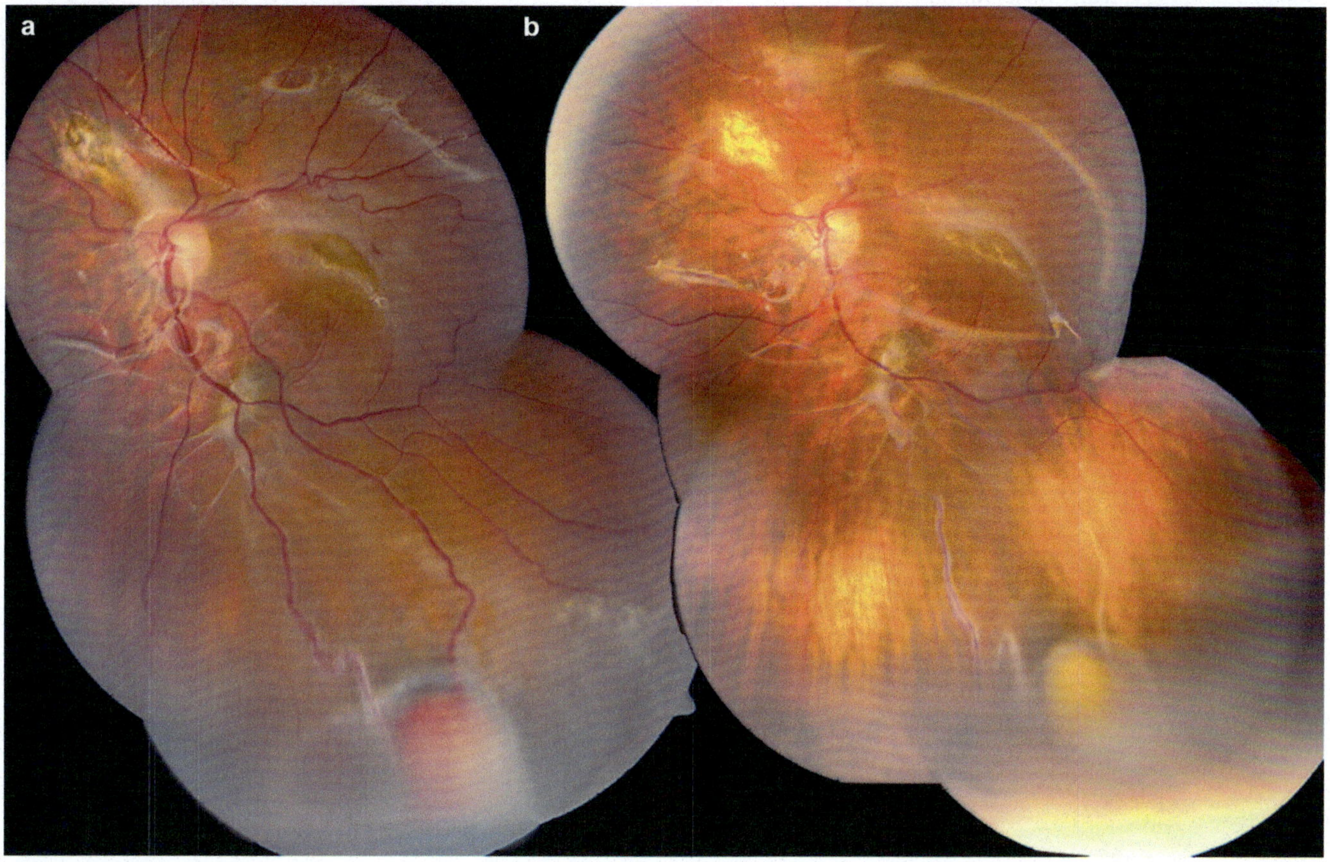

Fig. 5 Retinal hemangioblastoma following vitrectomy with silicone oil tamponade before (**a**) and after (**b**) photodynamic therapy

Retinal Cavernous Hemangioma

Retinal cavernous hemangioma is a vascular hamartoma with little potential for growth, but it can produce vitreous hemorrhage (Fig. 6). This can be a feature of a syndrome of cavernous hemangioma of the brain, skin, and eye. Management is typically observation.

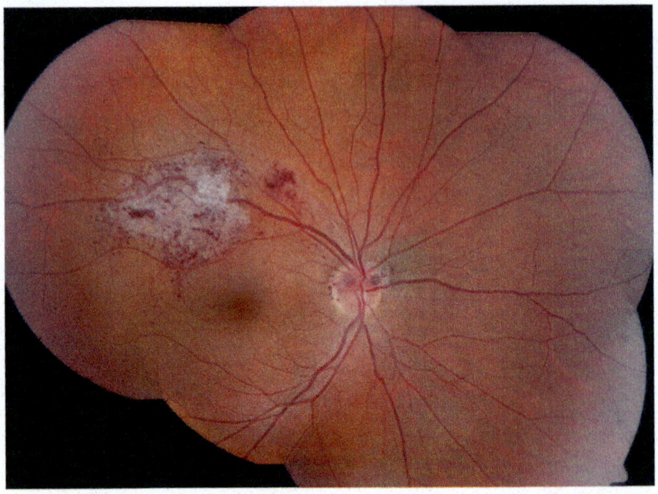

Fig. 6 Retinal cavernous hemangioma appearing like a "bunch of grapes" along the superotemporal vein with overlying preretinal fibrosis and over the optic disc

Retinal Racemose Hemangioma

Retinal racemose hemangioma is vascular malformation in which there is a dilated single or multiple retinal vessels without intervening capillary system, producing a vermiform vascular anomaly (Fig. 7). Occasionally, a vascular obstruction is noted. This lesion can be a feature of the Wyburn-Mason syndrome. Management is observation.

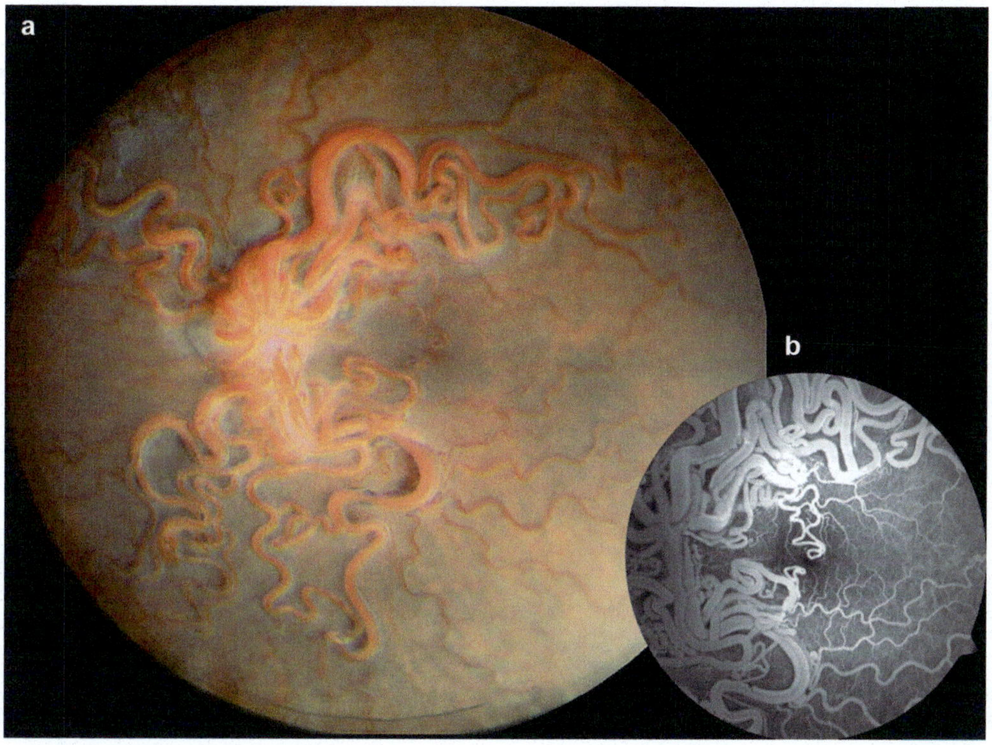

Fig. 7 Retinal racemose hemangioma shows the "vermiform" appearance without capillary bed (**a**), confirmed on fluorescein angiography (**b**)

Retinal Vasoproliferative Tumor

Retinal vasoproliferative tumor is an acquired, benign retinal mass, typically located in the inferotemporal periphery and with surrounding exudation and subretinal fluid (Fig. 8) [8–10]. This tumor is classified into primary or secondary lesions. Secondary lesions are found in eyes with retinitis pigmentosa, pars planitis, Coats disease, or other retinal scarring conditions. Management includes observation, laser photocoagulation, photodynamic therapy, cryotherapy, plaque radiotherapy, or anti-VEGF medications.

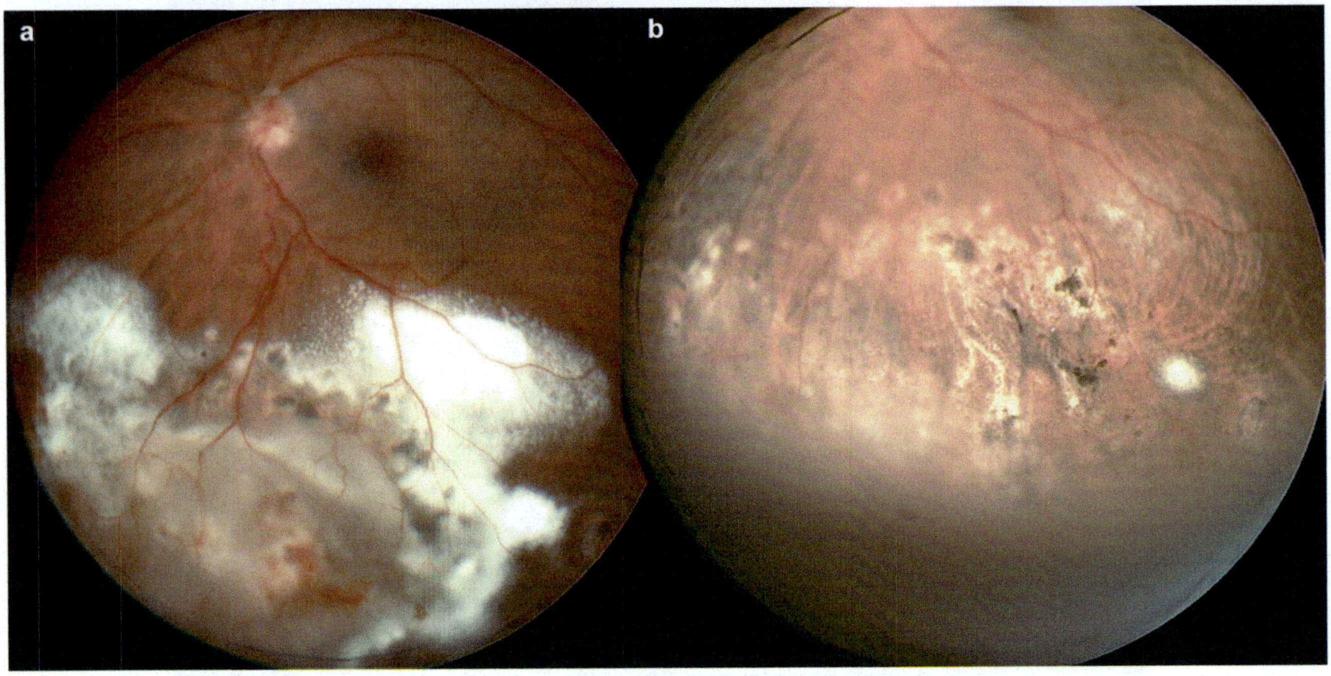

Fig. 8 Retinal vasoproliferative tumor appearing as an ill-defined mass with surrounding exudation, before (**a**) and after (**b**) photodynamic therapy

Retinal Lymphoma/Leukemia

Retinal involvement with lymphoma or leukemia can appear as a white infiltration, occasionally with surrounding hemorrhage [11]. Vitreoretinal lymphoma classically shows sub-RPE tumor and vitreous cells and can have central nervous system lymphoma. Retinal leukemia usually is a late finding with systemic leukemia. Management with systemic chemotherapy is indicated (Figs. 9 and 10).

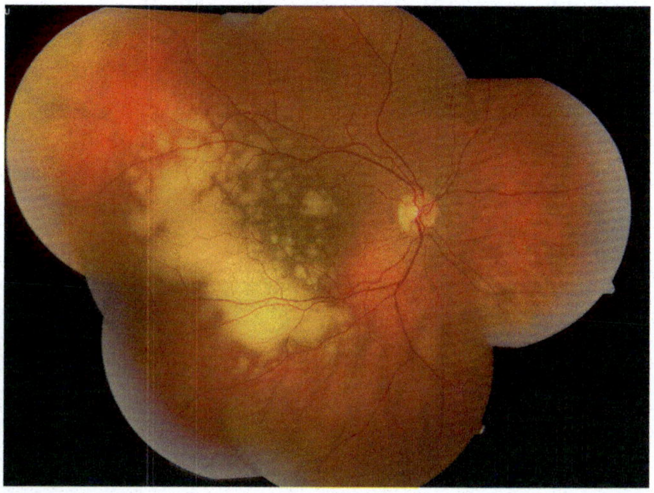

Fig. 9 Vitreoretinal lymphoma with sub-RPE lymphoma deposits in the right eye

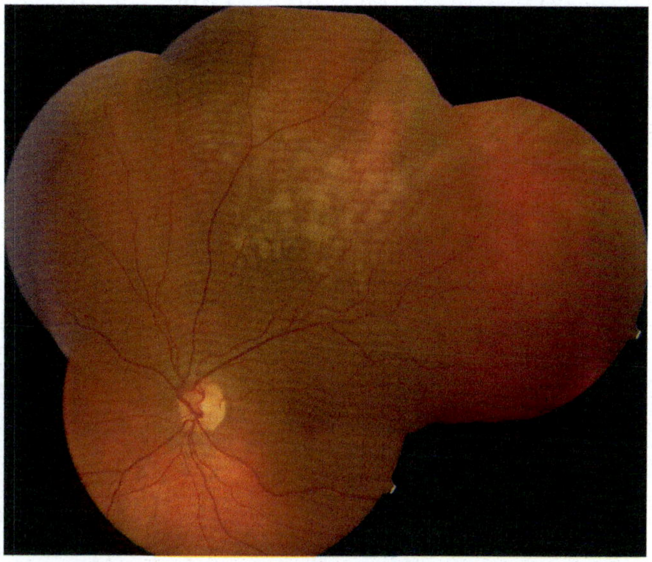

Fig. 10 Same patient as in Fig. 9 with vitreoretinal lymphoma and sub-RPE lymphoma deposits in the left eye

Tumors of the RPE

The RPE is a single-layer epithelium and can spawn several tumors including congenital hypertrophy of the RPE (CHRPE), congenital RPE markers of familial adenomatous polyposis (FAP), congenital simple hamartoma of the RPE, combined hamartoma of the retina and RPE, and adenoma/adenocarcinoma of the RPE.

Congenital Hypertrophy of the RPE

CHRPE is a flat, heavily pigmented benign lesion that classically occurs in the peripheral fundus [12]. The diameter of CHRPE varies from a tiny flat spot to large flat lesion of up to 13 mm with geographic margins and central hypopigmented lacunae [12]. This lesion classically displays sharp margins and can be associated with a surrounding nonpigmented and a complementary pigmented halo [12]. Multifocal CHRPE is known as "bear tracks." Optical coherence tomography (OCT) of CHRPE shows complete lack of photoreceptors over the lesion, and autofluorescence shows complete lack of lipofuscin (Figs. 11 and 12) [13–15].

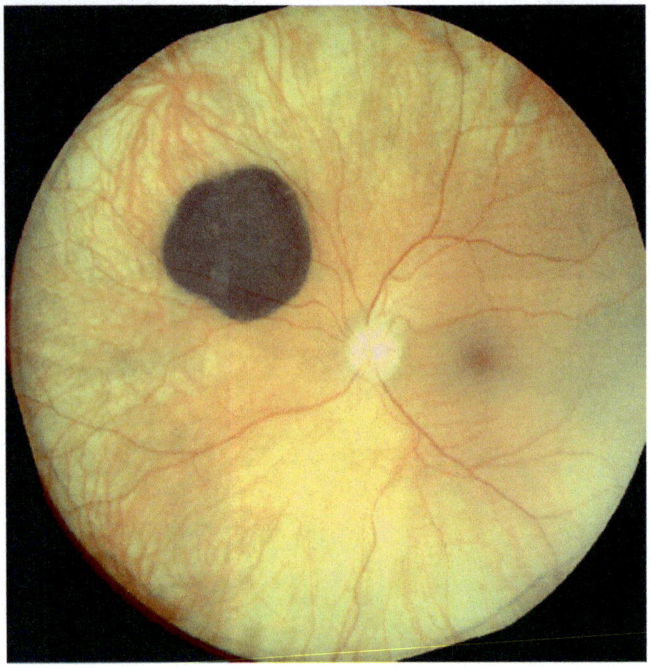

Fig. 11 Solitary congenital hypertrophy of the RPE appearing as a flat black mass

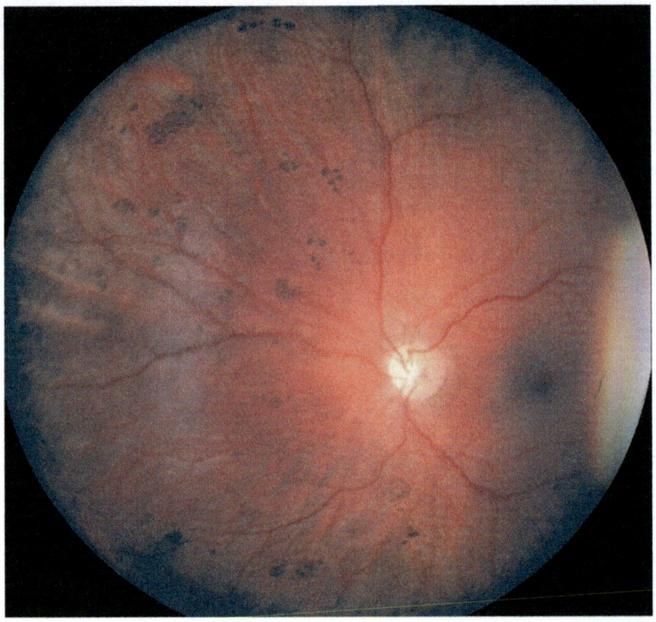

Fig. 12 Multifocal CHRPE appearing as "bear tracks"

Congenital RPE Markers of FAP

Congenital RPE lesions that show pisciform (fishlike) configuration, depigmented tail, or even focal RPE dot can serve as a marker of FAP, especially if the patient has four or more lesions in both eyes (Fig. 13) [16]. These lesions remain stable and require no ophthalmic intervention.

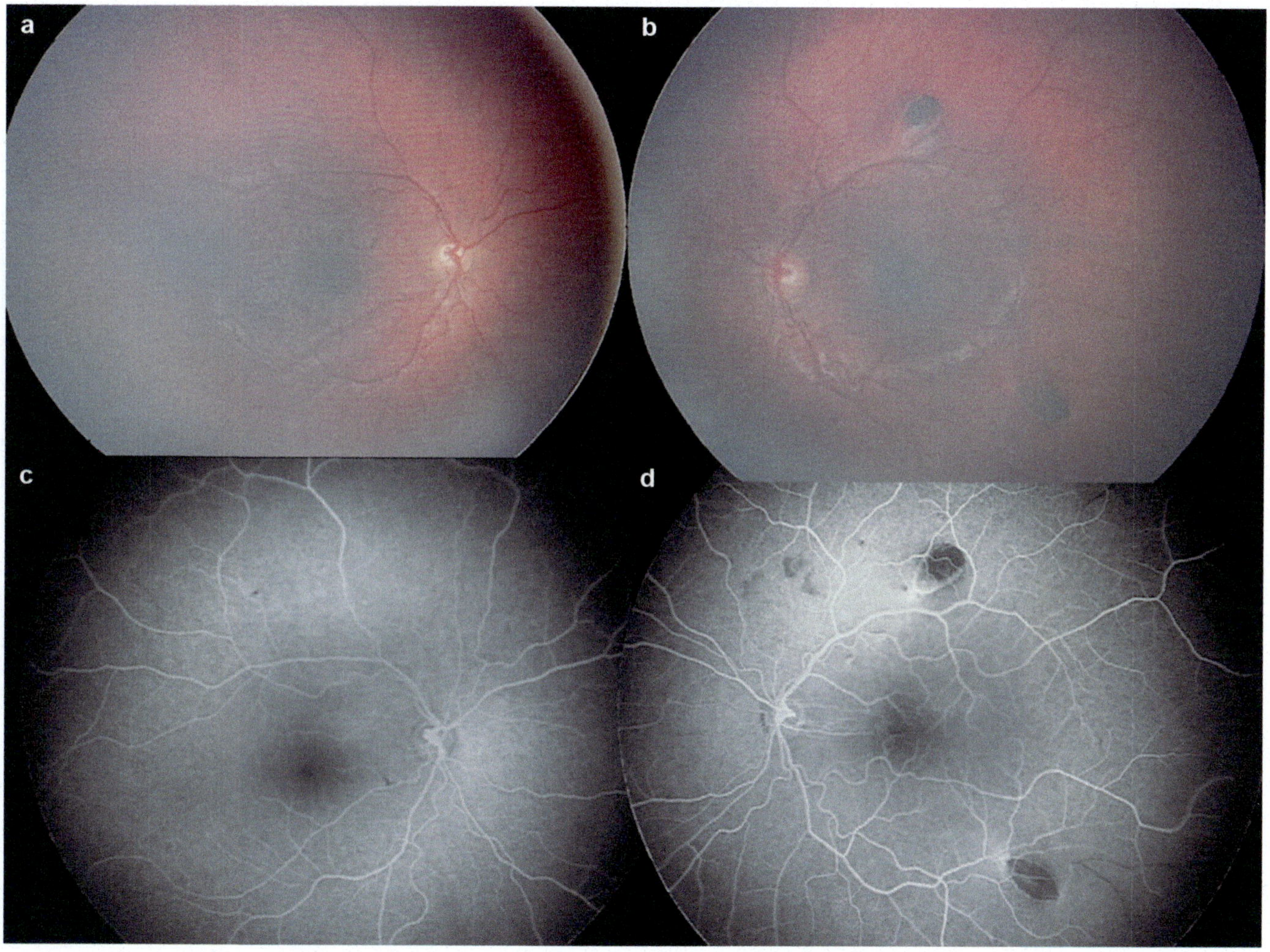

Fig. 13 Congenital RPE markers of FAP show the irregular "pisciform" RPE lesions (**a**, **b**), better seen on fluorescein angiography as focal hypofluorescent spots and dots in both eyes (**c**, **d**)

Congenital Simple Hamartoma of the RPE

Congenital simple hamartoma of the RPE is a dark black, round mass located in the parafoveal region (Fig. 14) [17]. In most cases, visual acuity is normal. This lesion rarely enlarges and requires no intervention.

Combined Hamartoma of the Retina and RPE

Combined hamartoma of the retina and RPE is a benign, presumed congenital condition that can manifest in the papillomacular region or more peripheral near the equator of the eye [18, 19]. This mass displays a mossy green color with retinal traction and tortuosity as well as vitreoretinal traction. Association with neurofibromatosis type 2 and brachial cleft syndrome is occasionally noted (Fig. 15).

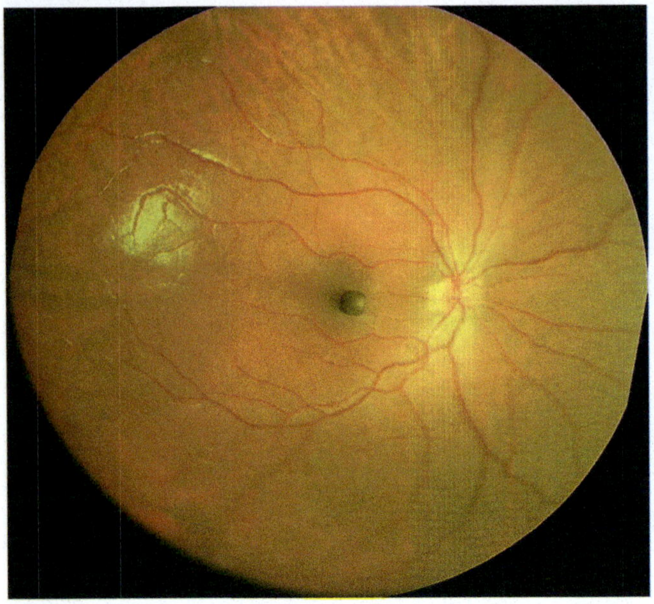

Fig. 14 Congenital simple hamartoma of the RPE appearing as a solitary black lesion near the foveola

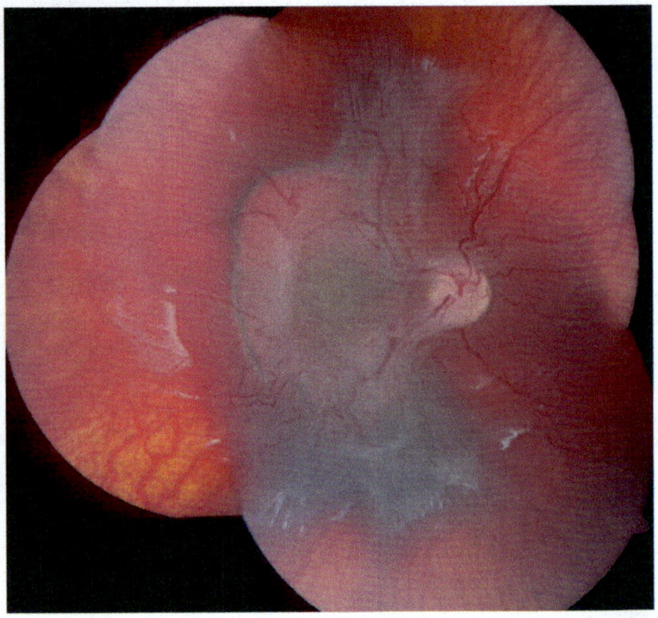

Fig. 15 Combined hamartoma of the retina and RPE appearing as a dark gray mass with extensive retinal traction

Adenoma/Adenocarcinoma of the RPE

The RPE can proliferate into a nodular mass composed of benign (adenoma) or malignant (adenocarcinoma) epithelial cells. Occasionally, surrounding exudation and vitreous hemorrhage is found (Fig. 16).

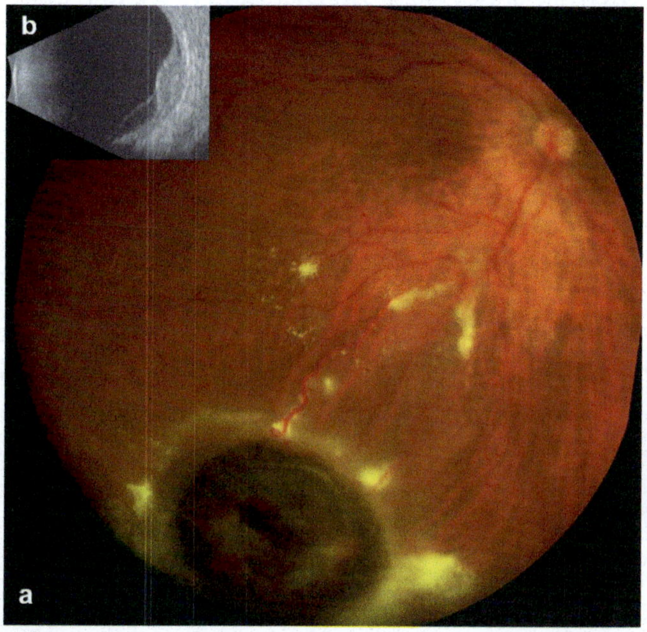

Fig. 16 Adenocarcinoma of the RPE with surrounding exudation (**a**) and appearing echodense with retinal detachment (**b**) on ultrasonography

Tumors of the Ciliary Body Epithelium

The ciliary body epithelium can produce benign or malignant medulloepithelioma of childhood or adenoma/adenocarcinoma of adulthood.

Medulloepithelioma

Medulloepithelioma is a benign or malignant proliferation of the nonpigmented ciliary epithelium that is believed to be a congenital tumor that continues to proliferate after birth. Lens coloboma and neovascular glaucoma are also found in some cases (Fig. 17). Management includes plaque radiotherapy or enucleation.

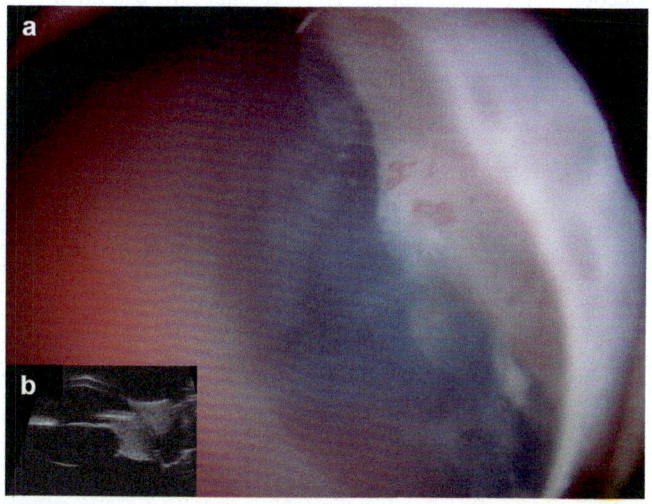

Fig. 17 Medulloepithelioma with intrinsic vascularity and vitreous involvement (**a**) and appearing echodense with posterior cyst (**b**) on ultrasound biomicroscopy

Adenoma/Adenocarcinoma of the Ciliary Body Pigmented or Nonpigmented Epithelium

Adenoma or adenocarcinoma of the ciliary body epithelium typically arises in midadult or older adults as a pigmented or nonpigmented mass located immediately behind the lens. Surgical resection is the treatment of choice.

Tumors of the Choroid

The choroid is composed of melanocytes, vascular elements, and neural tissue, each of which can produce tumors. The most common tumors of the choroid include nevus, metastasis, and melanoma. These lesions can be differentiated based on clinical and imaging evaluations. Occasionally, fine-needle aspiration biopsy is necessary to establish the diagnosis.

Choroidal Nevus

Choroidal nevus is a benign tumor found in approximately 7 % of the Caucasian population [20, 21]. In a population-based study, the mean diameter of choroidal nevus was 1.5 mm [20]. In an ocular oncology clinic-based study, the mean diameter was 5 mm [22]. Choroidal nevus is brown-pigmented in 80 %, and yellow-nonpigmented in 20 % [22]. Overlying drusen (40 %), RPE atrophy (13 %), RPE hyperplasia (9 %), orange pigment (10 %), and choroidal neovascularization (<1 %) can be seen [15]. Transformation into melanoma occurs 1 in 8,845 cases, often identified by risk factors including tumor thickness greater than 2 mm; overlying orange pigment; associated subretinal fluid; symptoms of flashes, floaters, or blurred vision; location of the mass within 3 mm of the optic disc; ultrasound evidence of tumor hollowness, and absence of halo or drusen [23, 24] (Figs. 18, 19, 20, 21, 22 and 23).

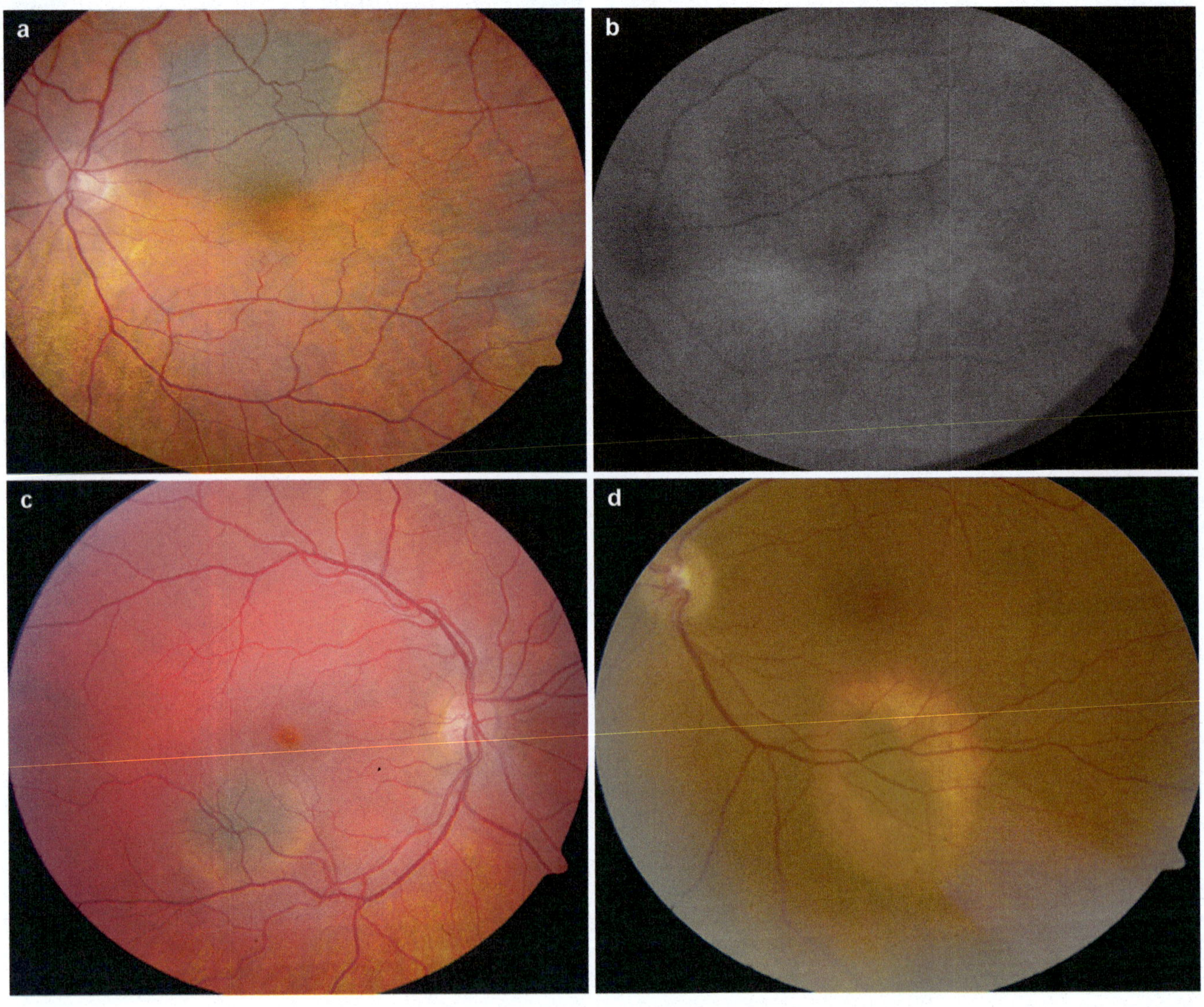

Fig. 18 Choroidal nevus shows dark brown mass (**a**) with hypoautofluorescence (**b**). Halo choroidal nevus in a right (**c**) and a left (**d**) eye of different patients

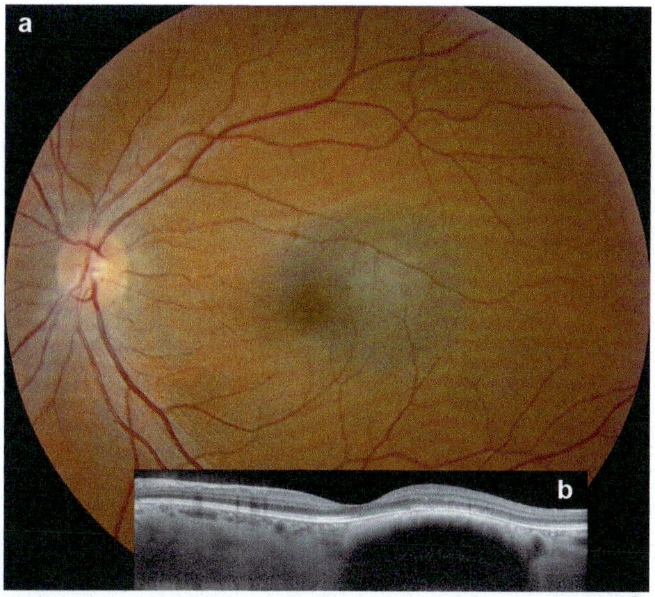

Fig. 19 Choroidal nevus with drusen over the subfoveal portion (**a**) shows optical coherence tomography (OCT) demonstrating optical density with shadowing and overlying RPE alterations (**b**)

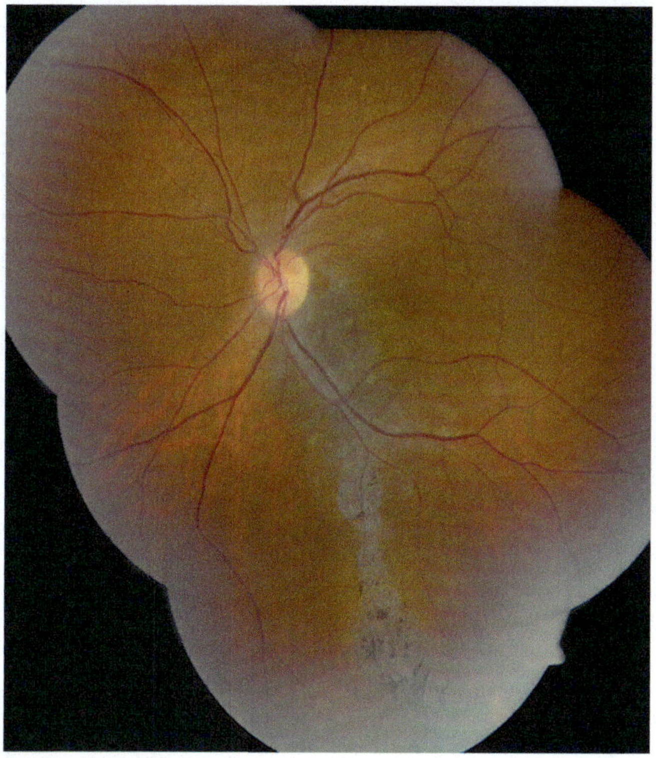

Fig. 20 Choroidal nevus in juxtapapillary region with an old trough of subretinal fluid

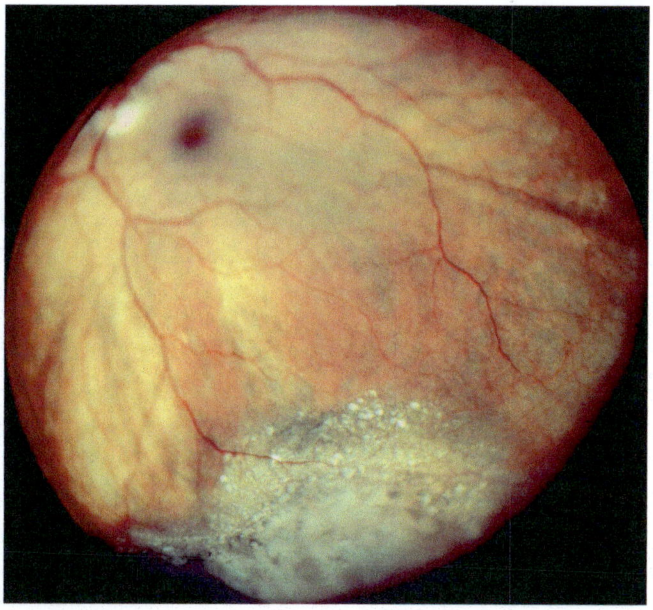

Fig. 21 Large peripheral choroidal nevus with overlying drusen

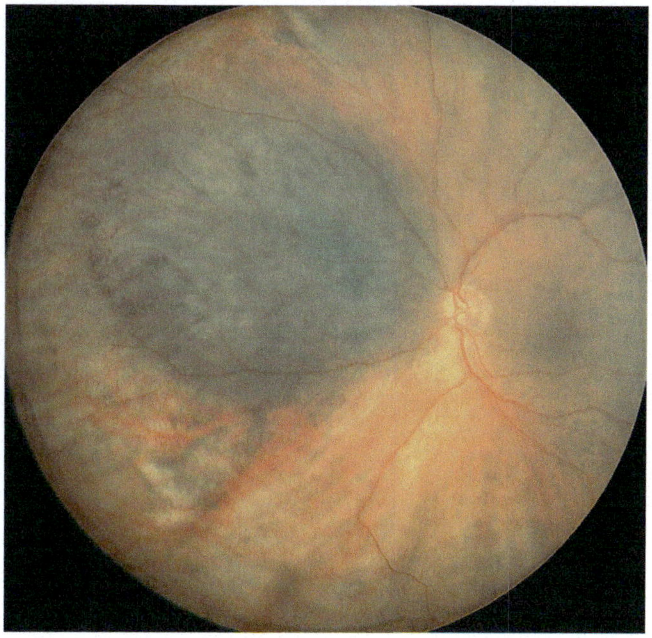

Fig. 22 Large juxtapapillary choroidal nevus with overlying RPE atrophy

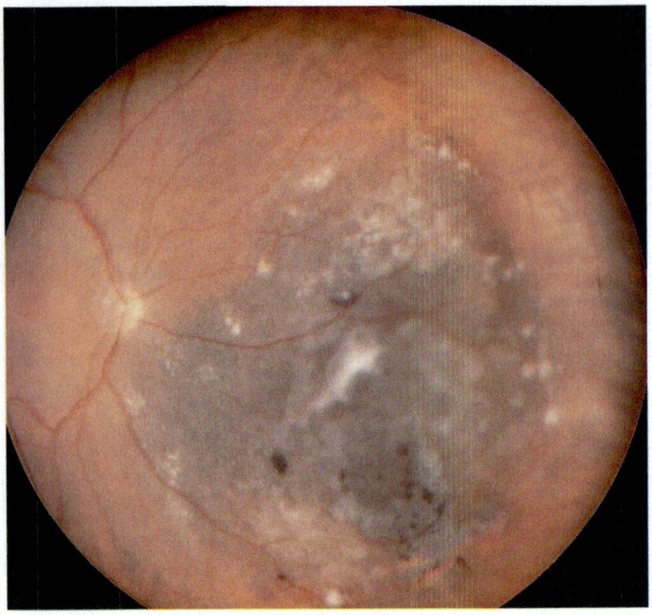

Fig. 23 Large equatorial choroidal nevus with overlying drusen and RPE fibrous metaplasia

Choroidal Melanoma

Choroidal melanoma is a serious, life-threatening intraocular malignancy that appears with a dome or mushroom configuration, often with surrounding subretinal fluid and occasional subretinal or vitreous hemorrhage [25]. Approximately six individuals per million population annually develop this malignancy, with roughly 2,000 new cases in the United States each year. Prognosis of melanoma depends on tumor thickness, with each increasing millimeter imparting 5 % increased risk for metastasis [26, 27]. Treatment includes enucleation, surgical resection, proton radiotherapy, plaque radiotherapy, or thermotherapy (Figs. 24, 25, 26, 27, 28, 29, 30, 31 and 32).

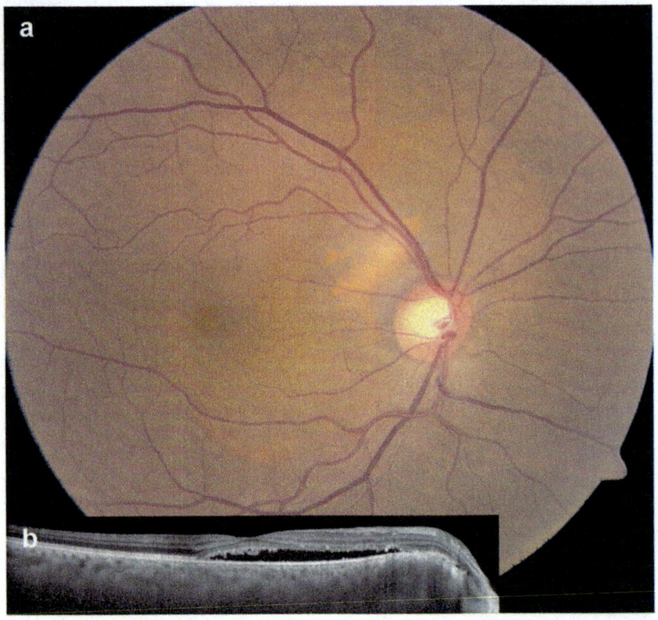

Fig. 24 Small juxtapapillary choroidal melanoma with overlying orange lipofuscin pigment (**a**) and subretinal fluid (**b**) on OCT

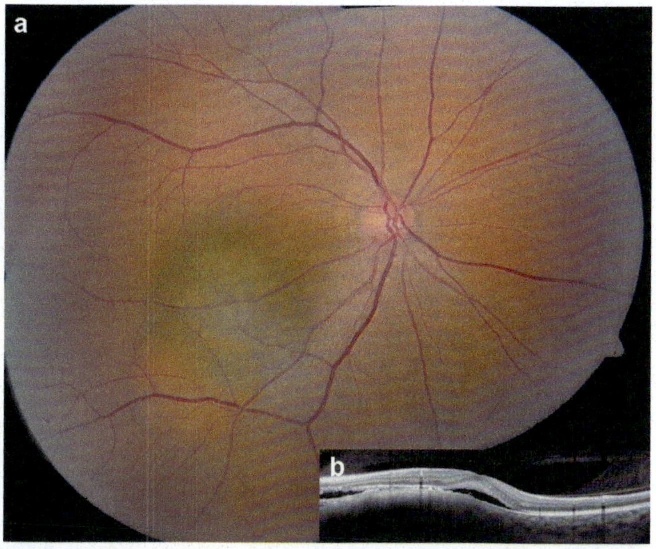

Fig. 25 Small macular choroidal melanoma with overlying and puddled orange lipofuscin pigment (**a**) and subretinal fluid (**b**) on OCT

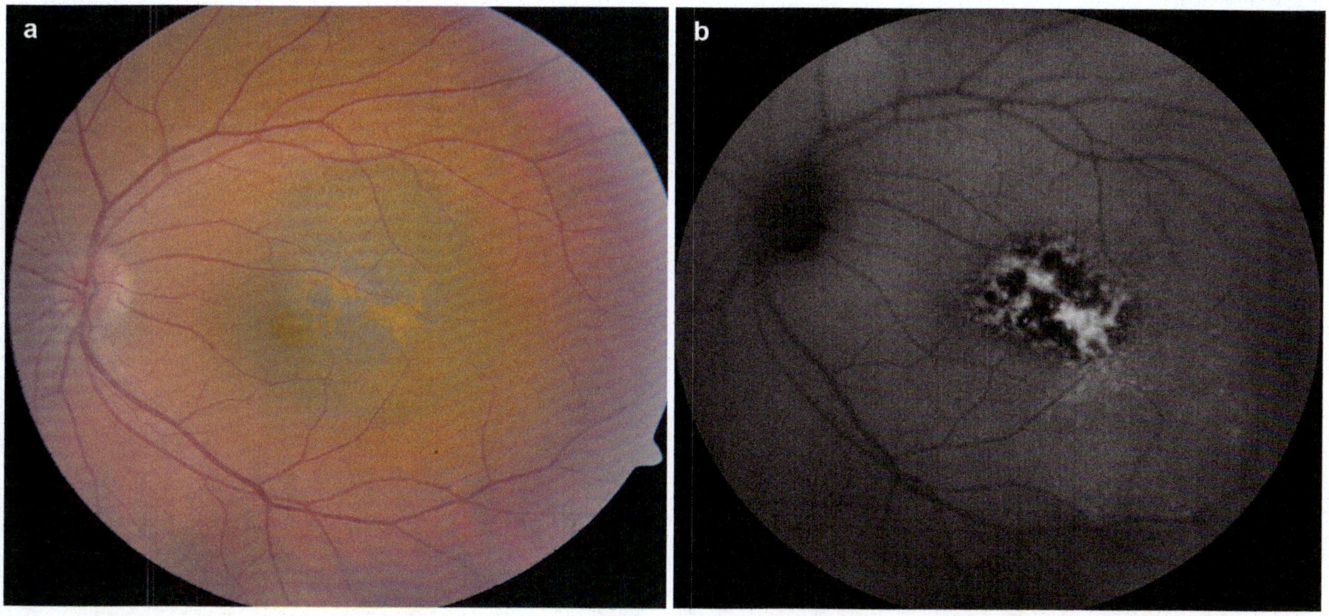

Fig. 26 Small macular choroidal melanoma with overlying orange lipofuscin pigment (**a**), confirmed as hyperautofluorescent (**b**)

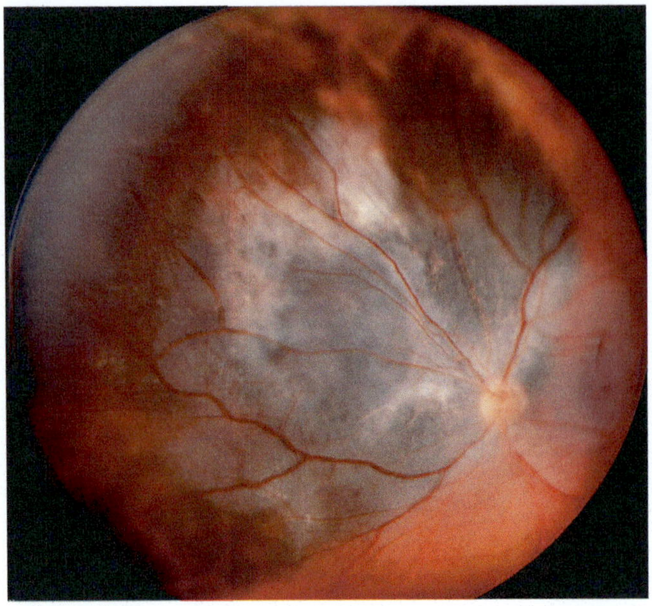

Fig. 27 Diffuse flat melanoma with overlying subretinal fluid and orange pigment

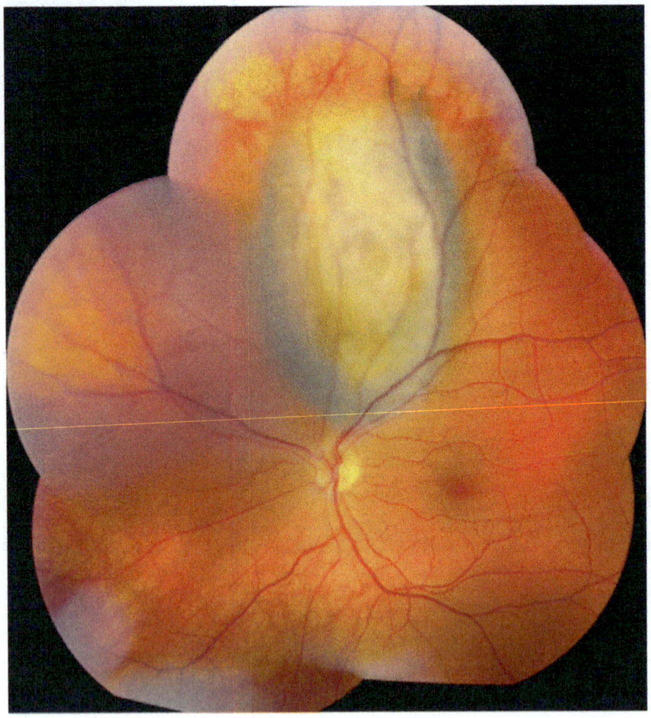

Fig. 28 Medium-size choroidal melanoma

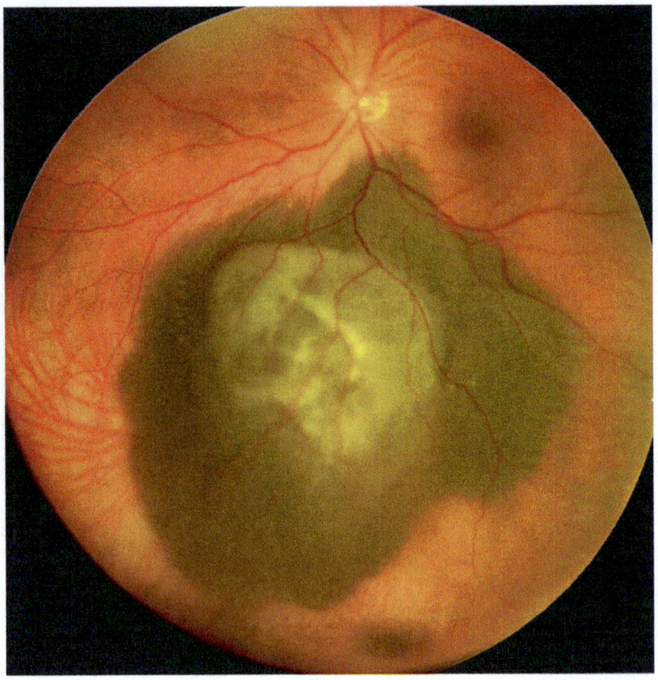

Fig. 29 Medium-size choroidal melanoma with minor overlying subretinal fluid

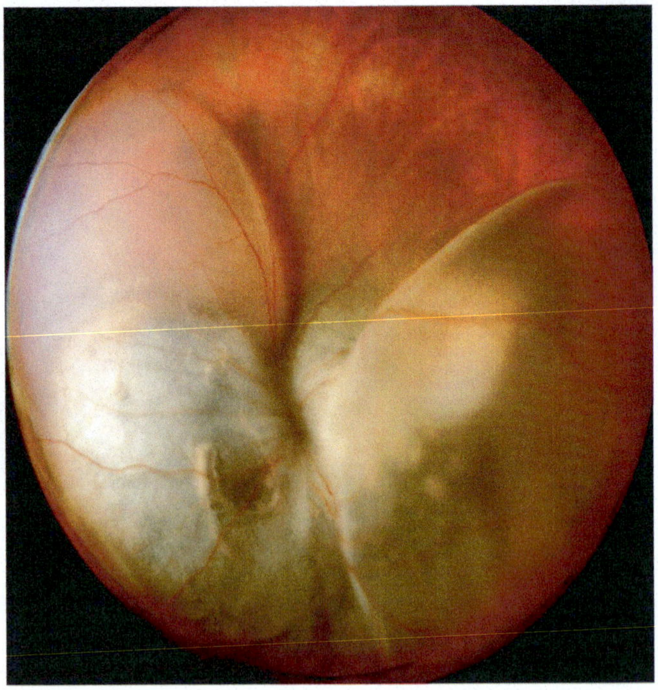

Fig. 30 Medium-size choroidal melanoma with extensive subretinal fluid

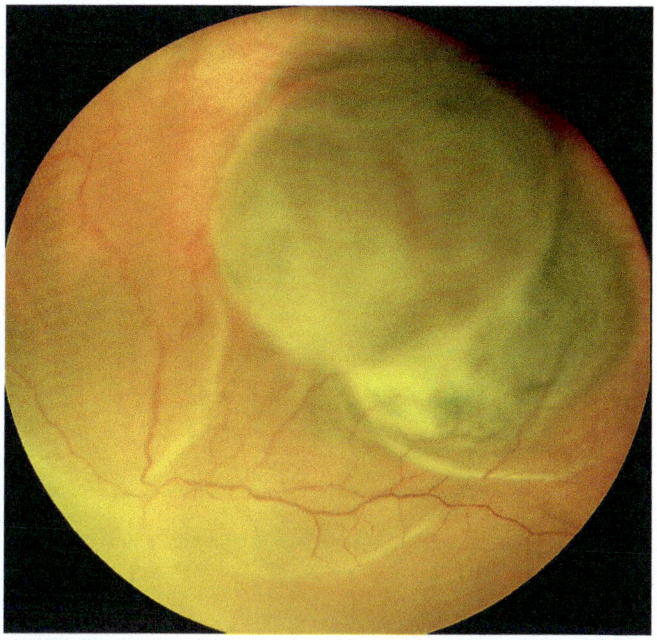

Fig. 31 Large choroidal melanoma with subretinal fluid

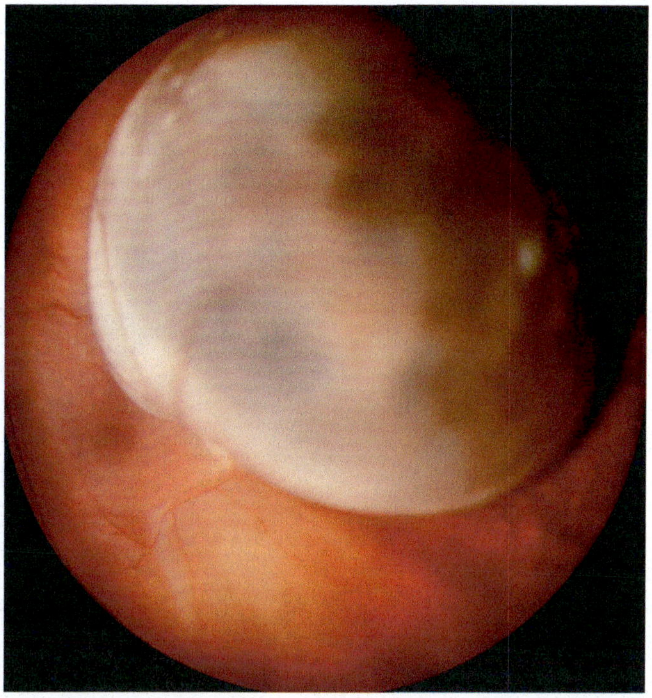

Fig. 32 Very large choroidal melanoma overhanging the optic disc and with subretinal fluid

Choroidal Metastasis

Choroidal metastases appear as a yellow mass, often with subretinal fluid. This malignancy originates from primary breast cancer in 53 %, lung cancer in 20 %, and others [28]. Bilateral metastases are most often secondary to breast carcinoma (70 %) (Figs. 33, 34, 35 and 36) [28].

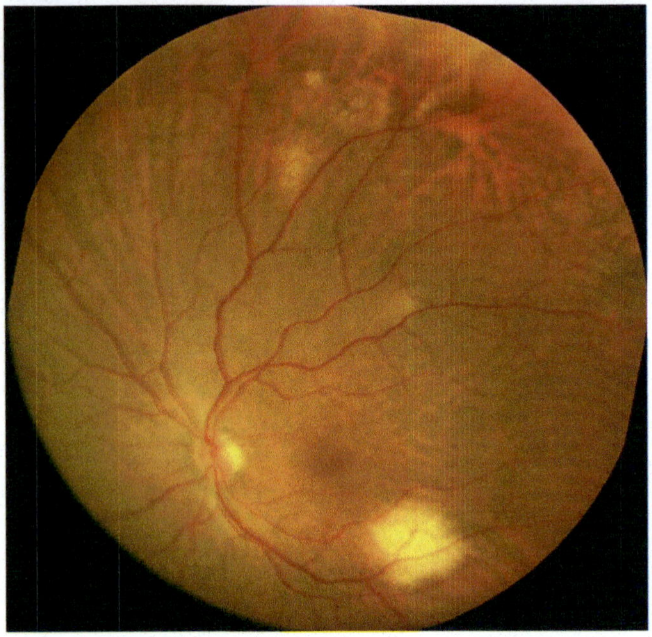

Fig. 33 Small choroidal metastasis inferior to the macular region and three small metastases superior to the macular region

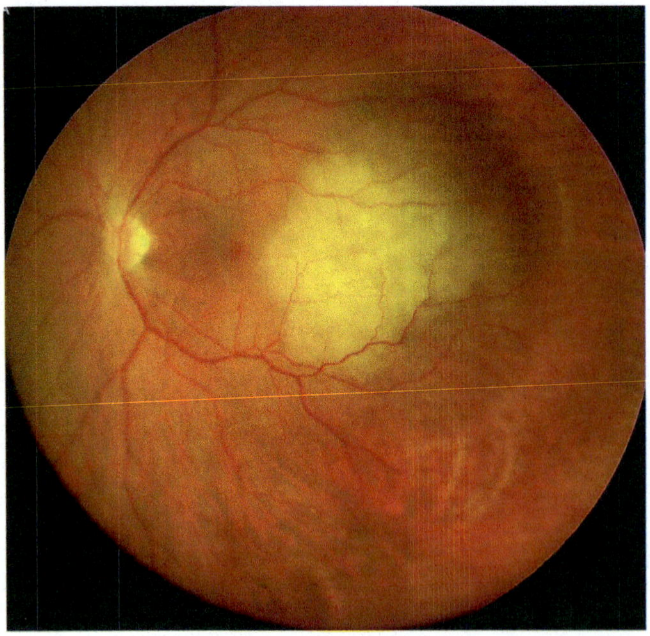

Fig. 34 Medium-size choroidal metastasis with minor subretinal fluid

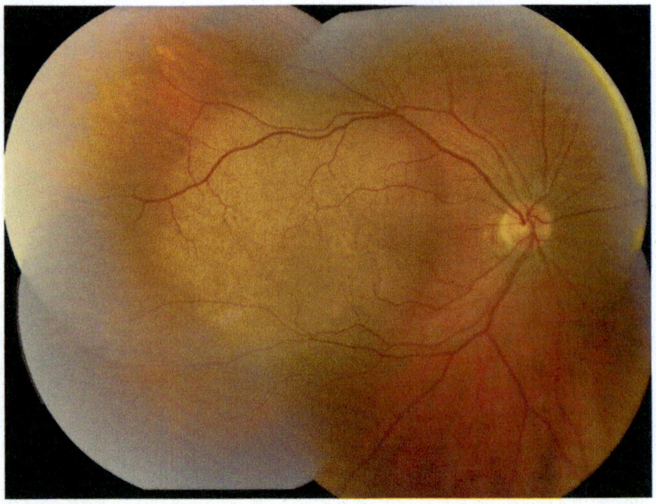

Fig. 35 Medium-size choroidal metastasis with minor subretinal fluid

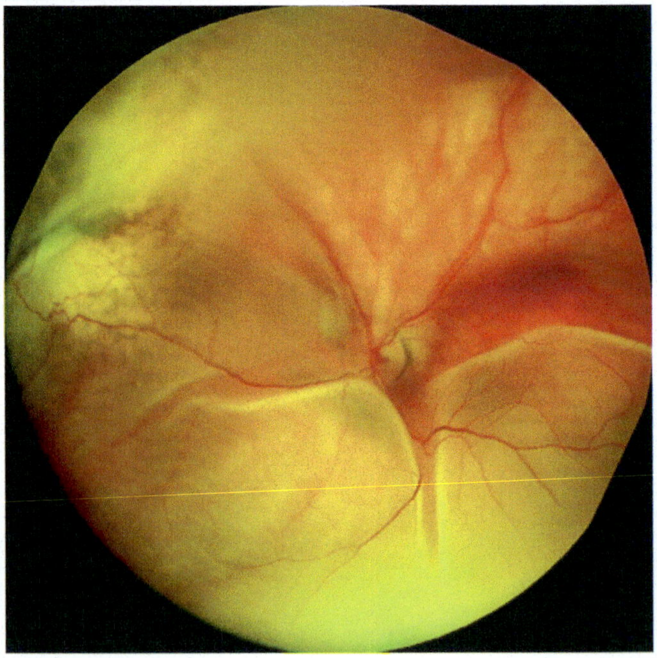

Fig. 36 Extensive choroidal metastasis with extensive subretinal fluid

Choroidal Hemangioma

Choroidal hemangioma can appear as a circumscribed or diffuse vascular mass. The circumscribed lesion appears as a circumscribed, round, slightly elevated orange mass of mean diameter 6 mm and thickness of 3 mm [29]. This tumor classically occurs in the postequatorial region and exhibits slow enlargement with progressive subretinal fluid or macular edema. The diffuse hemangioma occurs in patients with Sturge-Weber syndrome and can produce total retinal detachment. Management includes photodynamic therapy or radiotherapy (Figs. 37, 38, 39, 40 and 41) [30, 31].

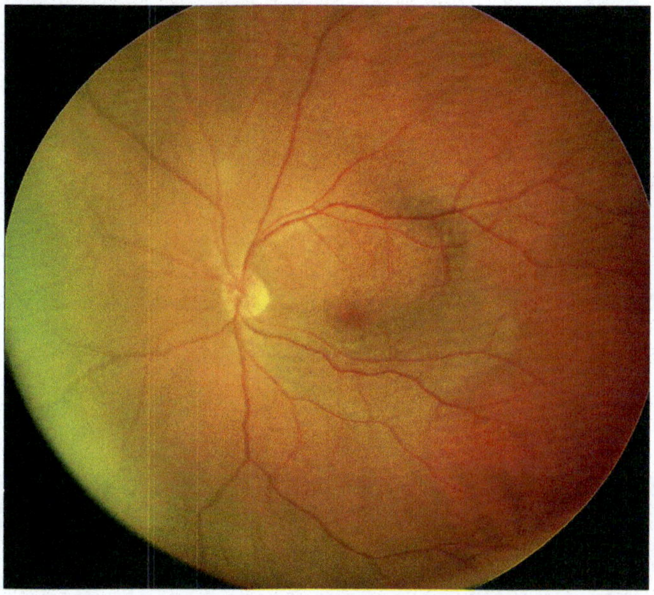

Fig. 37 Small submacular circumscribed choroidal hemangioma with subtle subretinal fluid

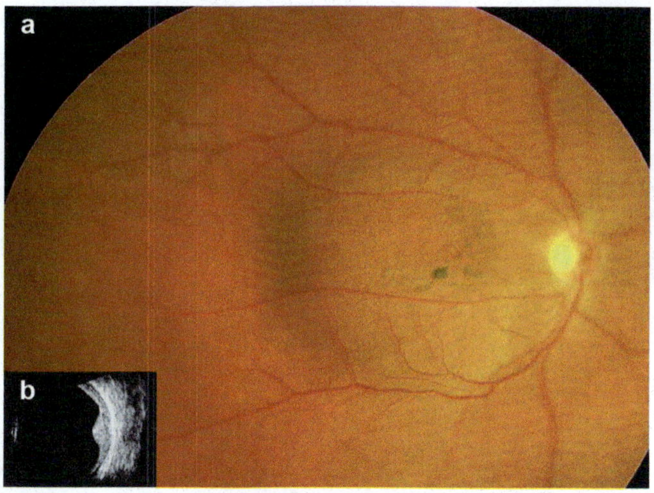

Fig. 38 Moderate submacular circumscribed choroidal hemangioma (**a**), appearing echodense (**b**) on ultrasonography

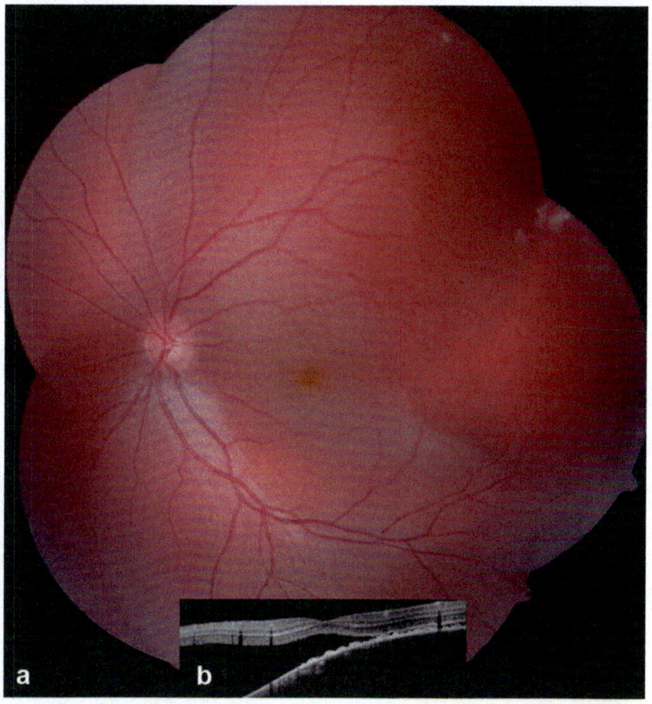

Fig. 39 Diffuse choroidal hemangioma of Sturge-Weber syndrome (**a**) with subretinal fluid (**b**) on OCT

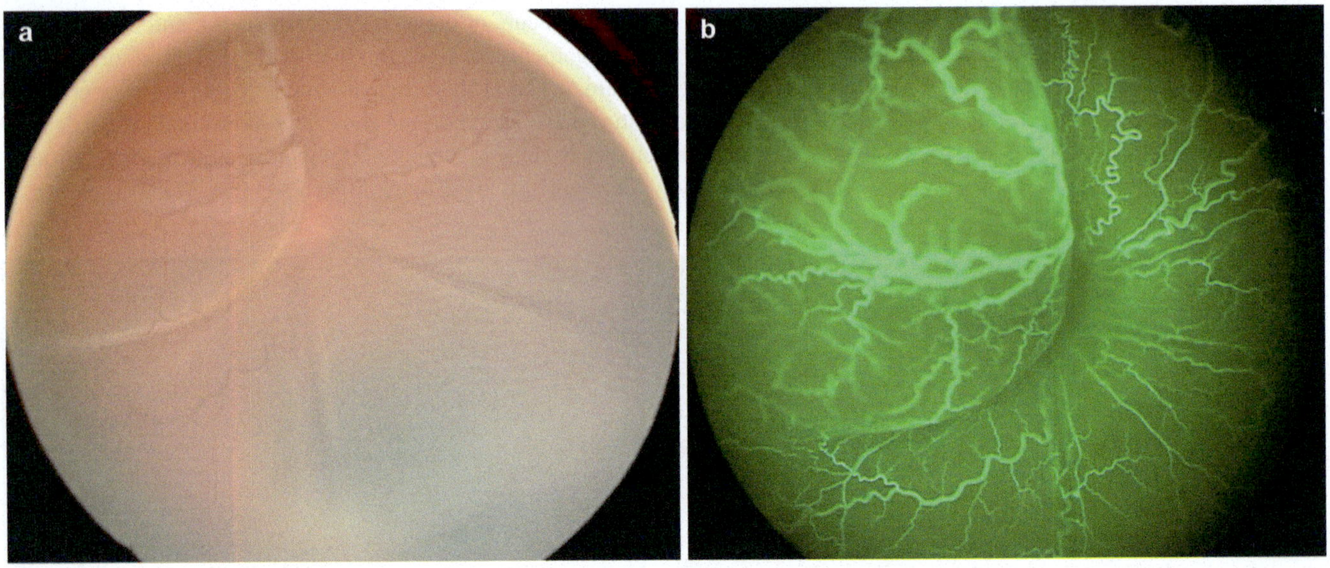

Fig. 40 Diffuse choroidal hemangioma of Sturge-Weber syndrome (**a**) with total retinal detachment (**b**) imaged with fluorescein angiography

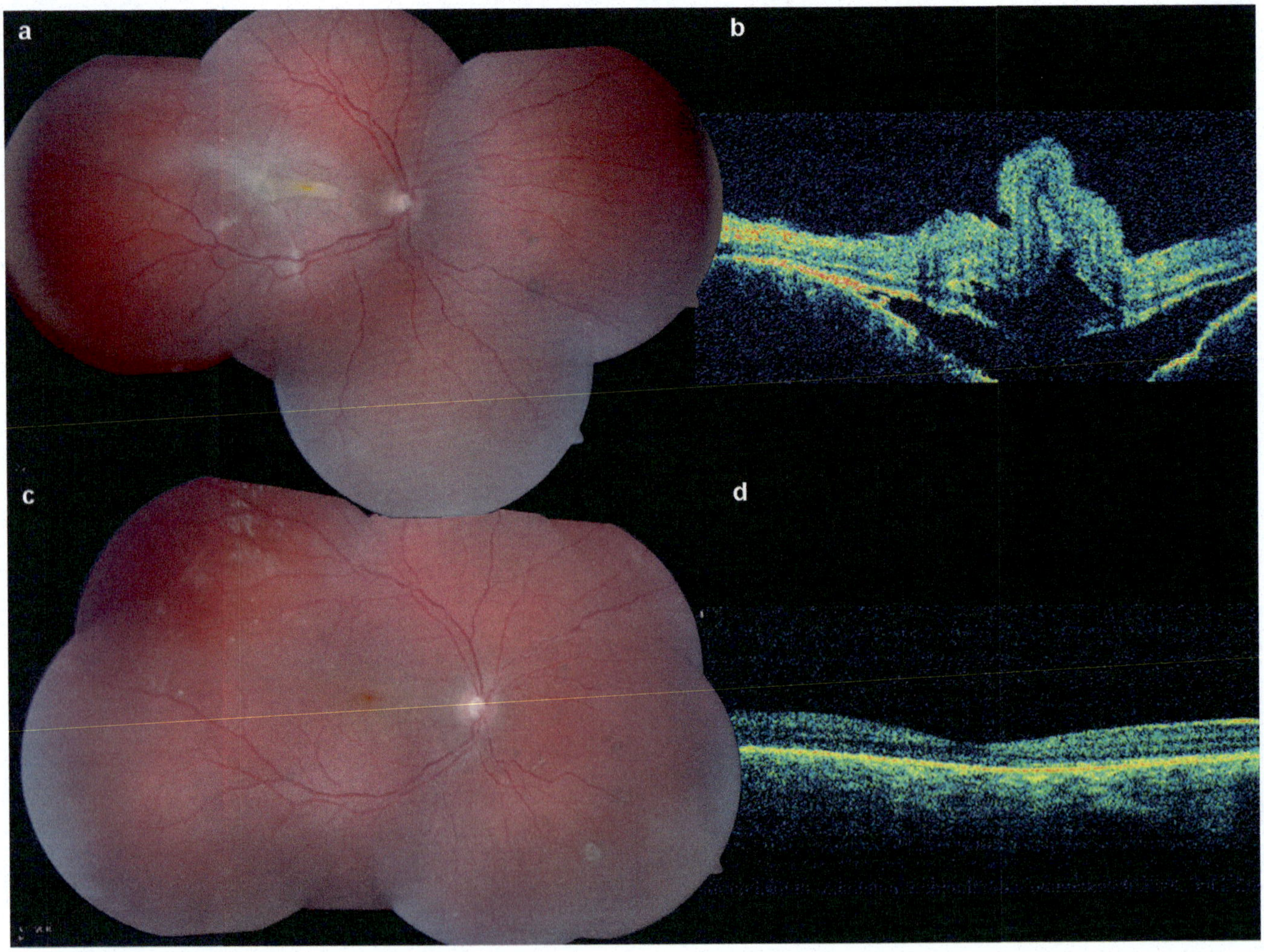

Fig. 41 Diffuse choroidal hemangioma with subretinal fluid before (**a**, **b**) and after (**c**, **d**) radiotherapy

Choroidal Osteoma

Choroidal osteoma is a benign intraocular tumor composed of mature bone [32, 33]. This tumor classically manifests as an orange-yellow plaque deep to the retina in the juxtapapillary or macular region of young women. This tumor can be unilateral (80 %) or bilateral (20 %). The cause and pathogenesis of this tumor are unknown. Ten-year probability for tumor growth is 51 %, tumor decalcification is 46 %, related choroidal neovascularization is 31 %, visual acuity loss of 3 or more Snellen lines is 45 % (Figs. 42, 43, 44 and 45) [33].

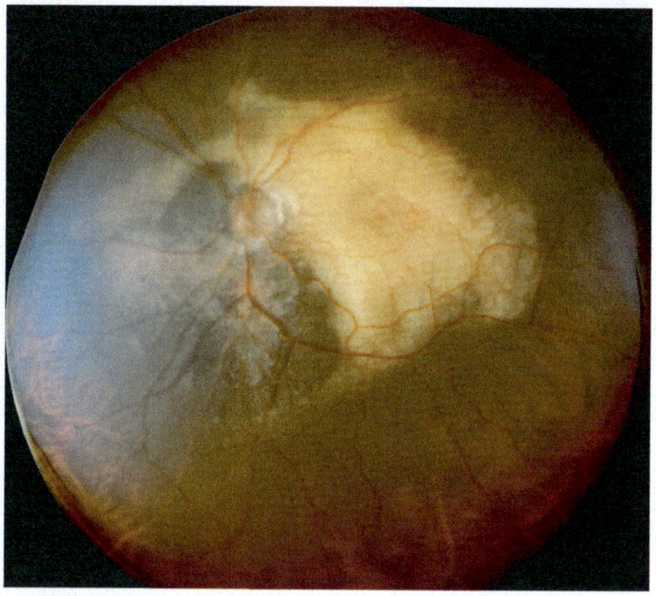

Fig. 42 Choroidal osteoma

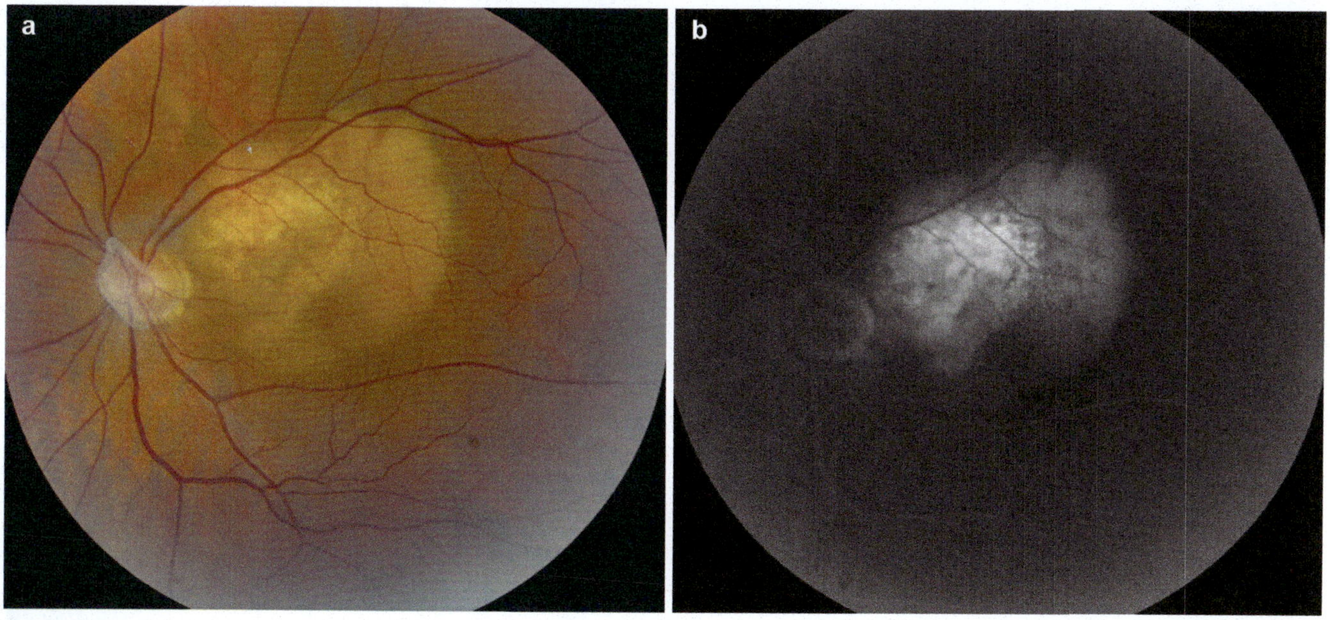

Fig. 43 Choroidal osteoma (**a**) shows hyperfluorescence (**b**)

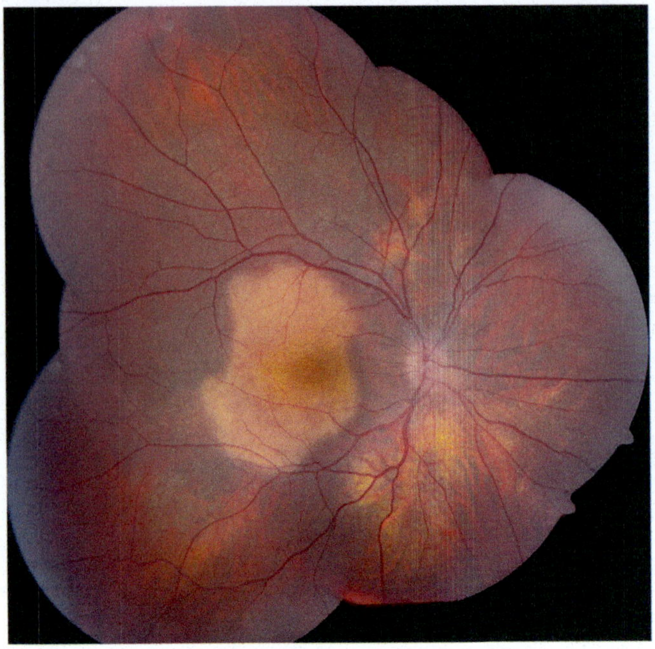

Fig. 44 Choroidal osteoma in the right macula

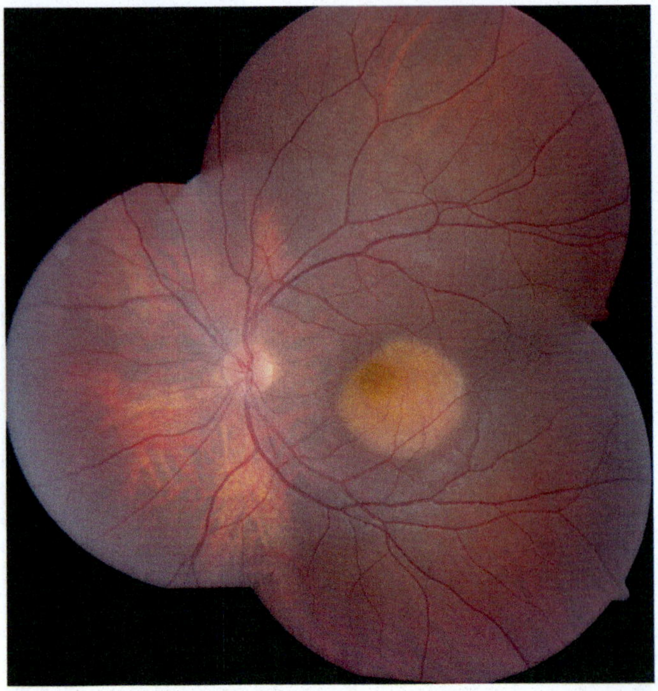

Fig. 45 Choroidal osteoma in the left macula of the patient in Fig. 44

Choroidal Leiomyoma

Ciliary body/choroidal leiomyoma is a benign tumor arising in the suprauveal space [34]. This tumor appears nonpigmented and most often is managed with surgical resection (Fig. 46).

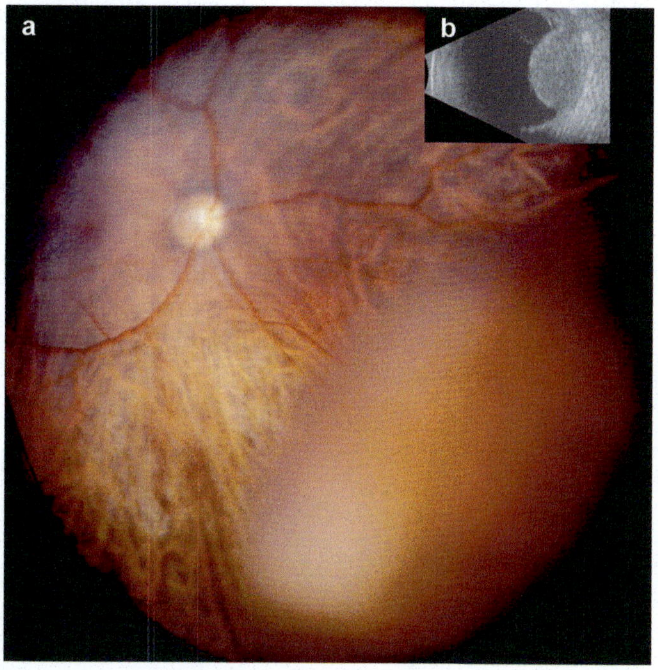

Fig. 46 Ciliochoroidal leiomyoma in the far periphery of the fundus (**a**) and echogenic (**b**) on ultrasonography

Choroidal Lymphoma

Intraocular lymphoma can be divided into uveal and vitreoretinal forms [35]. In the uveal form, the tumor is typically low grade and appears as a placoid thickening of the choroid with occasional overlying subretinal fluid. In the vitreoretinal form, the tumor is high-grade large cell lymphoma and can manifest with vitreous tumor, sub-RPE infiltration, and retinal infiltration. Definitive diagnosis is made through fine-needle aspiration biopsy (Figs. 47 and 48).

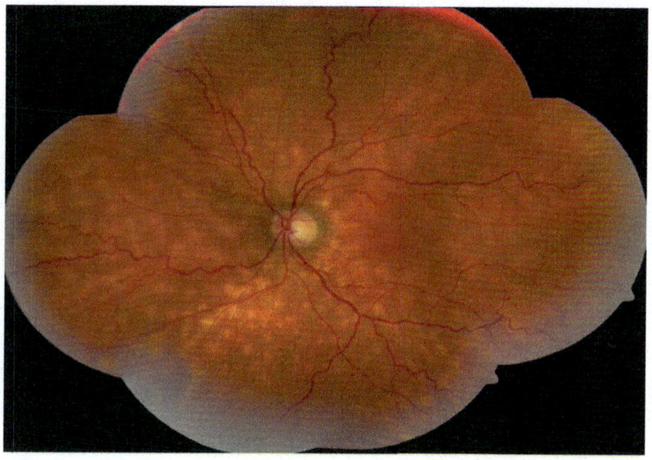

Fig. 47 Choroidal lymphoma with multifocal yellow spots of infiltration

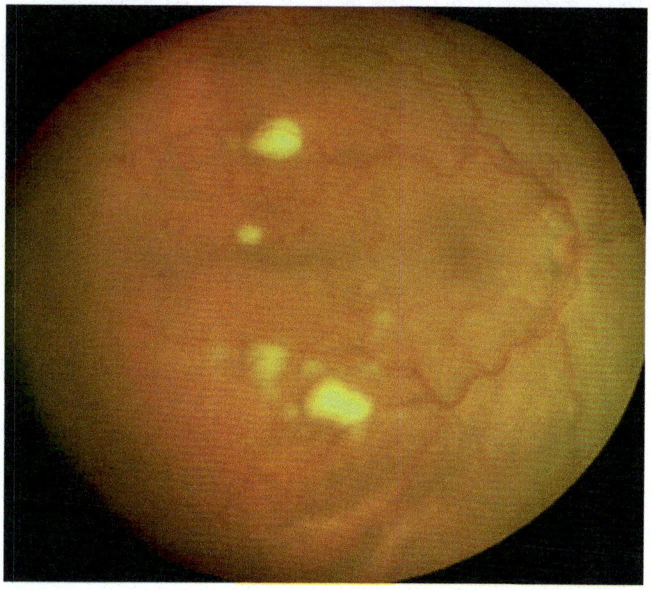

Fig. 48 Vitreoretinal lymphoma with sub-RPE infiltration of lymphoma

Tumors of the Disc

Optic Disc Melanocytoma

Optic disc melanocytoma is a darkly pigmented nevus obscuring the disc details and occasionally causing compression with visual acuity or visual field loss. This benign lesion can slowly grow in 14 % of cases and can rarely transform into melanoma [36]. Management is observation (Figs. 49 and 50).

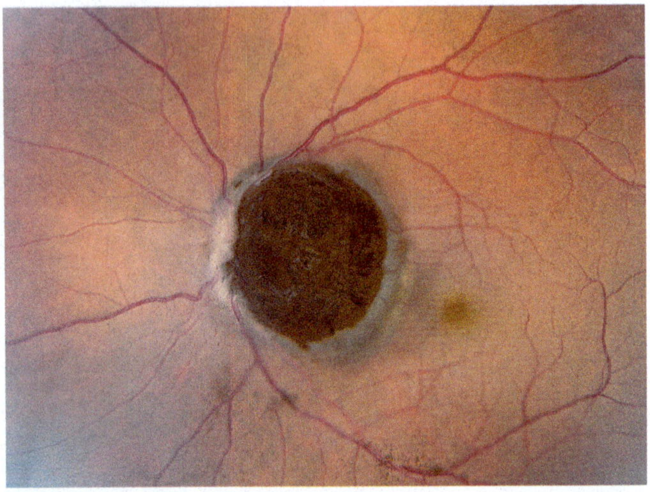

Fig. 49 Melanocytoma of the optic disc with minor vitreous seeding

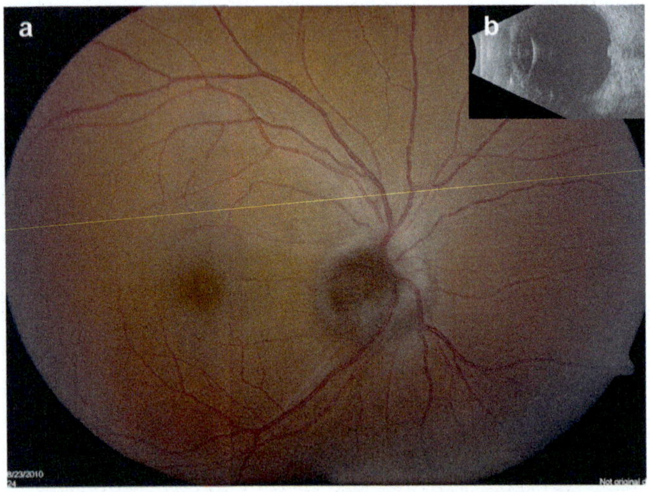

Fig. 50 Melanocytoma of the optic disc (**a**) appearing dense (**b**) on ultrasonography

Optic Disc Hemangioblastoma

Optic disc hemangioblastoma is a benign reddish mass of the disc, often with indiscrete margins that can produce subretinal fluid and exudation. Evaluation for von Hippel–Lindau disease is warranted. Management is challenging and includes laser photocoagulation, photodynamic therapy, plaque radiotherapy, external beam radiotherapy, or anti-VEGF medications (Fig. 51).

Optic Disc Metastasis

Optic disc metastasis appear as a yellow, pallid swelling of the disc with intrinsic vascularity, often in a patient with known cancer [37]. Typically, there are surrounding choroidal metastases. Management generally involves chemotherapy or ocular radiotherapy.

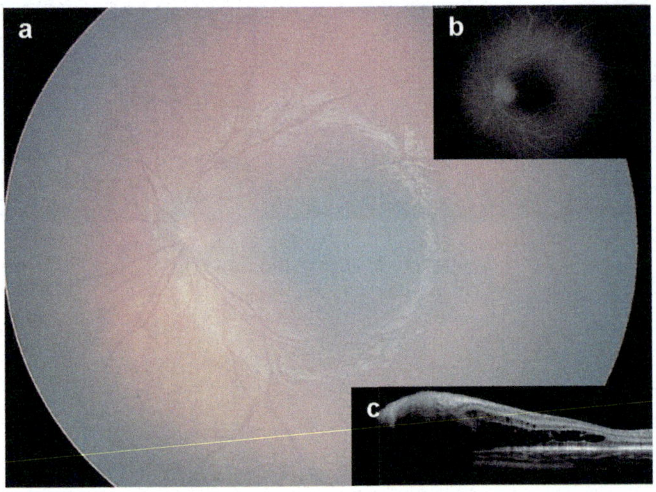

Fig. 51 Optic disc hemangioblastoma appearing as a subtle red mass along the superotemporal disc (**a**) with bright fluorescein angiographic enhancement (**b**) and evidence of subretinal and intraretinal fluid (**c**) on OCT

References

1. Wong JR, Tucker MA, Kleinerman RA, Sevesa SS. Retinoblastoma incidence patterns in the US Surveillance, Epidemiology, and End Results program. JAMA Ophthalmol. 2014;132:478–83.
2. Kivelä T. The epidemiological challenge of the most frequent eye cancer: retinoblastoma, an issue of birth and death. Br J Ophthalmol. 2009;93:1129–31.
3. Shields CL, Kaliki S, Rojanaporn D, Al-Dahmash S, Bianciotto CG, Shields JA. Intravenous and intra-arterial chemotherapy for retinoblastoma: what have we learned? Curr Opin Ophthalmol. 2012;23:202–9.
4. Shields CL, Fulco EM, Arias JD, Alarcon C, Pelligrini M, Rishi P, et al. Retinoblastoma frontiers with intravenous, intra-arterial, periocular and intravitreal chemotherapy. Eye. 2013;27:253–64.
5. Mennel S, Meyer CH, Eggarter F, Peter S. Autofluorescence and angiographic findings of retinal astrocytic hamartomas in tuberous sclerosis. Ophthalmologica. 2005;219:350–6.
6. Shields CL, Reichstein DA, Bianciotto CG, Shields JA. Retinal pigment epithelial depigmented lesions associated with tuberous sclerosis complex. Arch Ophthalmol. 2012;130:387–90.
7. Singh AD, Shields CL, Shields JA. Major review: von Hippel-Lindau disease. Surv Ophthalmol. 2001;46:117–42.
8. Shields JA, Decker WL, Sanborn GE, Ausberger JJ, Goldberg RE. Presumed acquired retinal hemangiomas. Ophthalmology. 1983;90:1292–309.
9. Shields CL, Shields JA, Barrett J, De Potter P. Vasoproliferative tumors of the ocular fundus. Classification and clinical manifestations in 103 patients. Arch Ophthalmol. 1995;113:615–23.
10. Shields CL, Kaliki S, Al-Dahmash S, Rajanaporn D, Shukla S, Reilly B, et al. Retinal vasoproliferative tumors: comparative clinical features of primary versus secondary tumors in 334 cases. JAMA Ophthalmol. 2013;131:328–34.
11. Guyer DR, Schachat AP, Vitale S, Markowitz JA, Braine H, Burke PJ, et al. Leukemic retinopathy. Relationship between fundus lesions and hematologic parameters at diagnosis. Ophthalmology. 1989;96:860–4.
12. Shields CL, Mashayekhi A, Ho T, Cater J, Shields JA. Solitary congenital hypertrophy of the retinal pigment epithelium: clinical features and frequency of enlargement in 330 patients. Ophthalmology. 2003;110:1968–76.
13. Shields CL, Materin MA, Walker C, Marr BP, Shields JA. Photoreceptor loss overlying congenital hypertrophy of the retinal pigment epithelium by optical coherence tomography. Ophthalmology. 2006;113:661–5.
14. Fung AT, Pellegrini M, Shields CL. Congenital hypertrophy of the retinal pigment epithelium: enhanced depth imaging optical coherence tomography in 18 cases. Ophthalmology. 2014;121:251–6.
15. Shields CL, Pirondini C, Bianciotto C, Harmon SA, Shields JA. Autofluorescence of congenital hypertrophy of the retinal pigment epithelium. Retina. 2007;27:1097–100.
16. Traboulsi EI, Apostolides J, Giardiello FM, Krush AJ, Booker SV, Hamilton SR, et al. Pigment ocular fundus lesions and APC mutations in familial adenomatous polyposis. Ophthalmol Genet. 1996;17:167–74.
17. Shields CL, Shields JA, Marr BP, Sperber DE, Gass JD. Congenital simple hamartoma of the retinal pigment epithelium: a study of five cases. Ophthalmology. 2003;110:1005–11.
18. Schachat AP, Shields JA, Fine SL, Sanborn GE, Weingeist TA, Valenzuela RE, et al. Combined hamartomas of the retina and retinal pigment epithelium. Ophthalmology. 1984;91:1609–15.
19. Shields CL, Thangappan A, Hartzell K, Valente P, Pirondini C, Shields JA. Combined hamartoma of the retina and retinal pigment epithelium in 77 consecutive patients. Visual outcome based on macular versus extramacular tumor location. Ophthalmology. 2008;115:2246–52.
20. Sumich P, Mitchell P, Wang JJ. Choroidal nevi in a white population: the Blue Mountains Eye Study. Retina. 1998;116:645–50.
21. Greenstein MB, Myers CE, Meuer SM, Klein BE, Cotch MF, Wong TY, et al. Prevalence and characteristics of choroidal nevi: the multi-ethnic study of atherosclerosis. Ophthalmology. 2011;118:2468–73.
22. Shields CL, Furuta M, Mashayekhi A, Berman EL, Zahler JD, Hoberman DM, et al. Clinical spectrum of choroidal nevi based on age at presentation in 3422 consecutive eyes. Ophthalmology. 2008;115:546–52.
23. Singh AD, Kalyani P, Topham A. Estimating the risk of malignant transformation of a choroidal nevus. Ophthalmology. 2005;112:1784–9.
24. Shields CL, Furuta M, Berman EL, Zahler JD, Hoberman DM, Dinh DM, et al. Choroidal nevus transformation into melanoma: analysis of 2514 consecutive cases. Arch Ophthalmol. 2009;127:981–7.
25. Shields CL, Kaliki S, Furuta M, Mashayekhi A, Shields JA. Clinical spectrum and prognosis of uveal melanoma based on age at presentation in 8033 cases. Retina. 2012;32:1363–72.
26. Shields CL, Furuta M, Thangappan A, Nagori S, Mashayekhi A, Lally DR, et al. Metastasis of uveal melanoma millimeter-by-millimeter in 8033 consecutive eyes. Arch Ophthalmol. 2009;127:989–98.
27. Margo CE. The Collaborative Ocular Melanoma Study: an overview. Cancer Control. 2004;11:304–9.
28. Shields CL, Shields JA, Gross NE, Schwartz GP, Lally SE. Survey of 520 eyes with uveal metastases. Ophthalmology. 1997;104:1265–76.
29. Shields CL, Honavar SG, Shields JA, Cater J, Demirci H. Circumscribed choroidal hemangioma: clinical manifestations and factors predictive of visual outcome in 200 consecutive cases. Ophthalmology. 2001;108:2237–48.
30. Blasi MA, Tiberti AC, Scupola A, Balestrazzi A, Colangelo E, Valente P, et al. Photodynamic therapy with verteporfin for symptomatic circumscribed choroidal hemangioma: five-year outcomes. Ophthalmology. 2010;117:1630–7.
31. Arepalli S, Shields CL, Kaliki S, Komarnicky L, Shields JA. Diffuse choroidal hemangioma management with plaque radiotherapy in 5 cases. Ophthalmology. 2013;120:2358–9.
32. Shields CL, Shields JA, Augsburger JJ. Choroidal osteoma. Surv Ophthalmol. 1988;33:17–27.
33. Shields CL, Sun H, Demirci H, Shields JA. Choroidal osteoma: factors predictive of tumor growth, tumor decalcification, choroidal neovascularization, and visual outcome in 74 eyes. Arch Ophthalmol. 2005;123:1658–66.
34. Shields JA, Shields CL, Eagle Jr RC, De Potter P. Observations on seven cases of intraocular leiomyoma. The 1993 Byron Demorest Lecture. Arch Ophthalmol. 1994;112:521–8.
35. Mashayekhi A, Shukla SY, Shields JA, Shields CL. Choroidal lymphoma: clinical features and association with systemic lymphoma. Ophthalmology. 2014;121:342–51.
36. Shields JA, Demirci H, Mashayekhi A, Shields CL. Melanocytoma of the optic disc in 115 cases. The 2004 Samuel Johnson Memorial Lecture. Ophthalmology. 2004;111:1739–46.
37. Shields JA, Shields CL, Singh AD. Metastatic neoplasms in the optic disc. The 1999 Bjerrum Lecture. Part 2. Arch Ophthalmol. 2000;118:217–24.

13 Wide-Field Retinal Imaging of Retinal and Choroidal Inflammatory Diseases

Keegan A. Harkins, Michael J. daSilva, Quan Dong Nguyen, and Diana V. Do

Diagnosis of uveitis can be challenging. Research in advanced imaging modalities is currently a very active field, with the promise of improving our ability to detect and treat the wide spectrum of uveitic disease.

Peripheral disease activity is present in many uveitides. Whereas an ophthalmologist may have previously performed montage photography or a peripheral sweep to aid its discovery, ultra-wide-field images allow for a more comprehensive depiction of disease severity and progression. Several recent studies have suggested the superiority of ultra-wide-field imaging, indicating that it may reveal disease beyond what is apparent in the initial clinical presentation.

K.A. Harkins, MD (✉)
Department of Ophthalmology and Visual Science, Stanley M. Truhlsen Eye Institute, University of Nebraska Medical Center, Omaha, NE, USA
e-mail: kharkins@unmc.edu

M.J. daSilva, MD • Q.D. Nguyen, MD, MSc • D.V. Do, MD
Department of Ophthalmology and Visual Science, Stanley M. Truhlsen Eye Institute, University of Nebraska Medical Center, Omaha, NE, USA
e-mail: michael.dasilva@unmc.edu; quan.nguyen@unmc.edu; diana.do@unmc.edu

I. Kozak, J.F. Arevalo (eds.), *Atlas of Wide-Field Retinal Angiography and Imaging*, DOI 10.1007/978-3-319-17864-6_13

Noninfectious (Autoimmune) Uveitis

Posterior Uveitis

Susac Syndrome (Fig. 1)
A 52-year-old woman with hearing loss, vertigo, and corpus callosum lesions on brain magnetic resonance imaging.

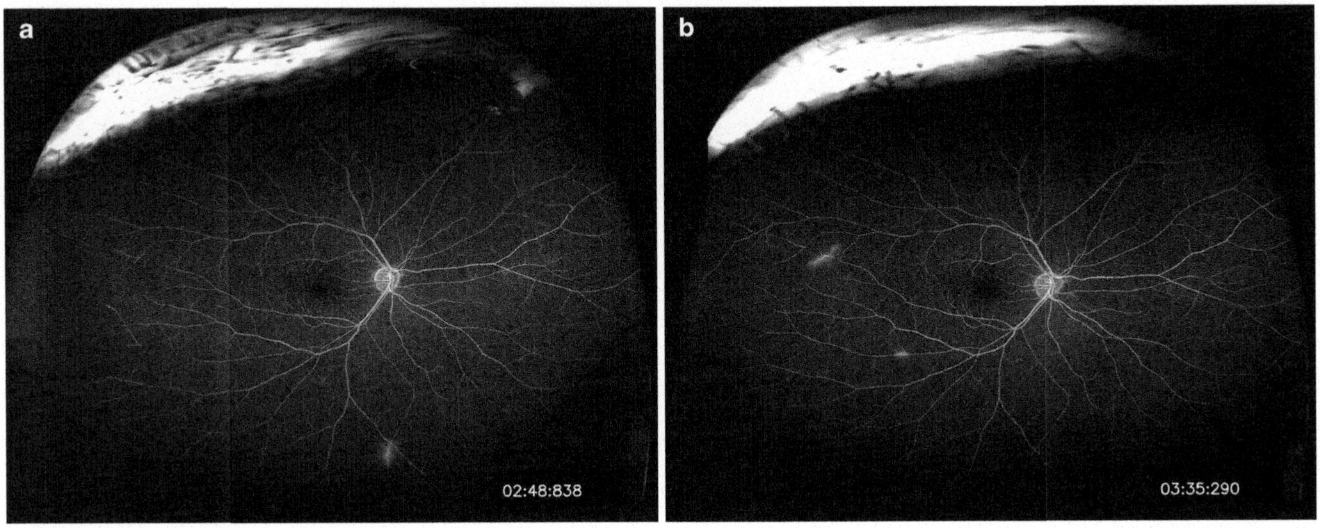

Fig. 1 (**a**) Wide-field fluorescein angiogram shows focal areas of nonperfusion in the inferotemporal arterioles with hyperfluorescent walls and areas of leakage. (**b**) Later frames of the same patient show more temporal leakage

Birdshot Choroidopathy (Figs. 2, 3, 4, 5, 6 and 7)

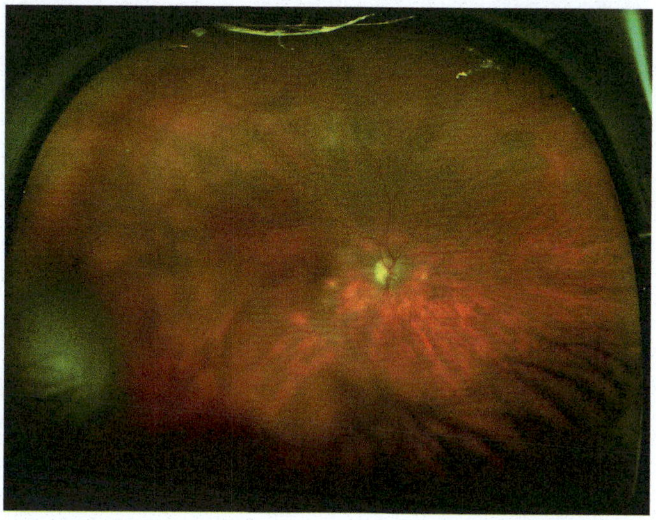

Fig. 2 Wide-field color fundus photograph of the right eye of a 62-year-old human leukocyte antigen (HLA)-A29–positive woman shows a few cream-colored ovoid chorioretinal lesions and a Retisert implant temporally

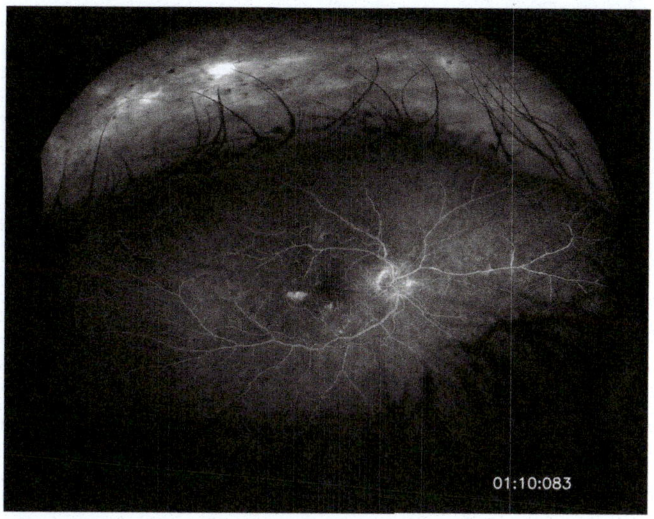

Fig. 4 Wide-field fluorescein angiogram of the right eye shows peripapillary and vascular leakage. Also apparent is the mottled hyperfluorescence of the peripheral chorioretinal changes

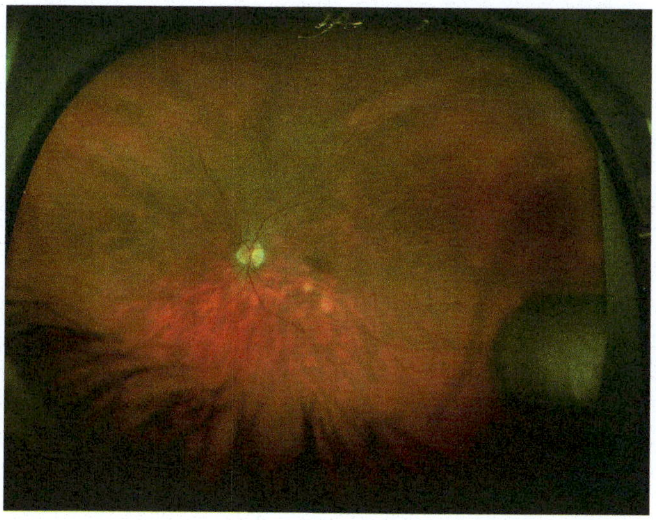

Fig. 3 Wide-field color fundus photograph of the left eye shows more chorioretinal lesions, peripapillary atrophy, and a Retisert implant temporally

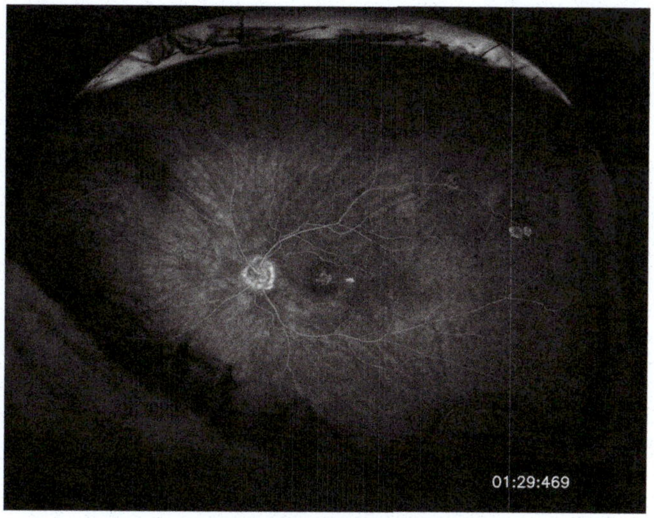

Fig. 5 Wide-field fluorescein angiogram of the left eye shows staining of the peripapillary atrophy and temporal lesions

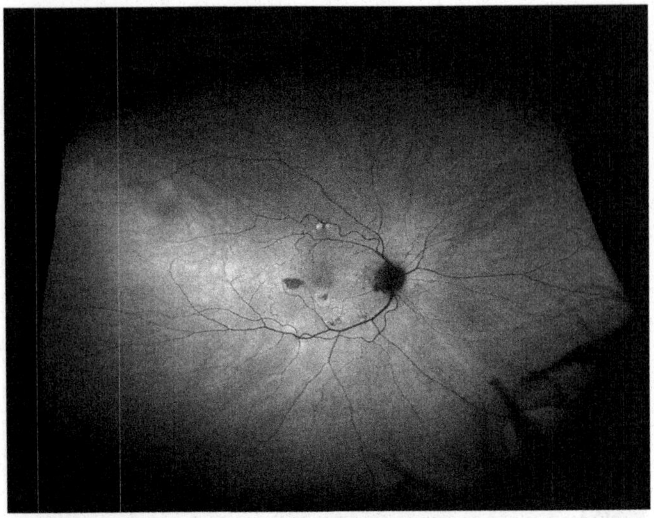

Fig. 6 Wide-field autofluorescence of the right eye shows hypofluorescence of the central lesions and mottled hyperfluorescence with the peripheral mottled hyperfluorescence

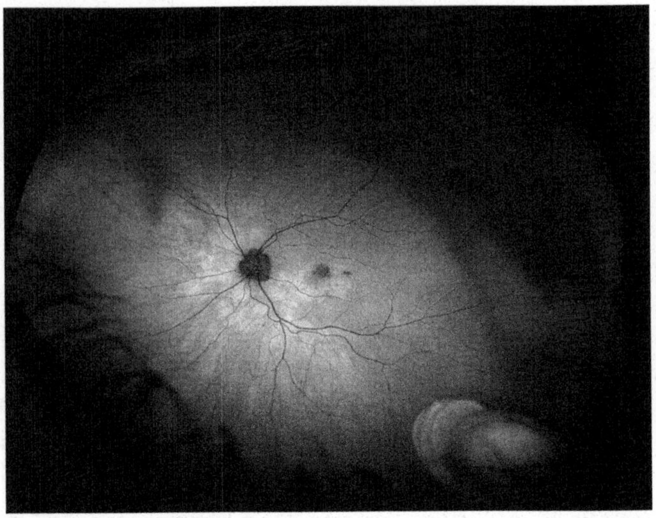

Fig. 7 Autofluorescence of the left eye shows more prominent peripheral changes

Serpiginous Choroiditis (Figs. 8 and 9)

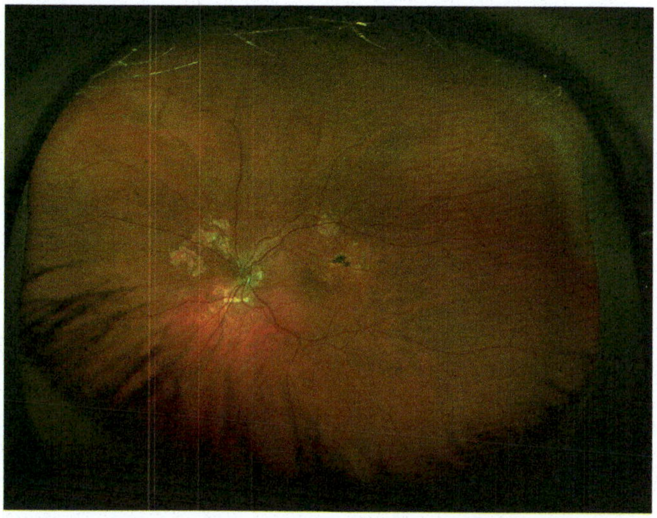

Fig. 8 Wide-field color fundus photograph shows peripapillary chorioretinal atrophy extending nasally

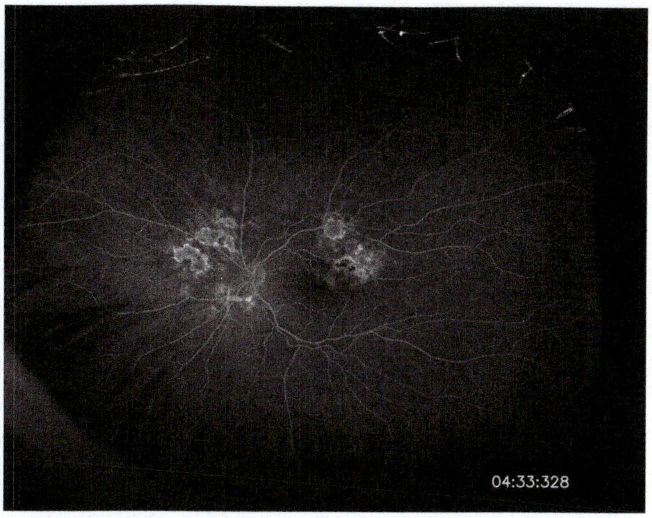

Fig. 9 Wide-field fluorescein angiogram shows staining of the areas of chorioretinal lesion

Multifocal Choroiditis and Panuveitis (MCP) (Figs. 10 and 11)

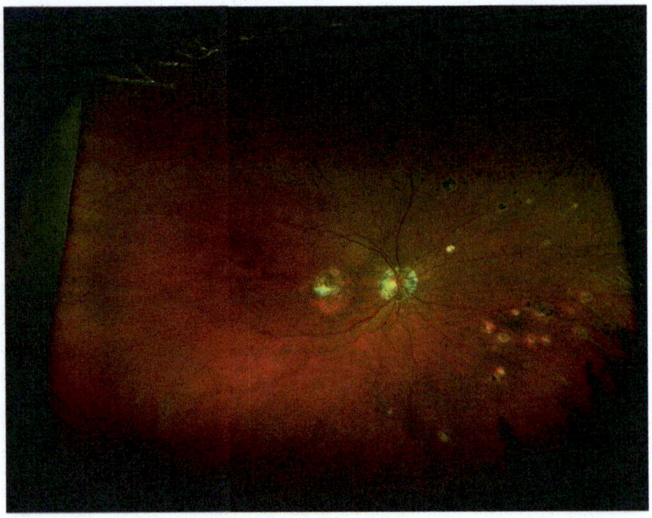

Fig. 10 A 61-year-old woman with MCP with foveal, subretinal fibrosis from a previous choroidal neovascularization and multiple peripheral punched-out white yellow spots with varying degrees of pigmentation

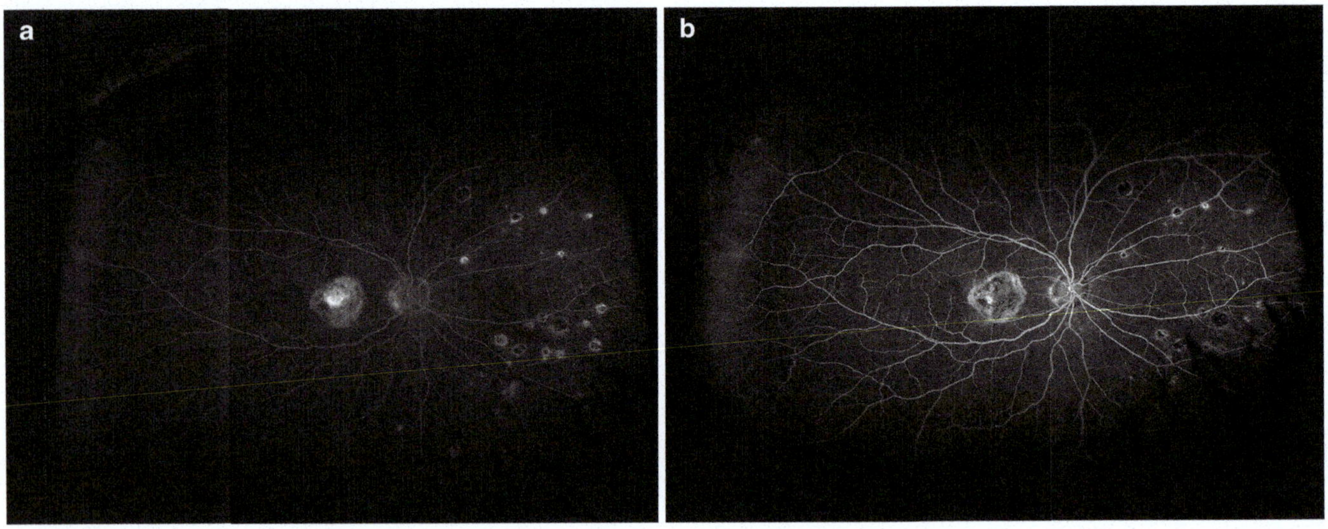

Fig. 11 Wide-field fluorescein angiogram shows staining of the central subretinal fibrosis and chorioretinal lesions in the AV phase (**a**) increasing in the later phase (**b**)

Punctate Inner Choroiditis (Figs. 12, 13 and 14)

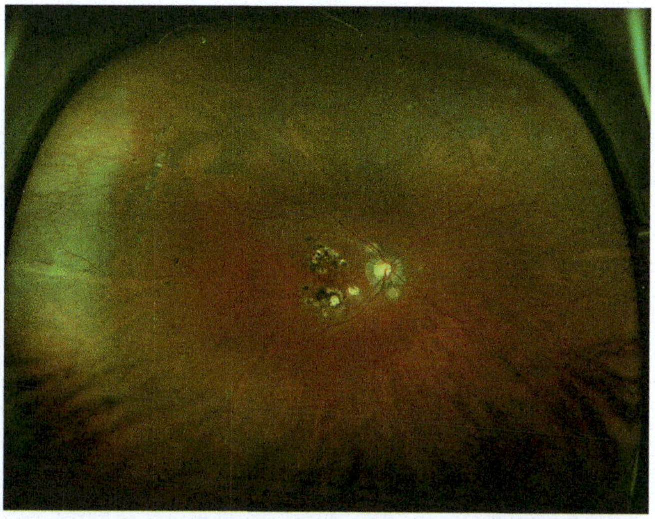

Fig. 12 Punctate inner choroiditis in a 36-year-old woman with multiple deep, punched-out atrophic lesions centrally and several smaller lesions in the temporal mid periphery

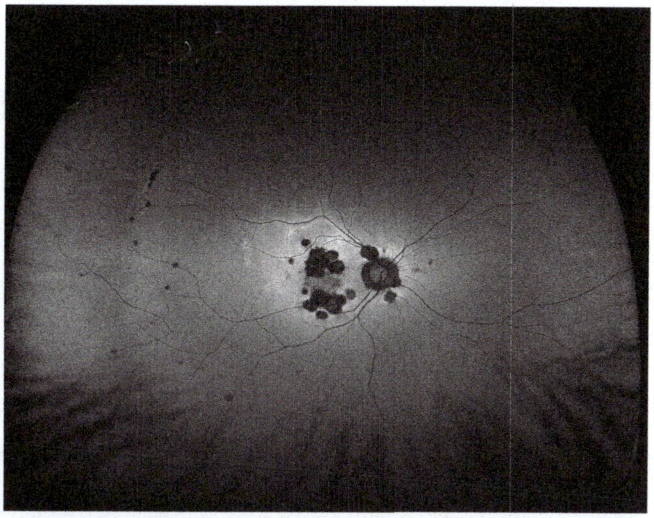

Fig. 14 Wide-field fundus autofluorescence shows decreased fluorescence of the central, peripapillary, and smaller temporal lesions

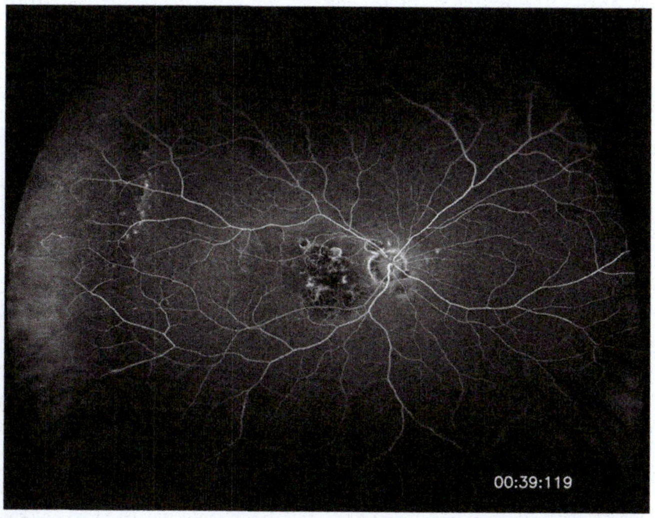

Fig. 13 Wide-field fluorescein angiogram shows blocked fluorescence from the scaring centrally and late, linear staining of the lesions

Acute Zonal Occult Outer Retinopathy (Figs. 15, 16, 17, 18, 19 and 20)

A 78-year-old woman with constricted visual fields and depressed rod and cone function on electroretinography.

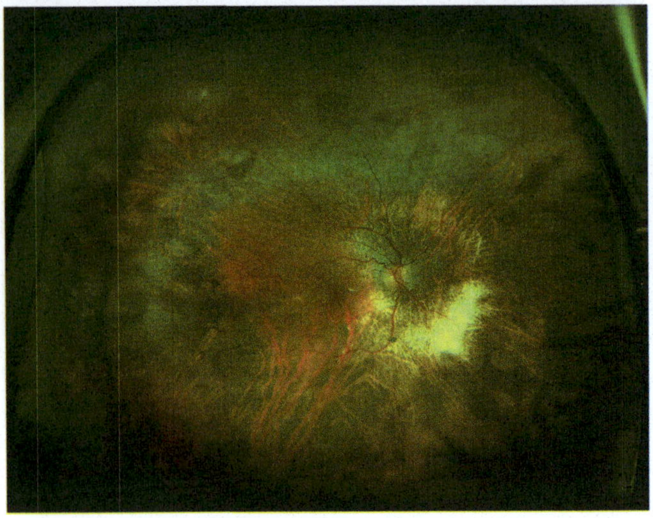

Fig. 15 Wide-field color fundus photograph shows extensive peripheral retinal pigment epithelium (RPE) changes as well as peripapillary RPE changes

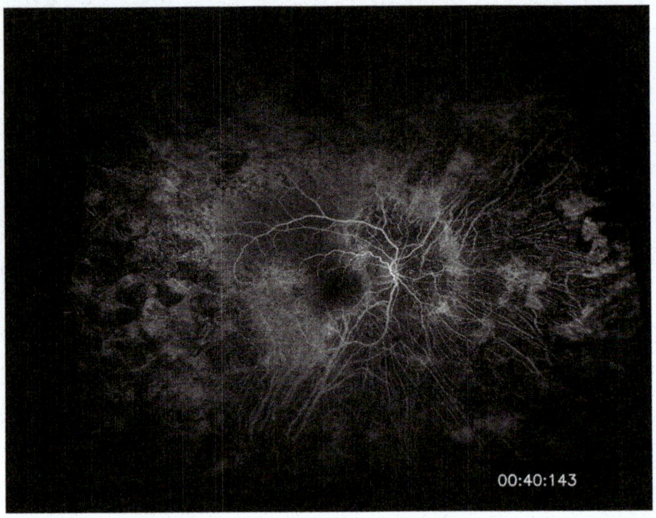

Fig. 17 Early-phase wide-field fluorescein angiogram of the right eye shows areas of peripheral hyperfluorescence corresponding to RPE atrophy and hypofluorescence corresponding to area RPE pigment clumping

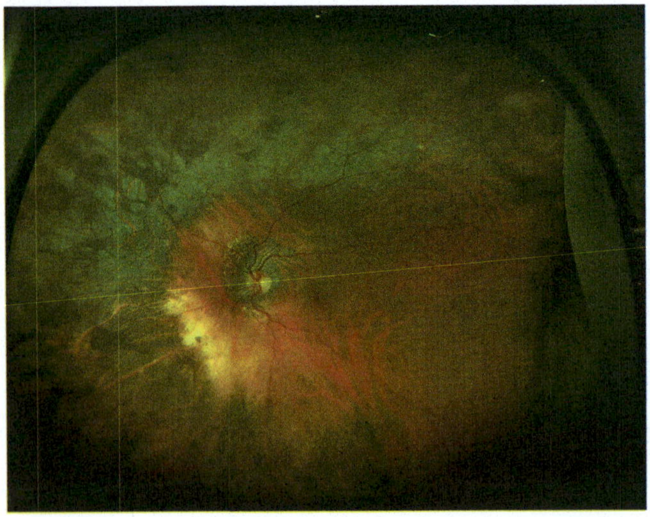

Fig. 16 The left eye in the same patient shows similar changes to the peripapillary and peripheral RPE

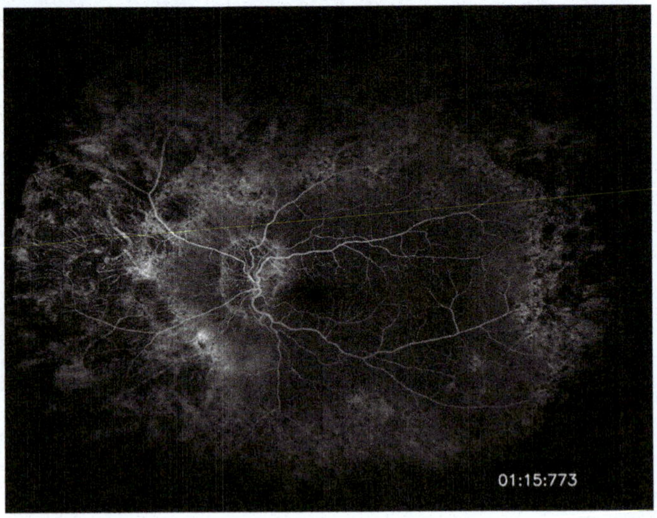

Fig. 18 Early-phase wide-field fluorescein angiogram of the left eye shows similar findings in the periphery

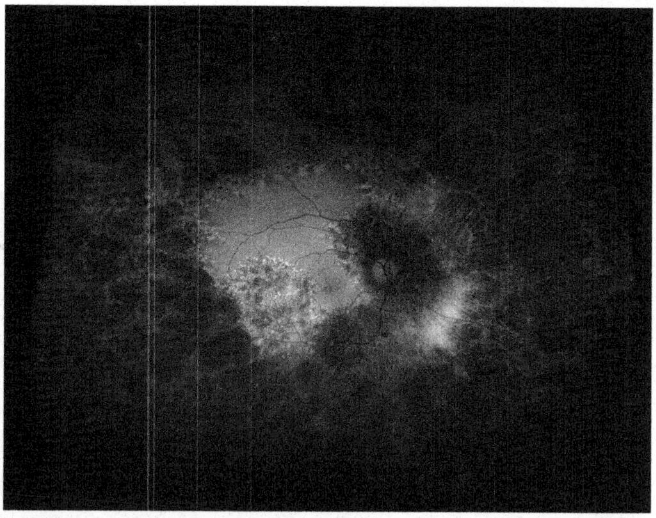

Fig. 19 Wide-field autofluorescence of the right eye shows extensive loss of peripheral and peripapillary autofluorescence corresponding to areas of RPE atrophy

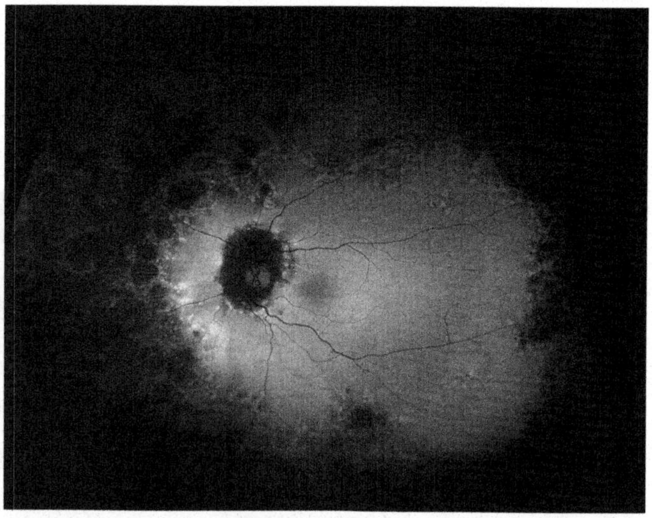

Fig. 20 Wide-field autofluorescence of the left eye shows less central involvement

Panuveitis

Sarcoidosis (Figs. 21, 22, 23, 24, 25 and 26)
A 56-year-old African American woman with lung as well as bilateral ocular involvement of sarcoidosis.

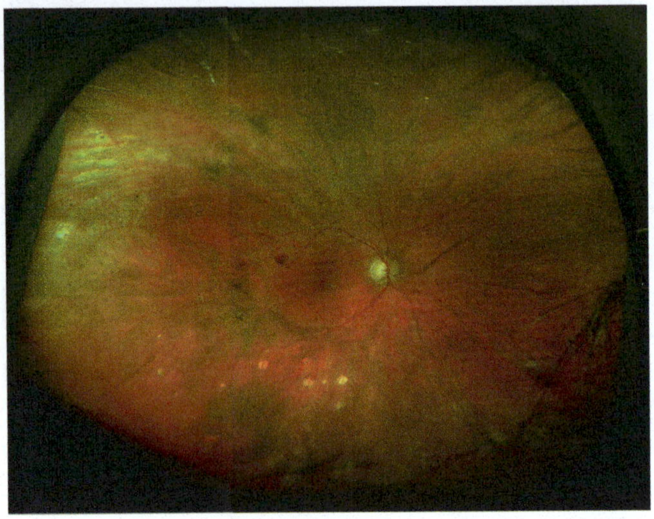

Fig. 21 Wide-field color fundus photograph of the right eye shows peripheral punctate chorioretinal lesions, vascular sclerosis and attenuation, and hemorrhage along the superior arcade

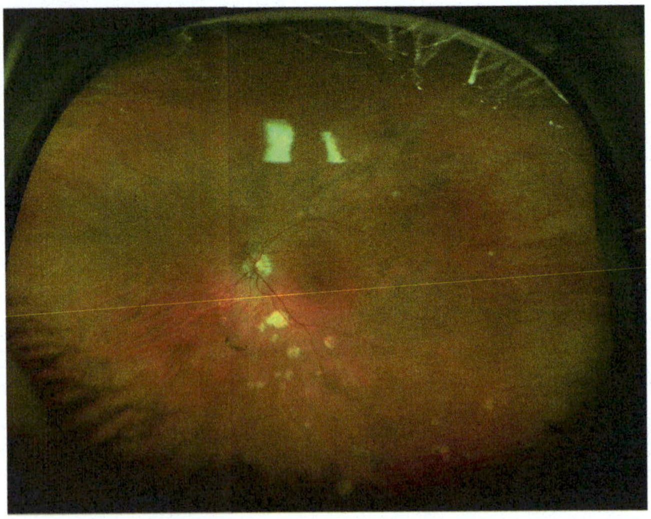

Fig. 22 Wide-field color fundus photograph of the left eye shows more punched-out peripheral chorioretinal lesions

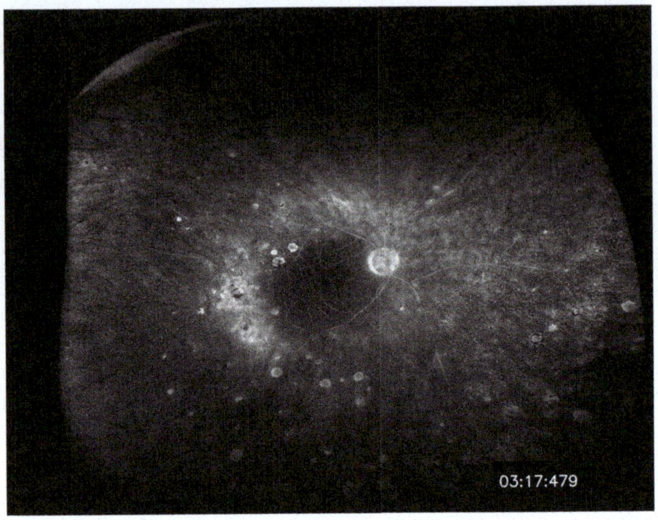

Fig. 23 Late-phase wide-field fluorescein angiogram of the right eye shows staining of the chorioretinal scars

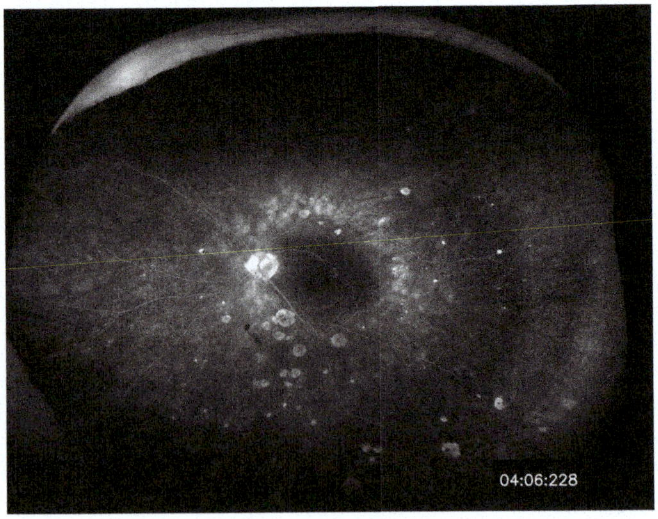

Fig. 24 Late-phase wide-field fluorescein angiogram of the left eye shows similar staining

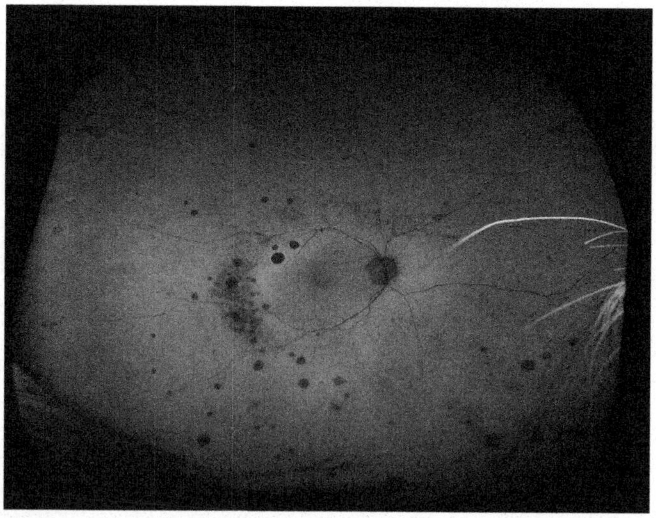

Fig. 25 Wide-field autofluorescence of the right eye shows an area of hypofluorescence corresponding to the chorioretinal lesions highlighting small lesions in the periphery not readily distinguished on the color photographs

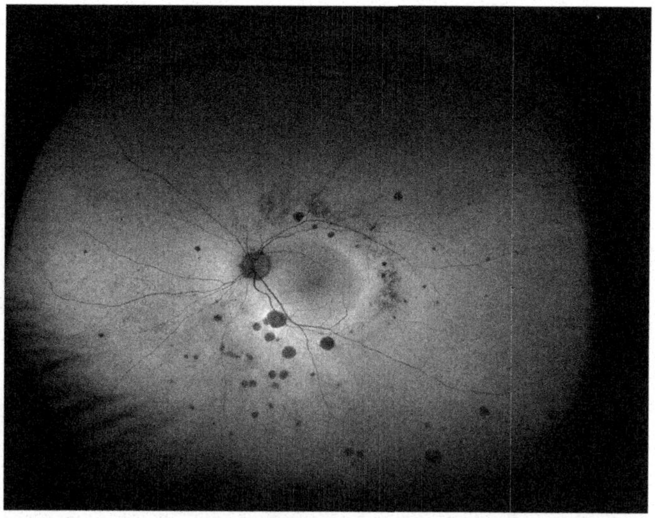

Fig. 26 Wide-field autofluorescence of the left eye shows similar areas of hypofluorescence corresponding to the chorioretinal lesions

Vogt-Koyangi-Harada (Figs. 27, 28 and 29)

A 46-year-old Asian woman with hearing loss and vitiligo.

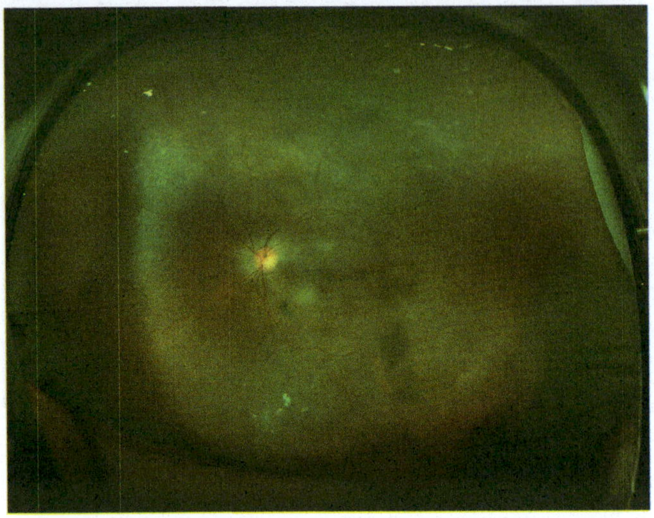

Fig. 27 Wide-field color fundus photograph of the left eye shows a dense vitritis, disc hyperemia, and chorioretinal lesions

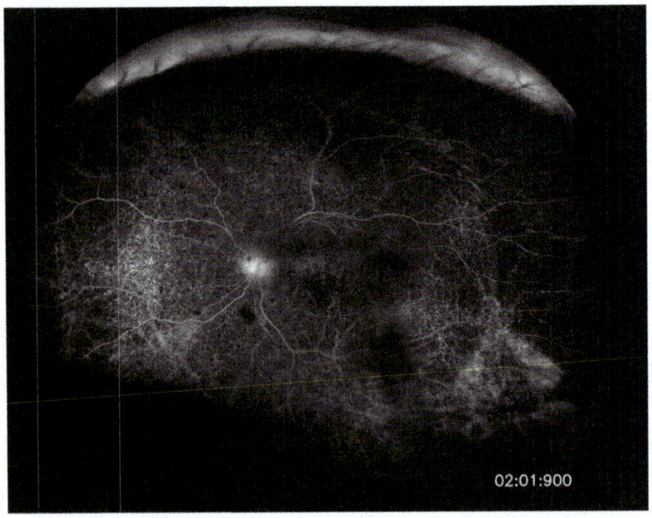

Fig. 28 Wide-field fluorescein angiogram of the left eye shows diffuse perivascular leakage and disc leakage

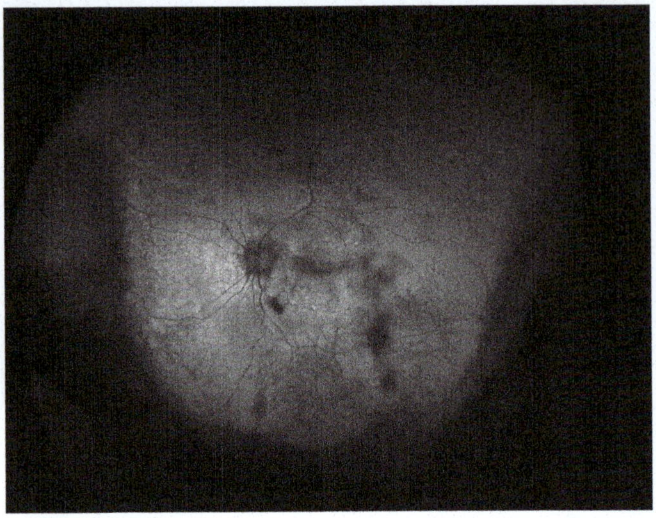

Fig. 29 Wide-field autofluorescence of the left eye shows hypofluorescence that corresponds to the chorioretinal lesions seen in the color fundus photographs

Amandiates-Behçet Disease (Figs. 30, 31, 32 and 33)

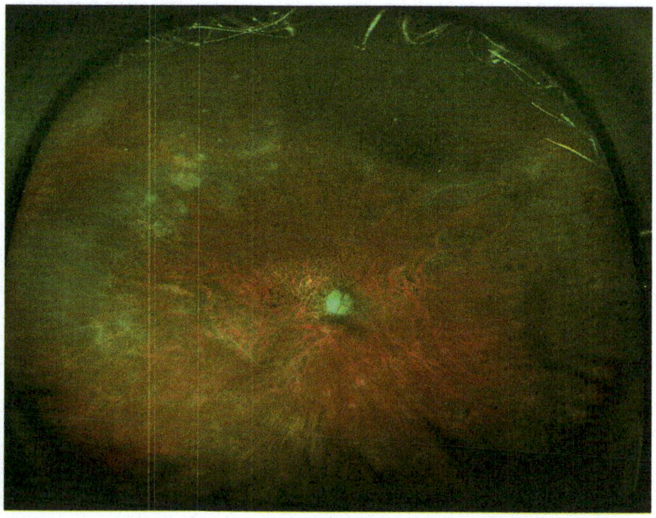

Fig. 30 A 48-year-old man with a diagnosis of Amandiates-Behçet. Wide-field color photographs of the right eye show arterial attenuation, chronic perivascular sheathing, optic nerve pallor, and diffuse retinal atrophy

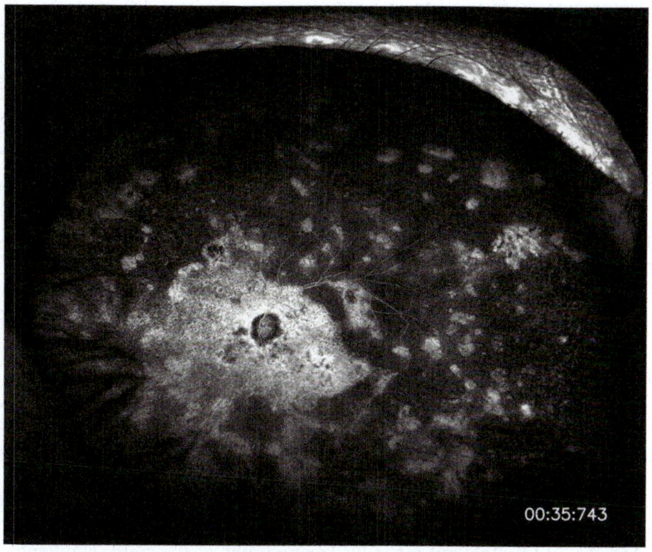

Fig. 32 Mid-phase wide-field fluorescein angiogram shows areas of hyperfluorescence consistent with window defects from retinal atrophy and areas of hypofluorescence corresponding to areas of nonperfusion

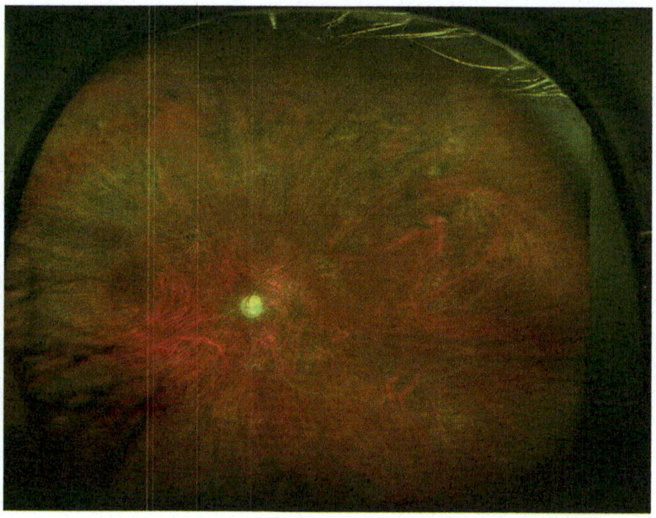

Fig. 31 Wide-field color photographs of the left eye also highlight arterial attenuation, chronic perivascular sheathing, optic nerve pallor, and retinal atrophy

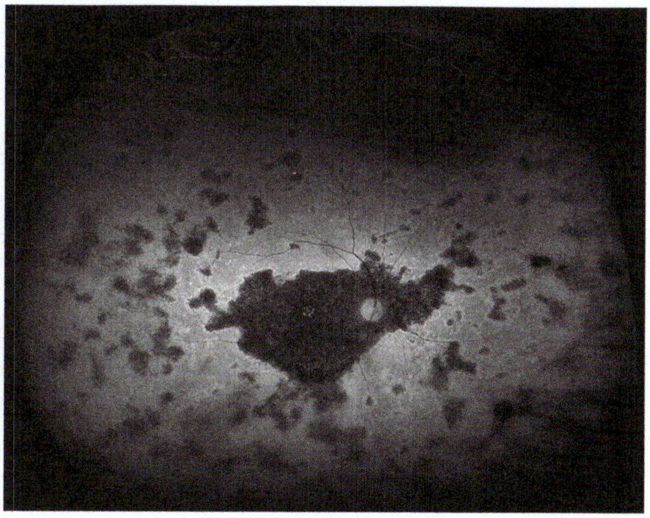

Fig. 33 Wide-field autofluorescence of the right eye shows patchy loss of autofluorescence peripherally and a more confluent loss centrally corresponding to the areas of retinal atrophy

Autoimmune Retinopathy (Figs. 34, 35, 36, 37, 38 and 39)

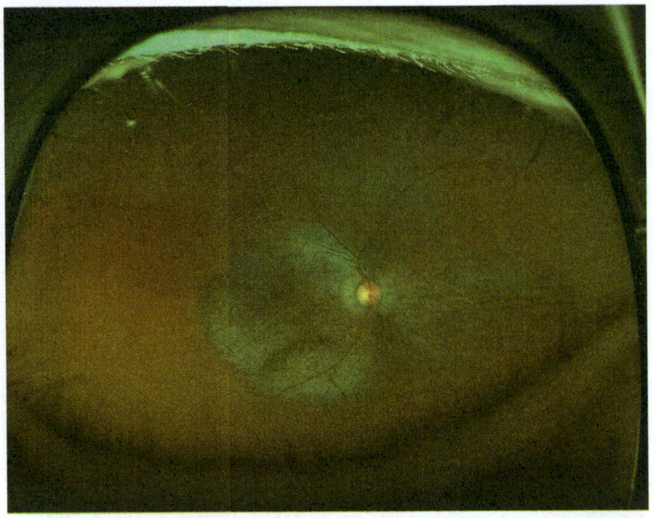

Fig. 34 Wide-field color fundus photographs of the right eye display central RPE changes and retinal pigment changes extending into the nasal and superior periphery

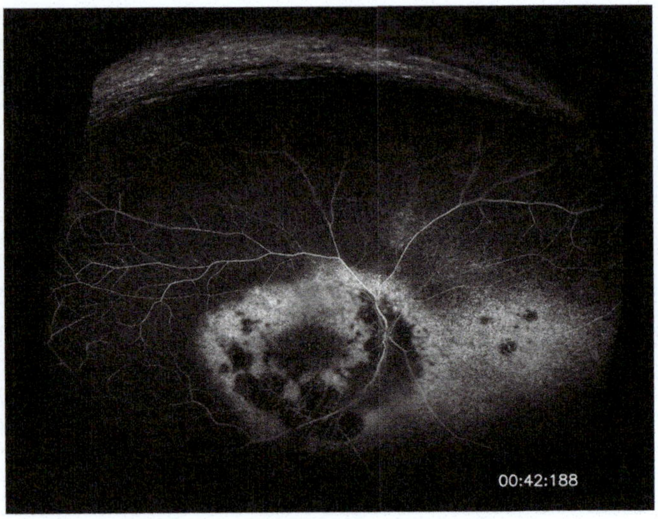

Fig. 36 Mid-phase wide-field fluorescein angiogram of the right eye shows hypofluorescence around the optic nerve and inferior arcade and mottled hyperfluorescence corresponding to the areas of retinal hypopigmentation

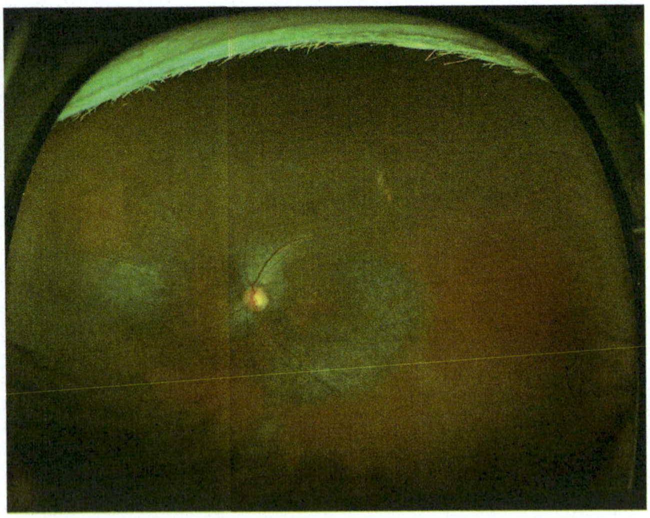

Fig. 35 Wide-field color fundus photographs of the left eye display similar RPE and pigmentary changes in the central macula and nasal periphery

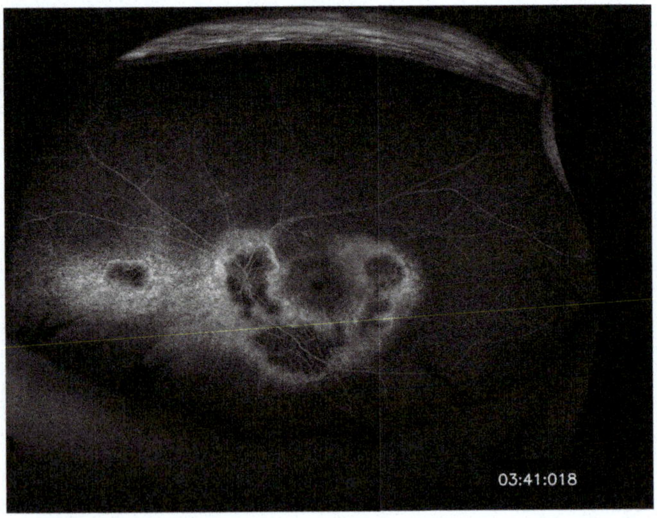

Fig. 37 Mid-phase wide-field fluorescein angiogram of the left eye also shows hypofluorescence around the optic nerve and inferior arcade and mottled hyperfluorescence

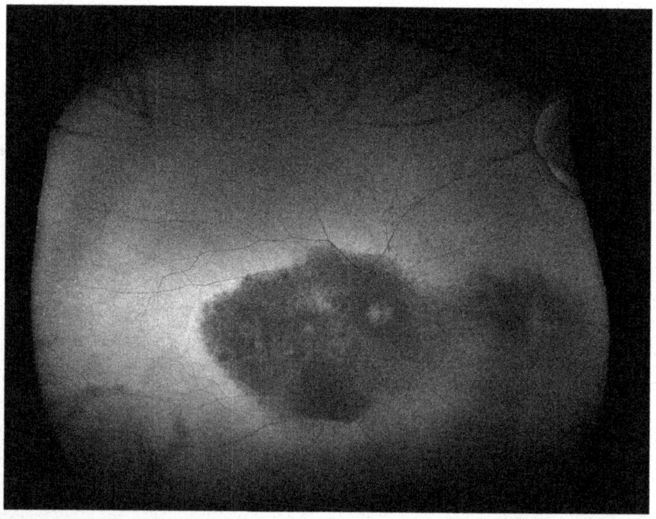

Fig. 38 Wide-field fundus autofluorescence of the right eye highlights the areas of RPE changes

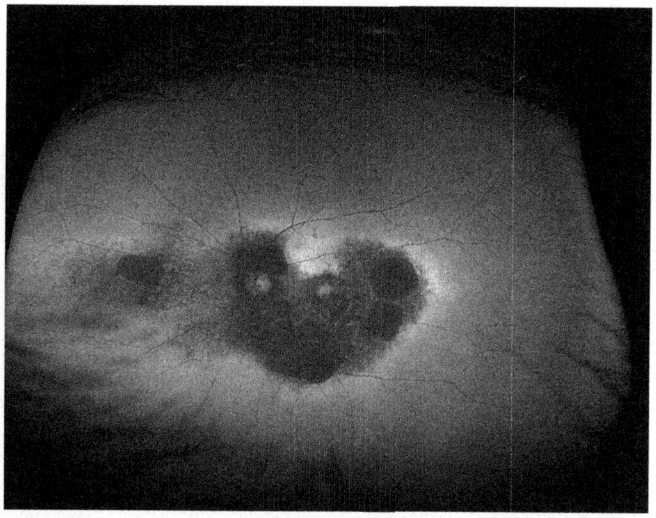

Fig. 39 Wide-field fundus autofluorescence of the left eye shows decreased autofluorescence along the inferior arcade and in the nasal periphery

Infectious Uveitis

Bacterial Tuberculosis (Figs. 40, 41 and 42)

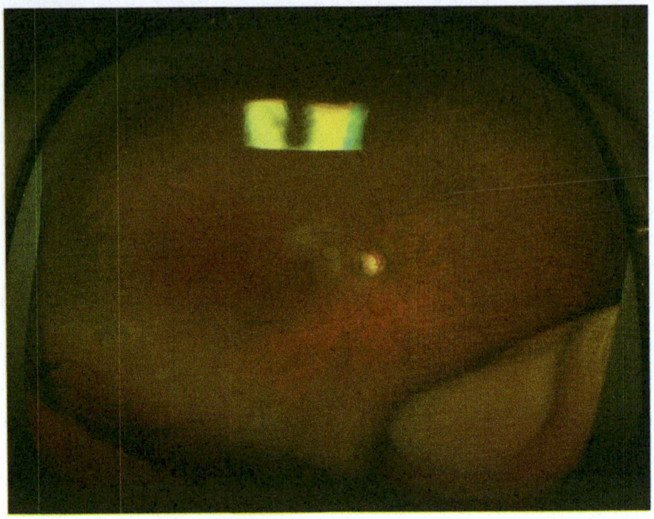

Fig. 40 A 78-year-old man was diagnosed with tuberculosis. Wide-field fundus photographs of the right eye show a solitary chorioretinal lesion in the temporal periphery

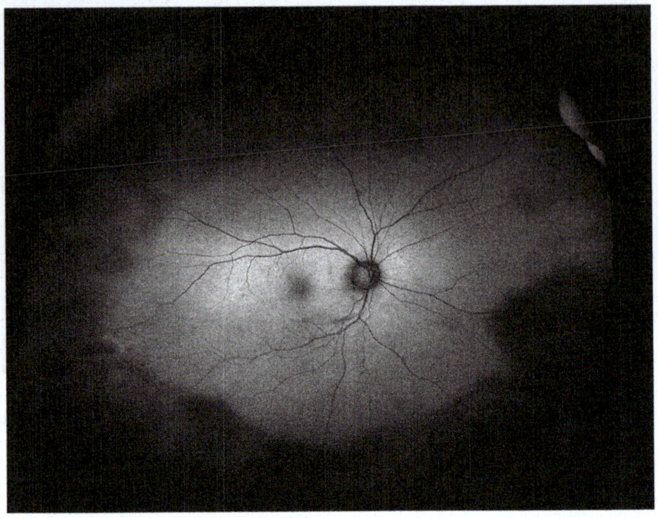

Fig. 42 Wide-field autofluorescence of the right eye shows hypofluorescence corresponding to the chorioretinal lesion

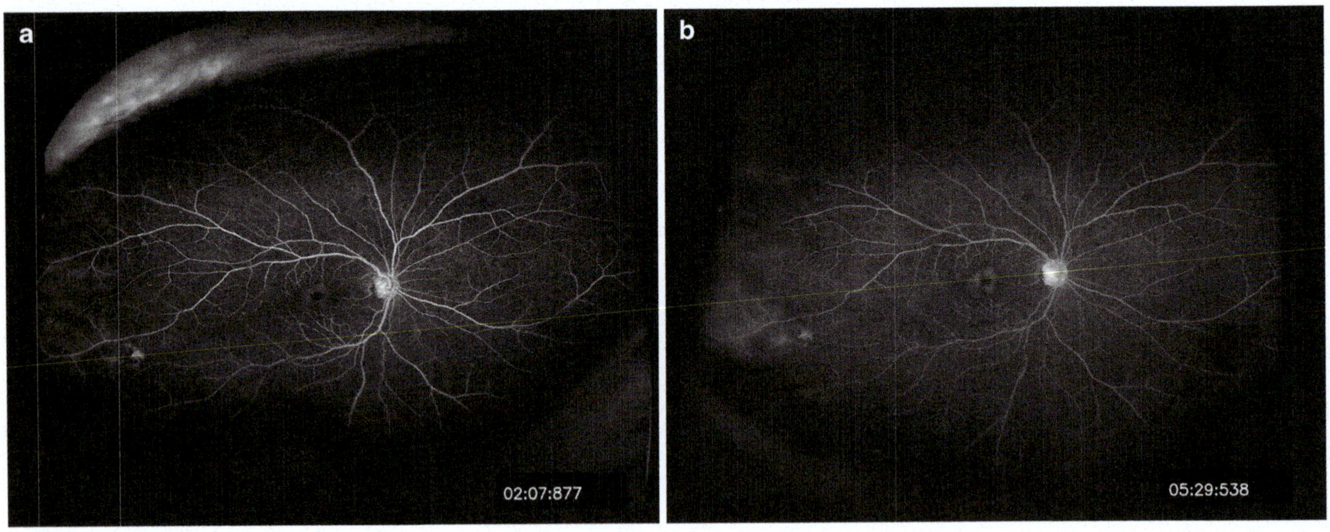

Fig. 41 (**a**) Wide-field fluorescein angiogram of the right eye shows early leakage perifoveally and in the temporal periphery. (**b**) Wide-field fluorescein angiogram of the left eye shows increased late leakage perifoveally and in the temporal periphery as well as staining of the temporal chorioretinal lesion

Syphilis (Figs. 43, 44, 45, 46 and 47)

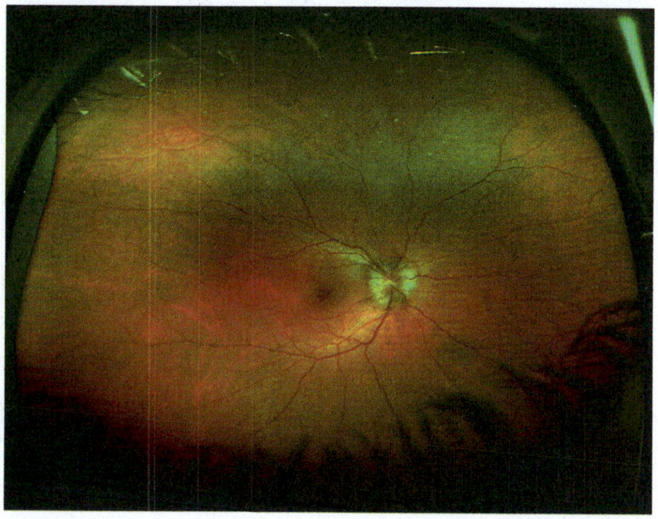

Fig. 43 A 40-year-old woman with bilateral uveitis that tested positive for syphilis. Wide-field color fundus photograph of the right eye shows prominent optic disc edema

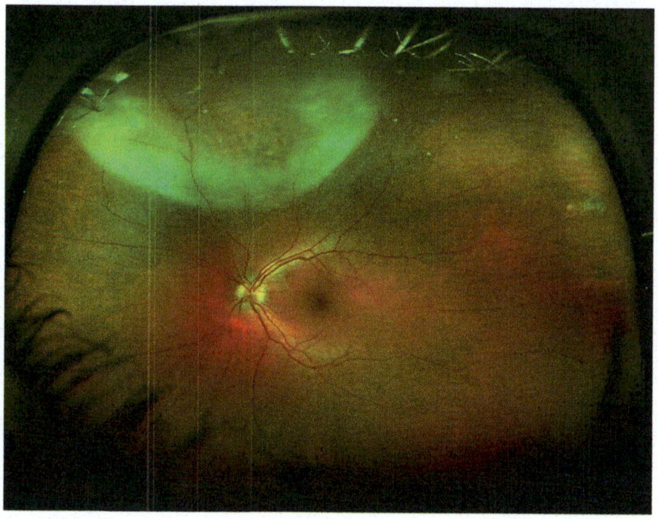

Fig. 44 Wide-field color photograph of the left eye shows peripheral chorioretinitis and optic disc edema

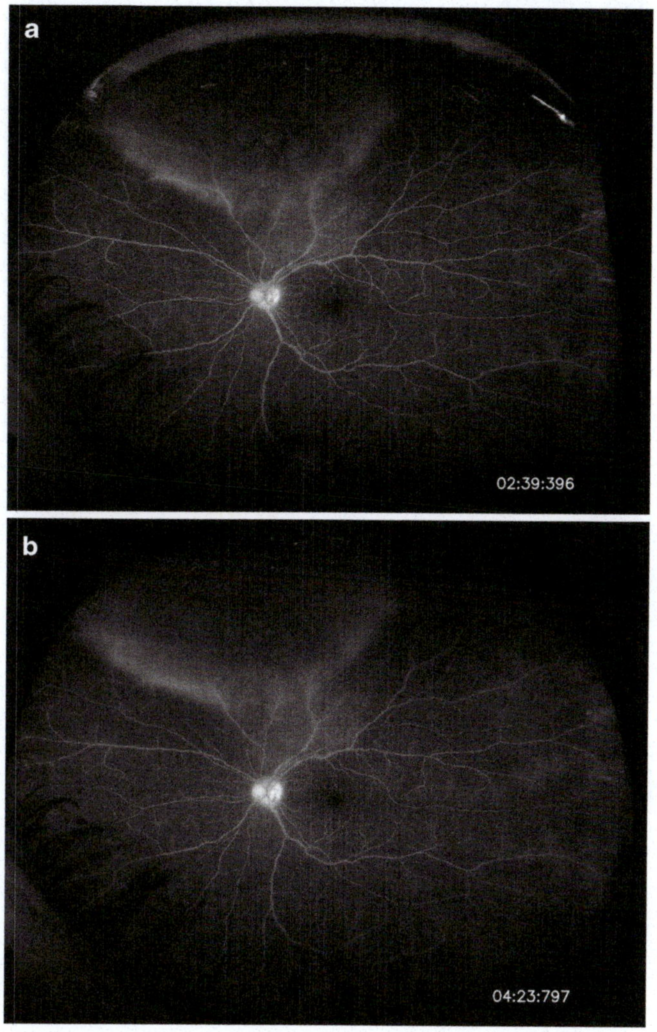

Fig. 45 (**a**) Wide-field fluorescein angiogram of the left eye shows early hyperfluorescence of superonasal periphery corresponding the area of chorioretinitis. (**b**) Wide-field fluorescein angiogram of the left eye shows late hyperfluorescence of the chorioretinitis and of the disc

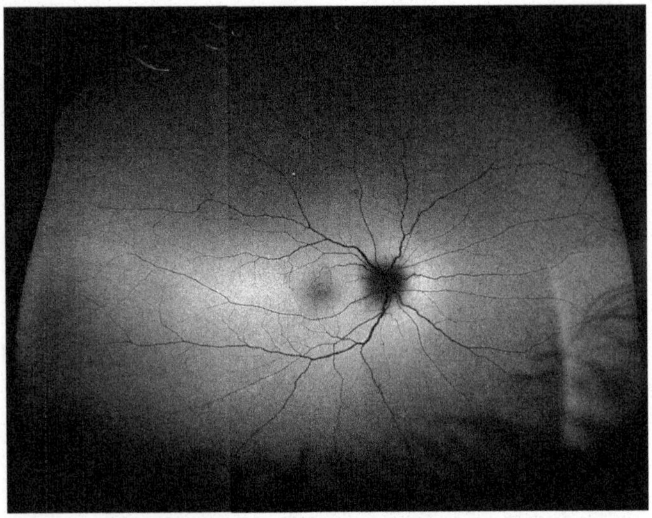

Fig. 46 Wide-field autofluorescence shows relative sparing of the RPE

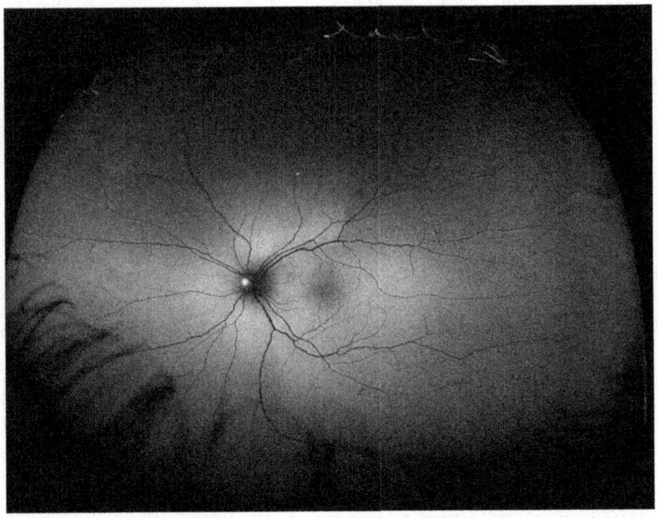

Fig. 47 Wide-field autofluorescence shows relative sparing of the RPE

Ocular Histoplasmosis Syndrome (Figs. 48, 49 and 50)

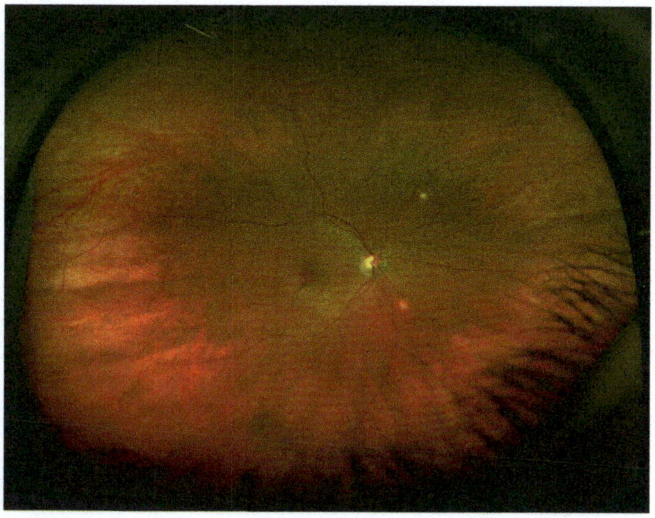

Fig. 48 Wide-field color fundus photographs of the right eye show several yellow-gray deep choroidal lesions and CNV along the inferotemporal arcade

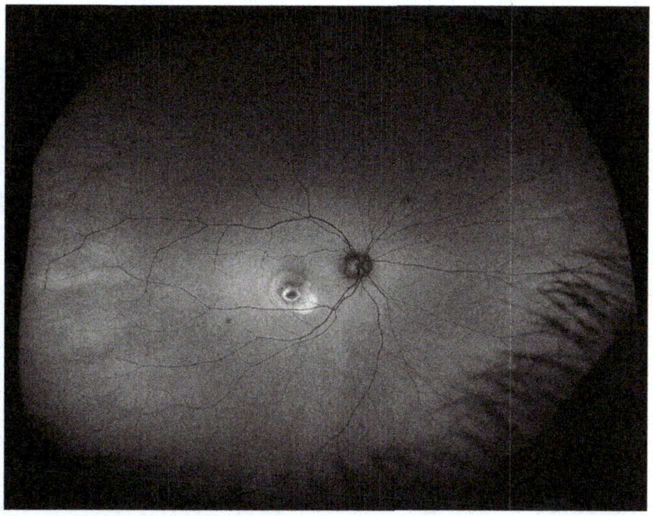

Fig. 50 Wide-field autofluorescence of the right eye shows a central area of hypoautofluorescence, a rim of hyperautofluorescence, and a surrounding area of hyperautofluorescence corresponding to the area of CNV

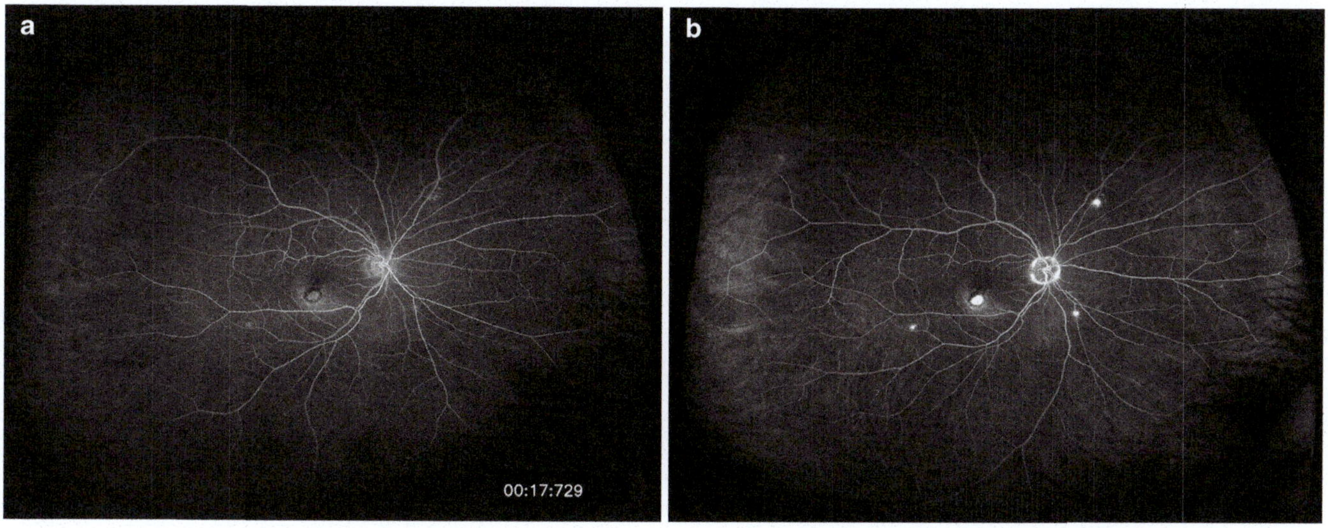

Fig. 49 (**a**) Early-phase wide-field fluorescein angiogram of the right eye shows hyperfluorescence in areas of leakage from the choroidal neovascularization. (**b**) Wide-field fluorescein angiogram of the right eye shows increased hyperfluorescence in the later phases

Cytomegalovirus (Figs. 51 and 52)

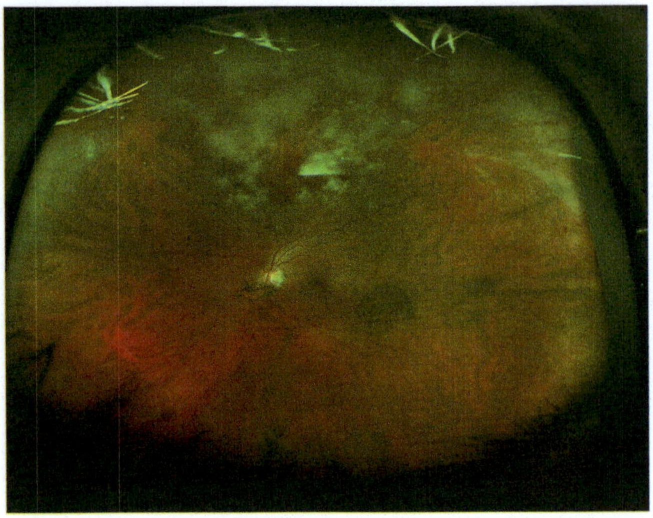

Fig. 51 Wide-field color fundus photograph of the right eye of 56-year-old man with vitritis and an area of hemorrhage and necrosis in the superior periphery

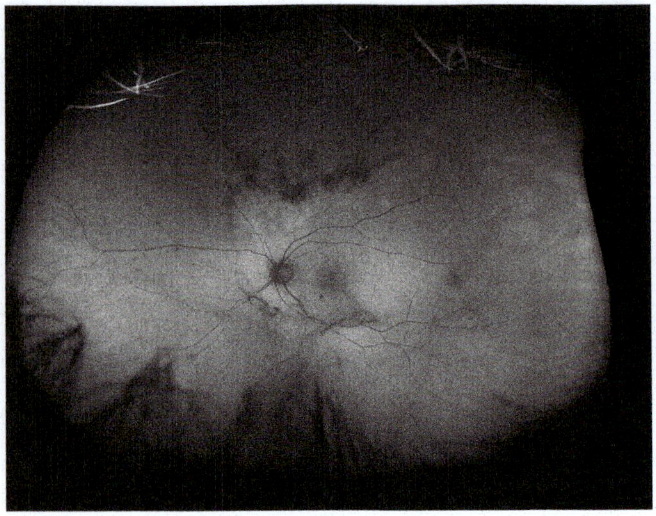

Fig. 52 Wide-field autofluorescence with an area of blocked autofluorescence corresponding to the areas of hemorrhage

Wide-Field Imaging in Infectious Uveitis

14

Alfredo Adán, Victor Llorenç, and Marina Mesquida

Introduction

Retinal and choroidal infectious diseases can be challenging to diagnose and treat. Diagnosis often requires careful clinical examination of the peripheral retina. Ultra-wide field (UWF) technology may add significantly to the sensitivity of detecting the presence of disease activity. Posterior uveitis can be associated with significant changes in the peripheral retina that may be missed by conventional, narrow-field fluorescein angiograms. However, those peripheral findings can be easily visualized using UWF fluorescein angiography (FA), which has been reported to be more useful than traditional FA and can be particularly helpful in following up patients with uveitis. Wide-field fundus autofluorescence (FAF) images may reveal more retinal or chorioretinal abnormalities in patients with posterior uveitis, with a farther extended demarcation than wide-field composite color fundus imaging.

Herpetic Retinal Diseases

Cytomegalovirus Retinitis

Fundus examination, the most common method for diagnosis in cytomegalovirus (CMV) retinitis, may reveal two characteristic fundus lesions [1]. The first one is a wedge-shaped or arcuate area of retinal infiltration that follows a vascular pattern and is often associated with intraretinal hemorrhages ("pizza fundus"). The other characteristic fundus appearance of CMV retinitis is seen more commonly in the retinal periphery and consists of a slowly expanding, yellow-white, granular lesion with active edges and a scarred center.

When assessing disease progression or response to therapy, important clinical findings are the size of the lesion and the appearance of its borders. Both characteristics can be evaluated and recorded with fundus photography. CMV retinitis lesions are often found in retinal periphery and they

A. Adán, MD, PhD (✉) • V. Llorenç, MD, PhD • M. Mesquida, MD, PhD
Ocular Iflammation Section,
Clínic Institute of Ophthalmology (ICOF),
Clínic Hospital of Barcelona, University of Barcelona,
Barcelona, Spain
e-mail: amadan@clinic.ub.es; llorens.victor@gmail.com;
mesquida@clinic.ub.es

I. Kozak, J.F. Arevalo (eds.), *Atlas of Wide-Field Retinal Angiography and Imaging*, DOI 10.1007/978-3-319-17864-6_14

may not be properly photographed with standard, 30° or 45° fundus camera. Standard photography missed peripheral CMV, whereas UWF imaging captured greater CMV retinitis lesion area than standard fundus montage photography (Fig. 1) [2]. The increased peripheral imaging of UWF technology may also help to assess disease progression and response to therapy in other peripheral retinal conditions (Figs. 2 and 3).

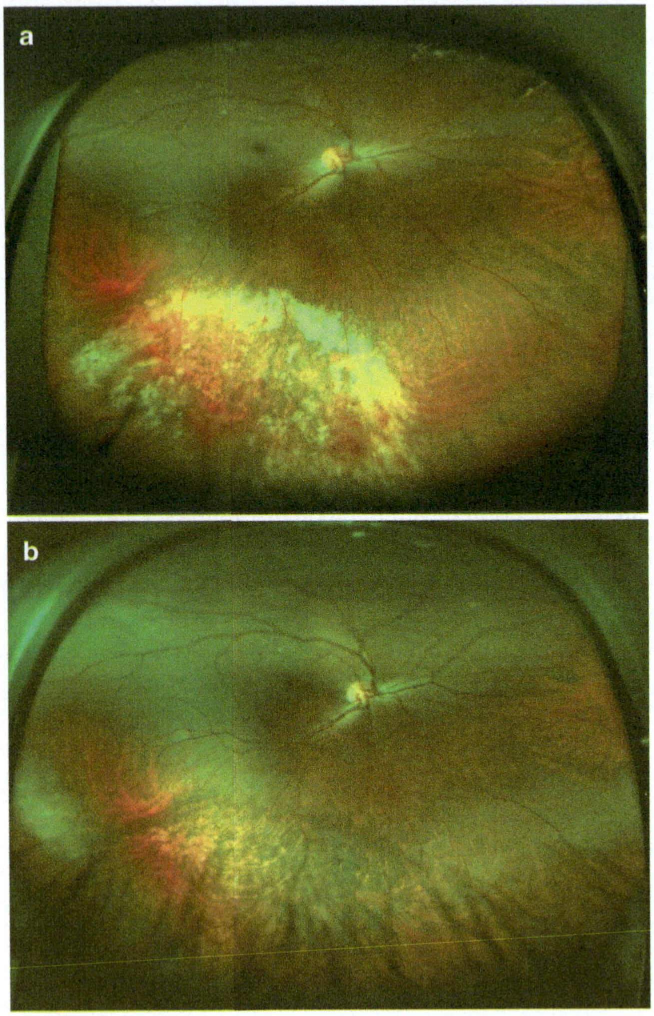

Fig. 1 An AIDS patient with peripheral, granular CMV retinitis in UWF retinography in the right eye (**a**). Lesion appearance after treatment with intravenous ganciclovir followed by oral valganciclovir (**b**)

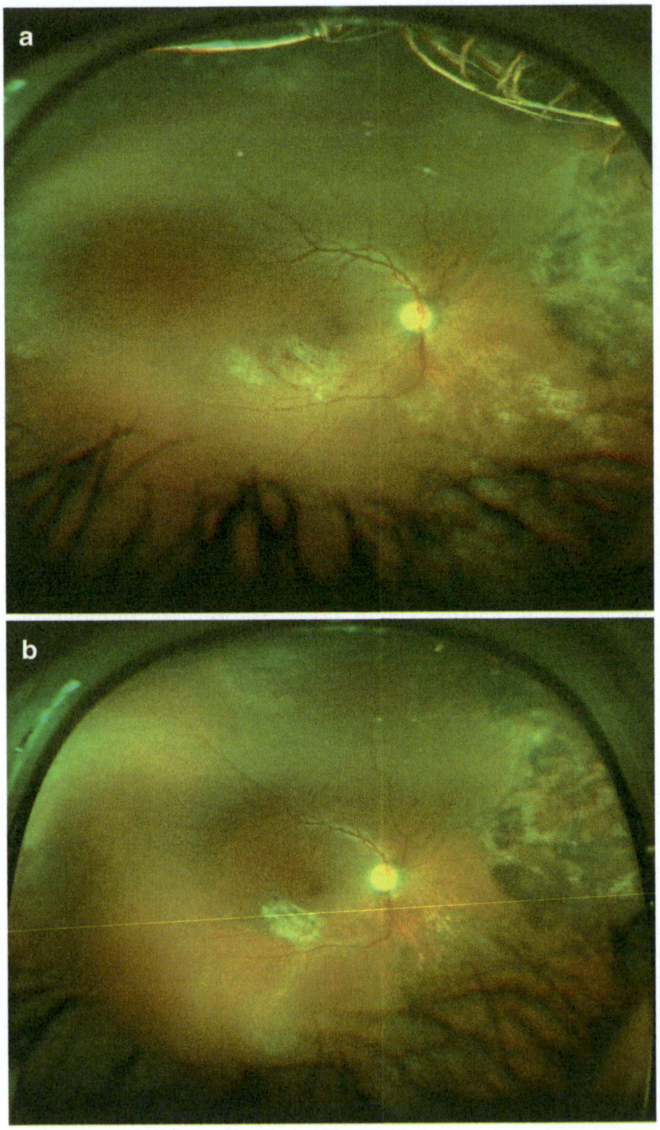

Fig. 2 A patient with chronic leukemia treated with bone marrow transplantation. UWF imaging in his right eye shows posterior active CMV retinitis and a peripheral inactive area (**a**). This patient was initially treated with intravenous ganciclovir with partial response Intravenous foscarnet was added afterward, with good response and inactivation of CMV lesions (**b**)

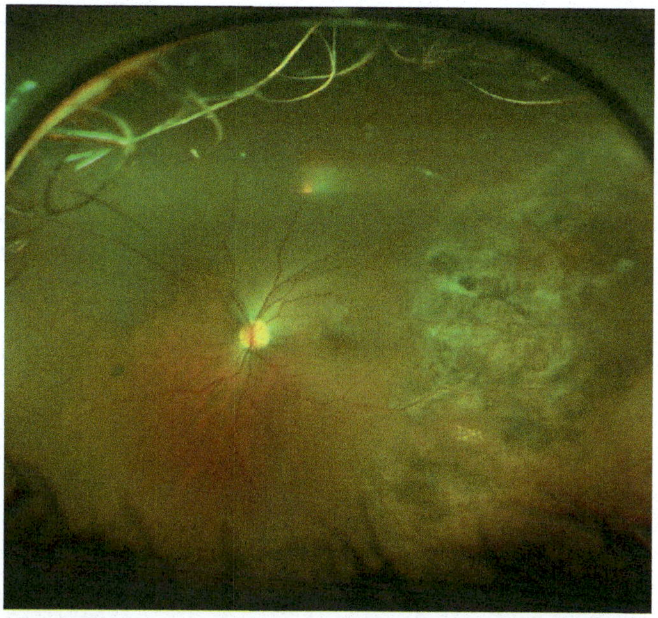

Fig. 3 UWF imaging of a patient with AIDS shows an inactive area of peripheral CMV retinitis

Immune Recovery Uveitis

Immune recovery uveitis (IRU) develops in patients with acquired immunodeficiency syndrome (AIDS) and inactive peripheral CMV retinitis that have experienced highly active antiretroviral therapy (HAART)–mediated increase in CD4+ T-lymphocyte levels. The current definition of IRU includes at least five main criteria: (1) being a patient with AIDS, (2) receiving HAART, (3) achieving an immune reconstitution indicated by increased CD4+ T cell count over 100 cells/mm^3 for at least 2 months, (4) having preexisting CMV retinitis that is currently in the inactive state, and (5) developing an intraocular inflammation that cannot be explained by drug toxicity or a new opportunistic infection [3]. IRU-related CMV retinitis is frequently localized in the periphery. UWF imaging can help detecting those peripheral CMV lesions and diagnose the IRU (Fig. 4).

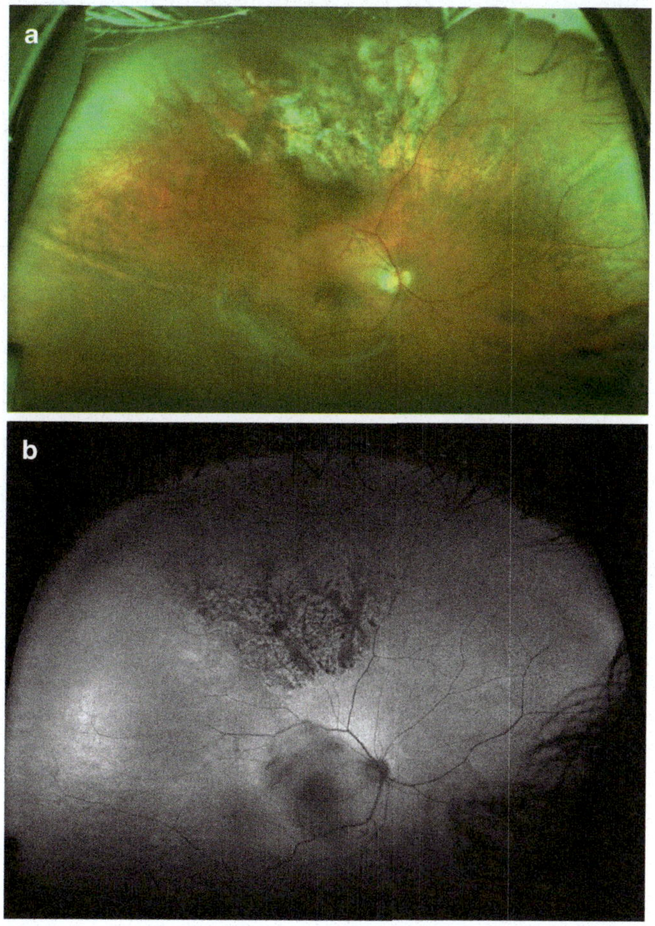

Fig. 4 An AIDS patient treated with HAART therapy. UWF fundus imaging disclosed a peripheral area of inactive CMV retinitis as well as a macular epiretinal membrane (**a**). Autofluorescence showed pigmentary changes with quiescence (**b**). This patient fulfilled IRU diagnosing criteria

Acute Retinal Necrosis

Acute retinal necrosis syndrome (ARNS) is an uncommon necrotizing, fulminant retinopathy caused by the herpes simplex virus (HSV) types 1 or 2 or by the varicella zoster virus (VZV) with visually devastating consequences. Generally, it occurs in patients who are systemically healthy, but occasionally, it appears in immunocompromised host. Examination of the posterior segment may reveal vitreous inflammation, arteritis, patchy full-thickness necrotising retinitis, and in certain cases, involvement of the optic disc. Typically, retinitis presents as either confluent or multifocal patches involving the peripheral retina. An occlusive periarteritis is often present [4].

With prompt initiation of treatment, progression of ARNS lesions can usually be halted within 2–4 weeks. As the active retinal infection and inflammation resolves, affected areas develop pigmentary changes, retinal thinning, and atrophy, often producing a scalloped appearance at the junction of involved and healthy retina (Fig. 5). Vitreous organization and traction may progress during this phase, producing retinal breaks, retinal detachment, and proliferative vitreoretinopathy. Rhegmatogenous retinal detachment occurs in a half to three-quarters of eyes with ARNS and may develop weeks to months after initial presentation of retinitis [5].

When retinal detachments do occur in the setting of ARNS, there are often both rhegmatogenous and tractional components, and management should address both contributing factors. Pars plana vitrectomy, lensectomy, scleral buckle, air-fluid exchange, endolaser, and long-acting gas or silicone oil tamponade have shown success in retinal reattachment repair and recovery of vision (Figs. 6 and 7).

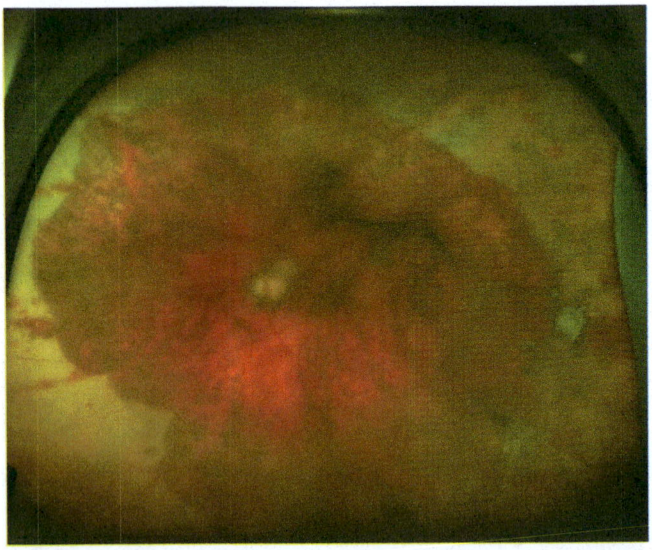

Fig. 5 A patient with a history of liver transplantation and VZV disseminated infection. He complained of visual loss in his left eye. UWF retinography showed peripheral 360° areas of active necrotizing retinitis, and vitreous cells suggestive of ARNS

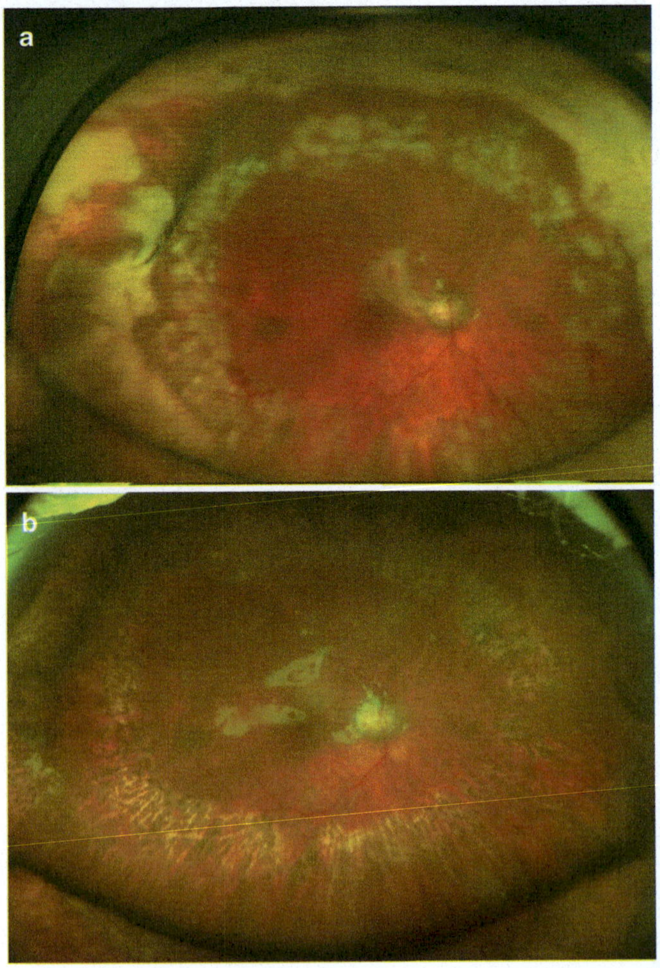

Fig. 6 UWF postoperative image of retinal detachment surgery of a patient with ARNS (**a**). The retina was attached with intravitreal silicone oil, 360° endophotocoagulation, and scleral buckle implant. The same patient's images 2 months after ocular surgery show attached retina and inactive retinitis lesions. Silicone oil had been removed (**b**)

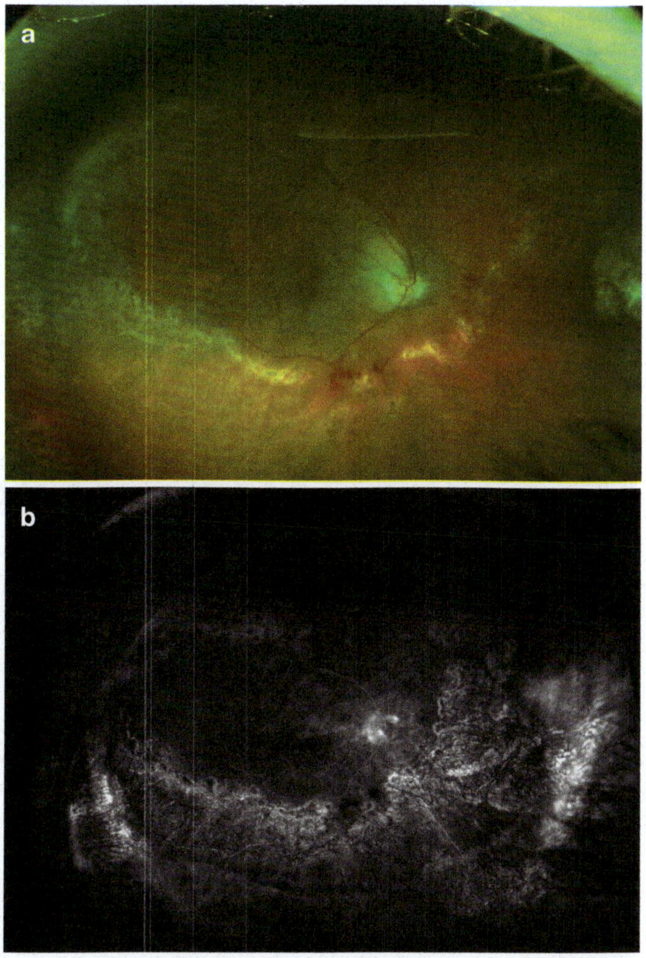

Fig. 7 UWF image of a patient diagnosed with retinal detachment secondary to ARNS (**a**). Atrophic peripheral areas of retinitis can be observed. The retina is attached. UWF-FA discloses macular edema (**b**)

Toxoplasmosis

Commonly, acute ocular toxoplasmosis appears as a well-defined focus of retinal necrosis accompanied by vitreous inflammatory reaction (Figs. 8 and 9) [6]. In addition, there is often diffuse inflammation close to retinal or choroidal tissue. Lack of visible chorioretinal scars and extensive areas of retinal involvement in immunocompromised patients can mimic ARNS or ocular lymphoma, leading to misdiagnosis of the disease (Figs. 10, 11 and 12) [7]. Retinal vasculitis may also be present associated with toxoplasmic retinitis (Fig. 13).

Retinal detachment is a severe complication that may occur in patients with ocular toxoplasmosis. The majority of retinal detachments observed in individuals with ocular toxoplasmosis are rhegmatogenous or tractional in nature. The pathogenesis of such types of retinal detachments may be associated with the severe inflammation of the vitreous that may lead to vitreous traction, causing not only the tractional but also a rhegmatogenous retinal detachment, particularly in patients in whom additional risk factors such as myopic retinal degenerations are present. Management of such complicated cases requires pars plana vitrectomy and scleral buckle and gas or silicone oil tamponade (Fig. 14) [8].

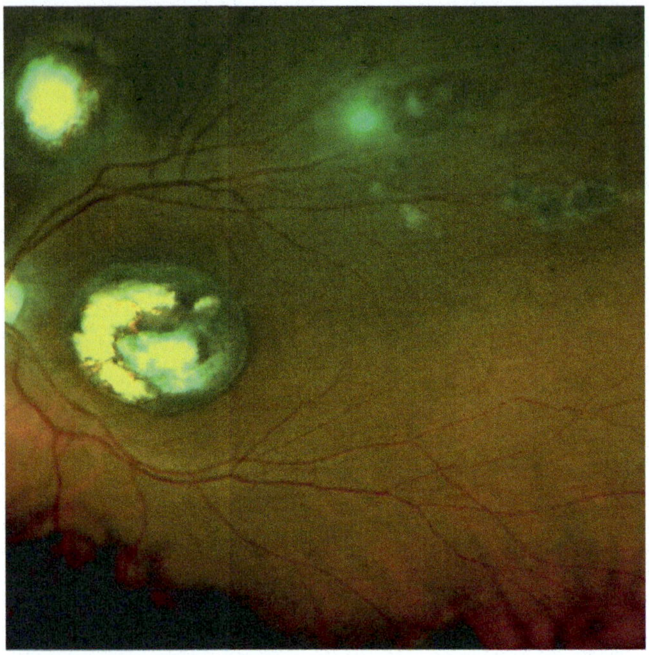

Fig. 8 UWF retinography in a patient with a history of congenital toxoplasmosis. A macular scar is observed along with other multiple retinal scars, with a new area of necrotizing retinitis

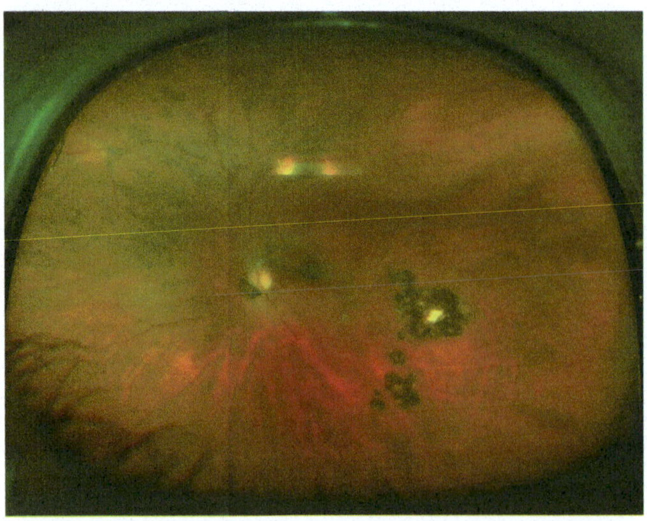

Fig. 9 UWF fundus image shows multiple areas of retinal scars located in the mid periphery in a patient with recurrent ocular toxoplasmosis

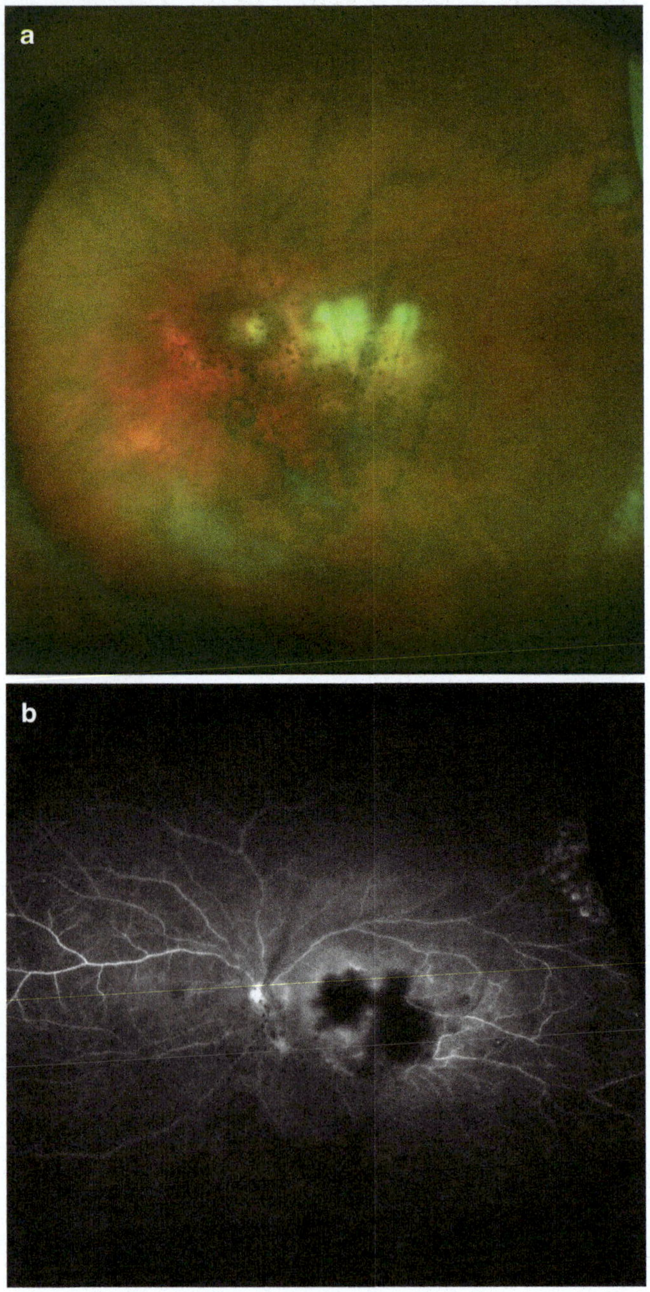

Fig. 10 UWF pseudocolor imaging of a 72-year-old man shows a large area of macular retinitis and vitreous cells (**a**). Macular hypofluorescence was noted with UWF-FA (**b**)

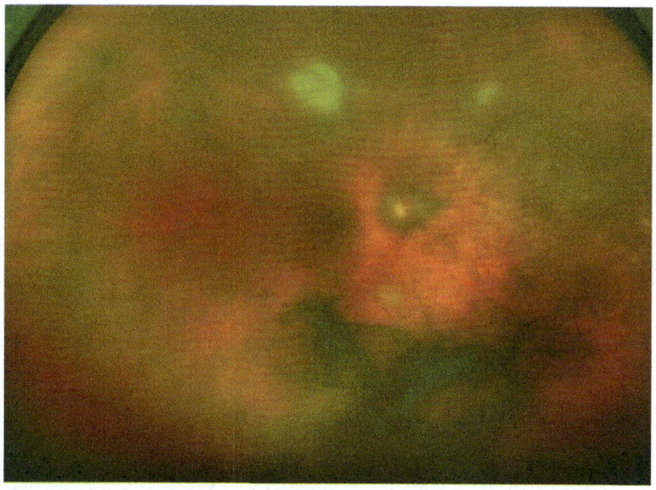

Fig. 11 UWF retinography shows multiple areas of toxoplasmic peripheral necrotizing retinitis and vitreous cells in a patient with splenic lymphoma

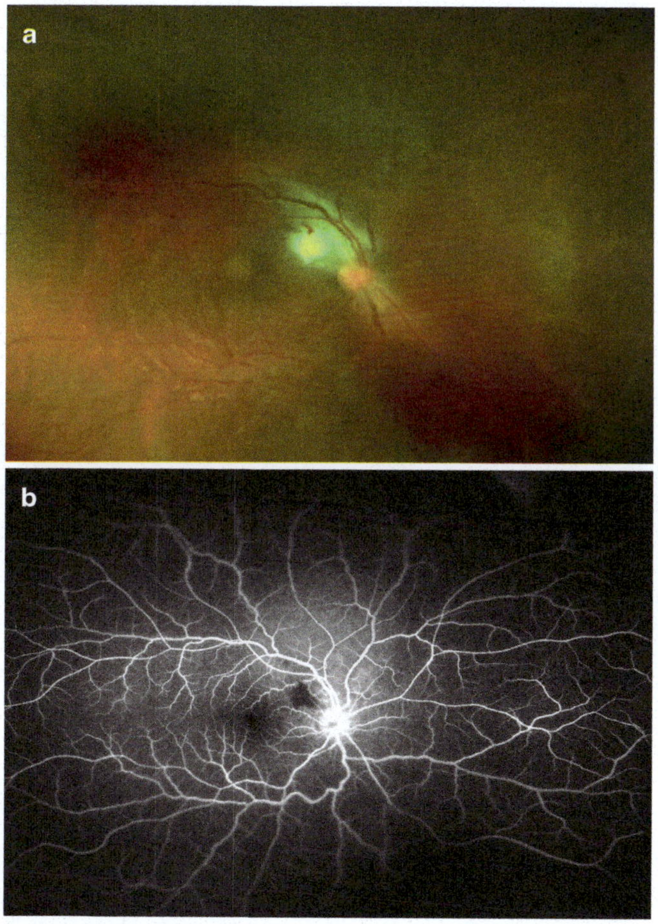

Fig. 12 UWF imaging shows toxoplasmic retinitis and retinal vasculitis (**a**). FA discloses a hypofluorescent area (**b**)

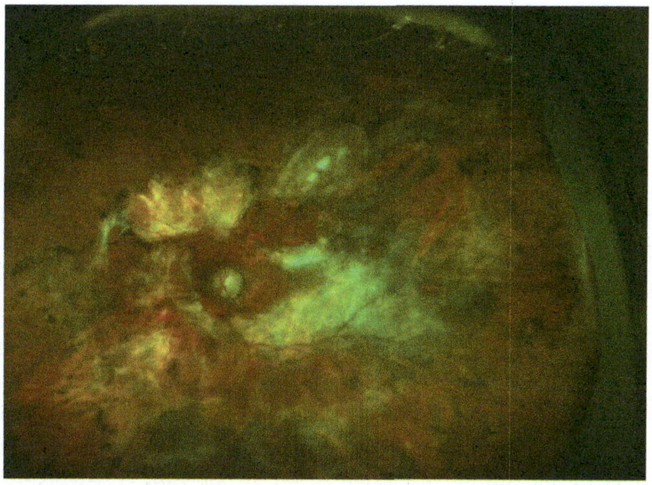

Fig. 13 UWF image shows diffuse scarring areas of toxoplasmic retinitis in a patient previously treated with periocular corticosteroids

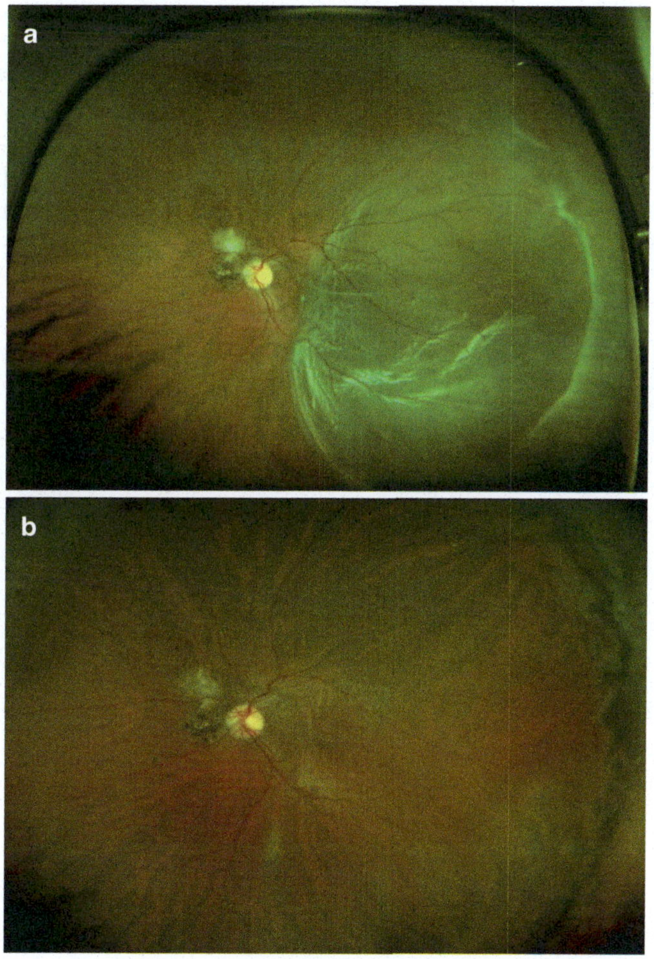

Fig. 14 UWF image of a patient with retinal vasculitis and rhegmatogenous retinal detachment associated with toxoplasmic retinitis (**a**). This patient was treated with pars plana vitrectomy, scleral buckle, endophotocoagulation, and gas injection. Postoperative imaging shows the retina to be well attached (**b**)

Tuberculosis-Related Uveitis

Tuberculosis-related uveitis (TRU) accounts for approximately 5 % of all uveitis cases in developed countries. There is a wide range of clinical forms of TRU. Although classical choroidal tubercles have been described as the principal forms, recognition of new patterns in recent years yielded to important therapeutic and prognostic improvements [9, 10].

Progressive multifocal choroiditis, so-called "serpiginous-like choroiditis," is a TRU form mimicking other noninfectious forms of serpiginous choroiditis. Differential diagnosis is the clue for therapeutic management, because TRU cases reach complete remission after antituberculous treatment (ATT) and initial moderate doses of steroids. Conversely, steroidal and immunosuppressive treatment leads to uveitis progression and blindness [11]. UWF imaging in serpiginous-like choroiditis is very helpful in detecting peripheral foci, a sign that may suggest a tuberculosis-related origin (Fig. 15) [12]. Autofluorescence is considered the monitoring examination of choice in serpiginous-like choroiditis. UWF fundus autofluorescence permits following up the healing process of the peripheral lesions, and even their complete resolution without sequelae if ATT is early instituted (Figs. 15 and 16). UWF red-free imaging enhances retinal involvement, which may be also helpful in monitoring the response to treatment (Fig. 17). Green-free images may show diffuse hyperreflective spots in the active lesions, disappearing after specific ATT, suggesting choroidal involvement (Fig. 18). UWF-FA in serpiginous-like choroiditis shows early hypofluorescence and late hyperfluorescence with dye leakage in fresh active lesions (Figs. 19 and 20).

Atypical and overlapped forms can be well characterized with the aid of UWF imaging. Rare cases starting with fibrosis surrounding the optic disc may be observed. Choroidal neovascularization in the peripapillary area can precede the serpiginous lesions for months to years (Figs. 21, 22, 23, 24 and 25). Overlapped serpiginous-like choroiditis and peripheral occlusive vasculitis may also be part of the tuberculosis-related uveitis spectrum, although they are rarely described [13, 14]. Wide-field multimodal imaging—including UWF fundus autofluorescence and FA—are extremely useful in the diagnosis and management of those infrequent cases (Figs. 26 and 27).

Tuberculosis-related vasculitis constitutes another important TRU entity. Chronic periphlebitis is frequently found, although occlusive and—less frequently—segmentary vasculitis can be also related to tuberculosis. Chronic vitreous inflammation with reactive hyalitis and small chorioretinal scars near affected veins are suggestive of its association to tuberculosis (Fig. 28) [9, 10, 15]. Chronic ischemia can be followed by retinal or optic disc neovascularization and hemovitreous in untreated cases. UWF-FA may allow defining the extent of peripheral ischemia and can disclose chorioretinal lesions in peripheral retina. Those wide-field findings are very useful for the adequate presumptive diagnosis and management of the case because specific ATT along with laser photocoagulation of the ischemic areas permits a definitive remission if instituted early [16].

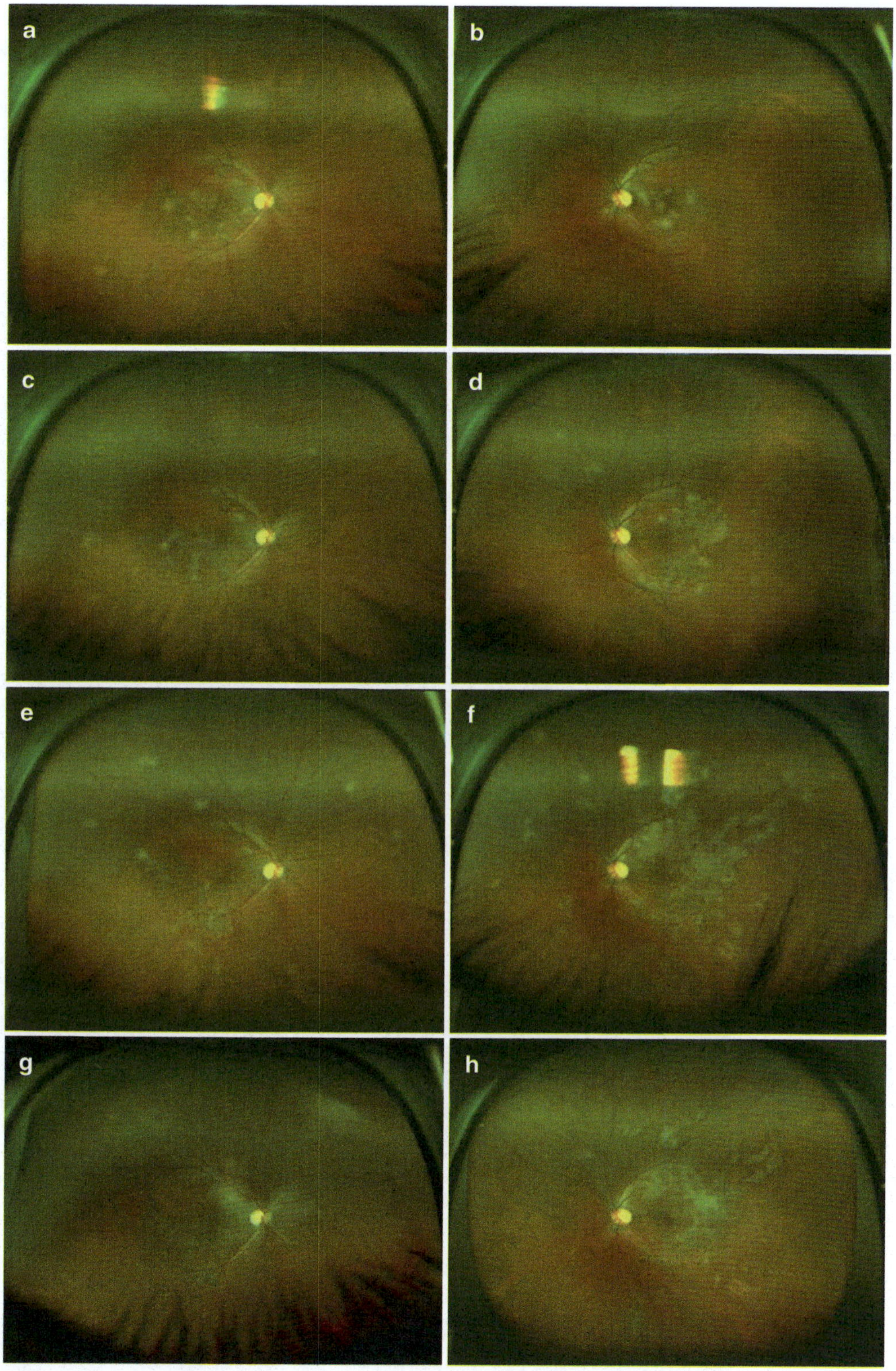

Fig. 15 UWF retinography. The patient is a Pakistan-born man, 33 years old, complaining of progressive visual loss in both eyes. The tuberculin skin test was 25 mm at 48 h; the quantiFERON-TB test was 22.8 U/mL. Extensive examinations, including chest computed tomography scan, were negative. Multifocal progressive choroiditis (serpiginous-like) in both eyes at presentation (**a**, **b**). Initial treatment with oral prednisone only led to the development of multiple peripheral creamy foci in both eyes (**c**–**f**). After adding full-course ATT for 9 months, a complete regression of fresh peripheral foci and healing of central lesions was observed (**g**, **h**). Visual acuity improved from 20/40 to 20/20 in the right eye and from 20/60 to 20/20 in the left eye

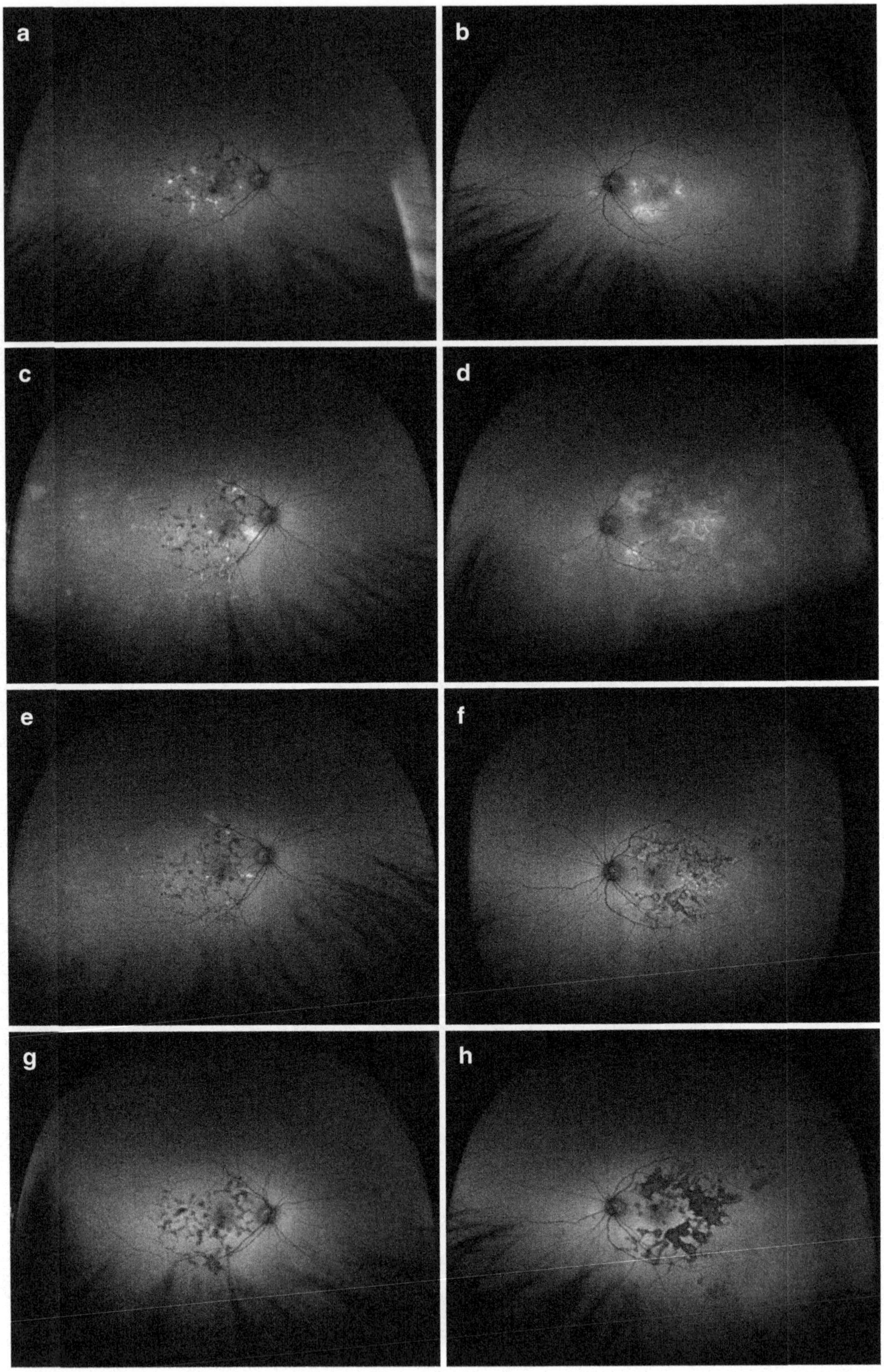

Fig. 16 UWF fundus autofluorescence of the patient described in Fig. 15. Hyperautofluorescent central lesions in both eyes along with healed central spiculated hypoautofluorescent old lesions in the right eye can be observed at baseline (**a**, **b**). Multiple hyperautofluorescent peripheral foci after steroid therapy led to disease progression (**c**, **d**). After ATT commencement, peripheral new lesions disappeared and central lesions became centripetally hypoautofluorescent at 1 month (**e**, **f**) and 9 months, a healing sign (**g**, **h**)

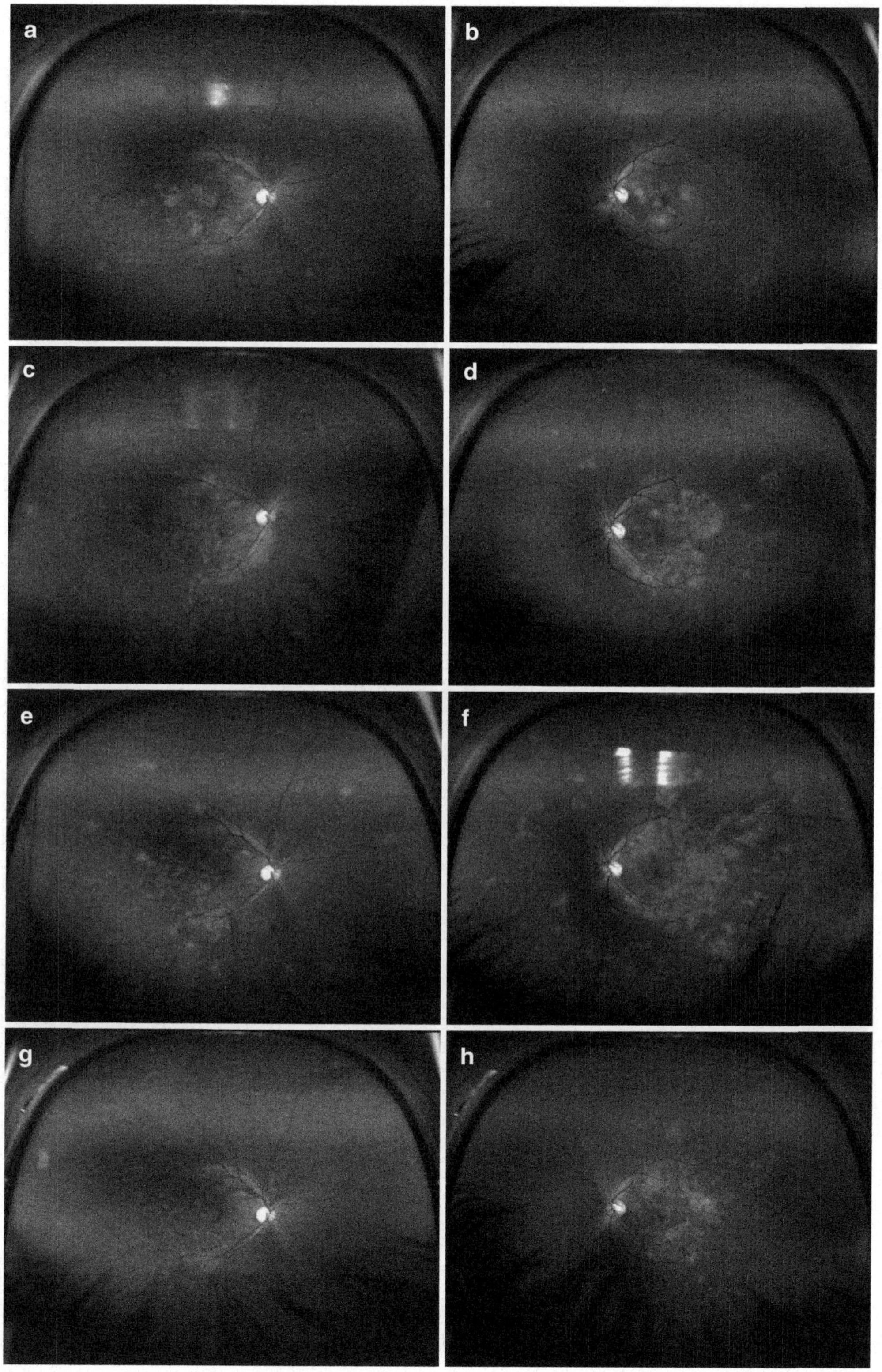

Fig. 17 UWF red-free retinography of the patient described in Fig. 15. Baseline findings (**a**, **b**). Red-free imaging enhances new retinal lesions appearing after steroidal treatment (**c**–**f**). Note that most peripheral new foci completely healed after ATT, whereas central healed lesions appearance was reduced (hyperreflective red-free zones) (**g**, **h**)

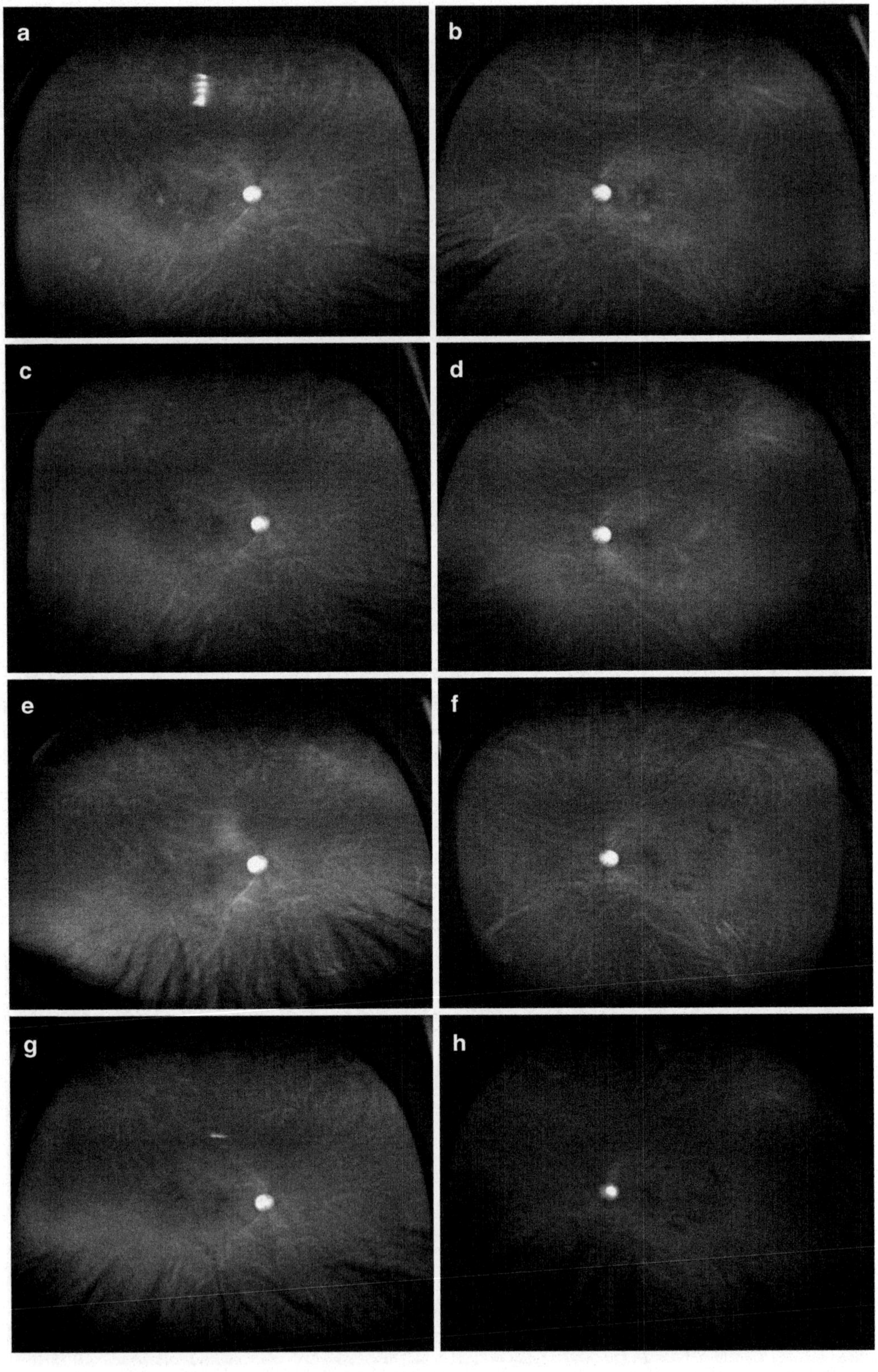

Fig. 18 UWF green-free retinography of the patient described in Fig. 15. Green-free imaging enhances choroid visualization. Active foci appear as hyperreflective spots in the center (at baseline: [**a**, **b**]) and extended to the periphery after steroid treatment (**c**, **d**). After ATT, peripheral lesions disappeared (**e**, **f**), whereas central old lesions become hyporeflective and were partly masked by retinal pigment epithelium hyperplasia (**g**, **h**)

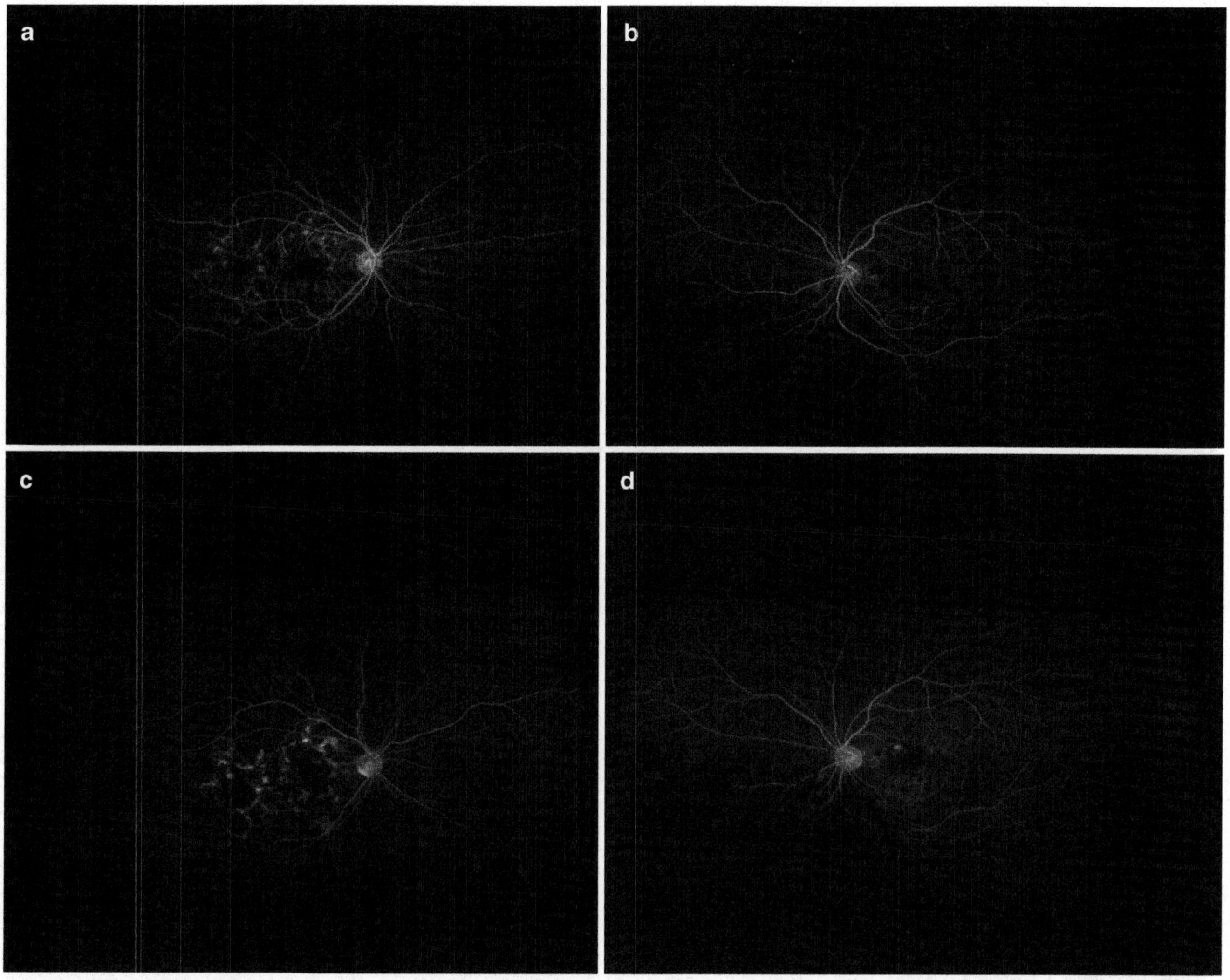

Fig. 19 UWF-FA of the patient described in Fig. 15. New active lesions are hypofluorescent in early frames (**a**, **b**), becoming centripetally hyperfluorescent with diffuse edges in later frames (**c**, **d**). Old fibrotic lesions in the right eye are hyperfluorescent from early frames and enhanced afterward with well-defined edges (**c**)

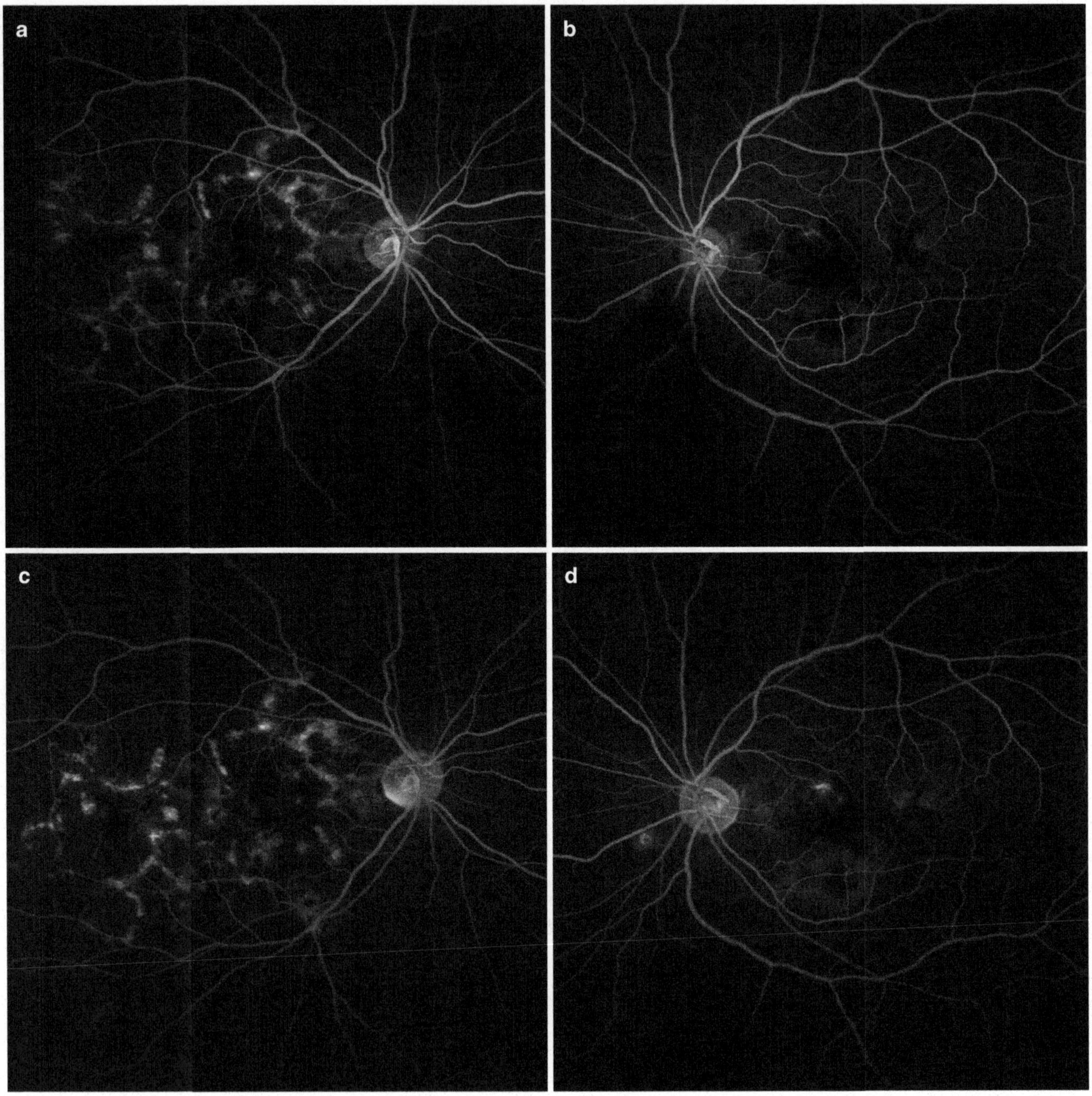

Fig. 20 Central-field focused angiography of the patient described in Fig. 15 at presentation. Wide-field imaging can be focused in the posterior pole. New active lesions appear hypofluorescent in early frames (**a**, **b**), becoming centripetally hyperfluorescent in the later frames (**c**, **d**). Old fibrotic lesions in the right eye are hyperfluorescent from early frames and enhanced afterward (**c**). Note that perivascular inflammation in third order lower-temporal vessels in the right eye can be appreciated in detail

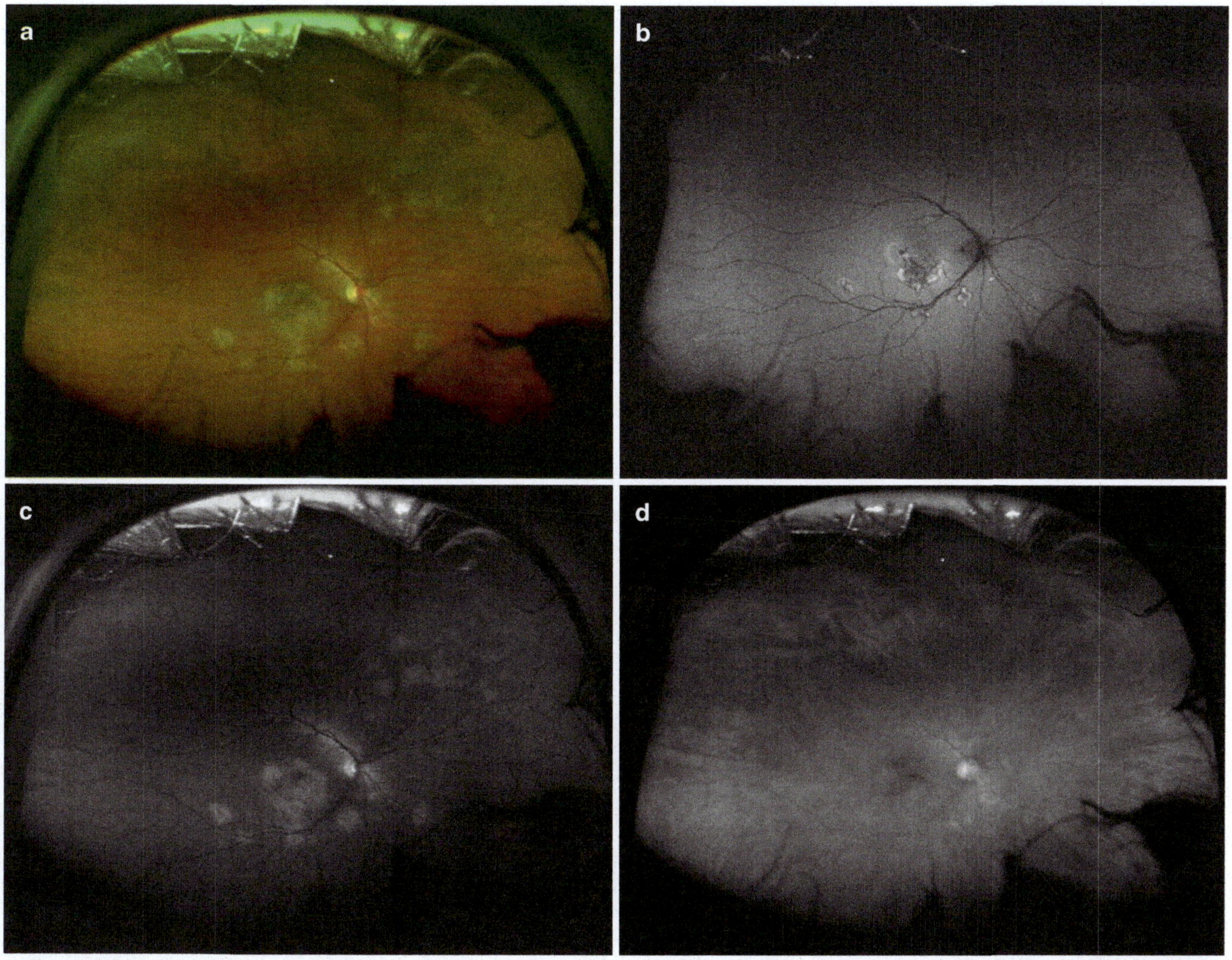

Fig. 21 UWF multimodal imaging. Presumed progressive multifocal choroiditis (serpiginous-like choroiditis) observed in a 73-year-old Caucasian man. The tuberculin skin test was greater than 15 mm at 48 h, and the quantiFERON-TB test was 19.97 IU/ml. Extensive examination was negative. UWF retinography shows central and peripheral serpiginous yellow-creamy foci (**a**). UWF fundus autofluorescence disclosed macular and mid-peripheral serpiginous-like lesions with hyperautofluorescent edges (**b**). Of note, upper-nasal lesions are isoautofluorescent and can be easily enhanced with red-free retinography (**c**). Green-free imaging showed slightly hyperreflective macular dots, suggesting choroidal involvement (**d**)

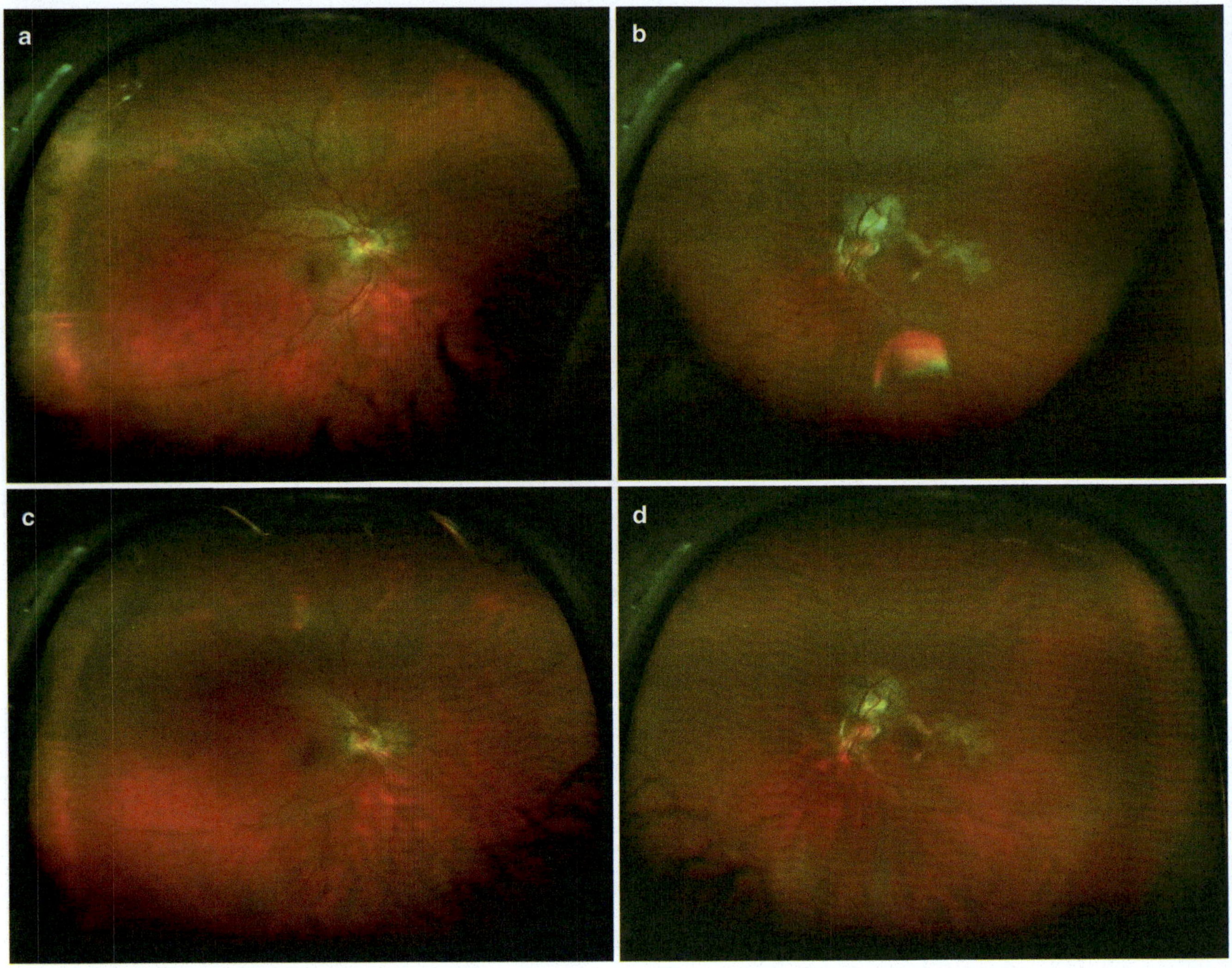

Fig. 22 UWF retinography of an atypical form of serpiginous-like choroiditis. A 40-year-old woman who was diagnosed with relapsing neovascular choroidal membranes around the optic disc of both eyes was successfully treated with anti–vascular endothelial growth factor (anti-VEGF) intravitreal therapy. Peripapillary involvement in both eyes shows fibrotic changes (**a**, **b**). A serpiginous spared focus appeared in the left eye 3 years later (**b**). QuantiFERON-TB test was positive, with tuberculin skin test at 0 mm. At 2 months of follow-up with ATT plus oral prednisone 30 mg/day, no progression is observed (**c**, **d**)

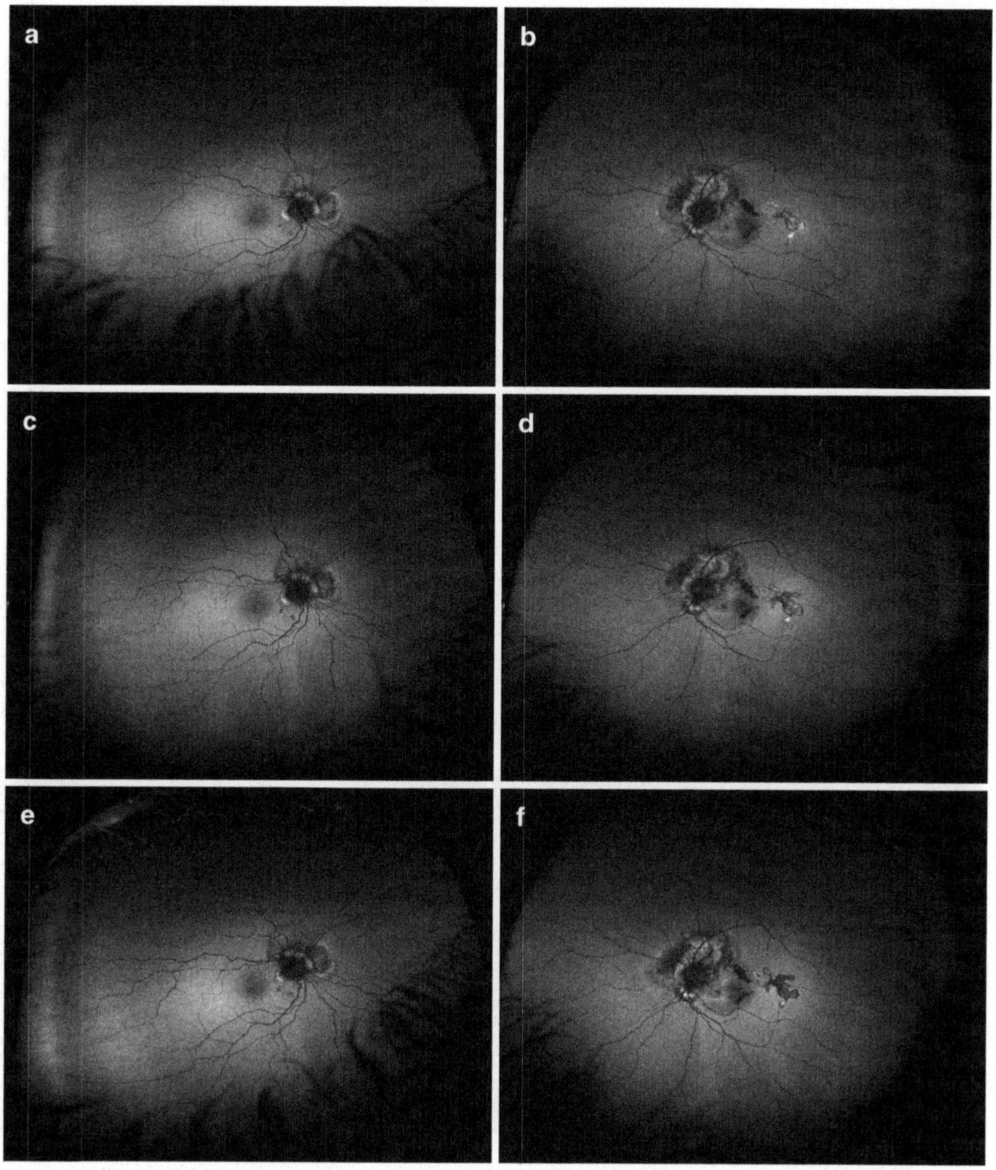

Fig. 23 UWF fundus autofluorescence of the patient described in Fig. 22. Hyper-/hypoautofluorescent peripapillary lesions in both eyes show fibrotic changes (**a**–**f**). In the left eye, a new hyperautofluorescent serpiginous lesion located temporal to the macula is observed (**b**). During follow-up with ATT plus oral prednisone, no changes are observed in peripapillary lesions, but the serpiginous focus shows progressive central hypoautofluorescence that indicates healing at 1 month (**d**) and 2 months (**f**)

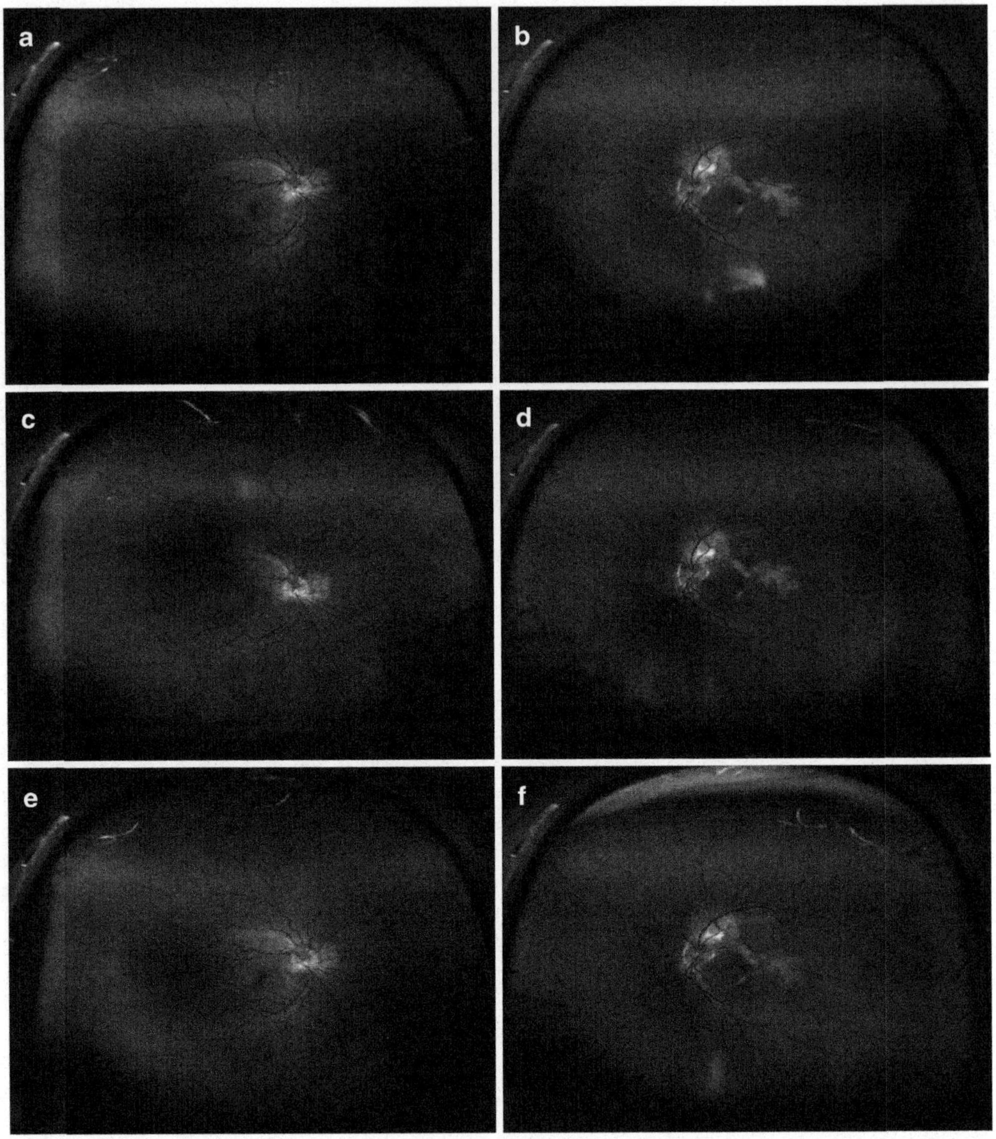

Fig. 24 UWF red-free retinography of the patient described in Fig. 22. Enhanced retinal images showed no changes in peripapillary and perifoveal lesions (**a**, **b**) at 1 month (**c**, **d**) and 2 months (**e**, **f**) of ATT and tapering oral prednisone doses. However, new serpiginous lesion in the left eye (**b**) appeared less hyperreflective, indicating response to specific treatment (**d**, **f**)

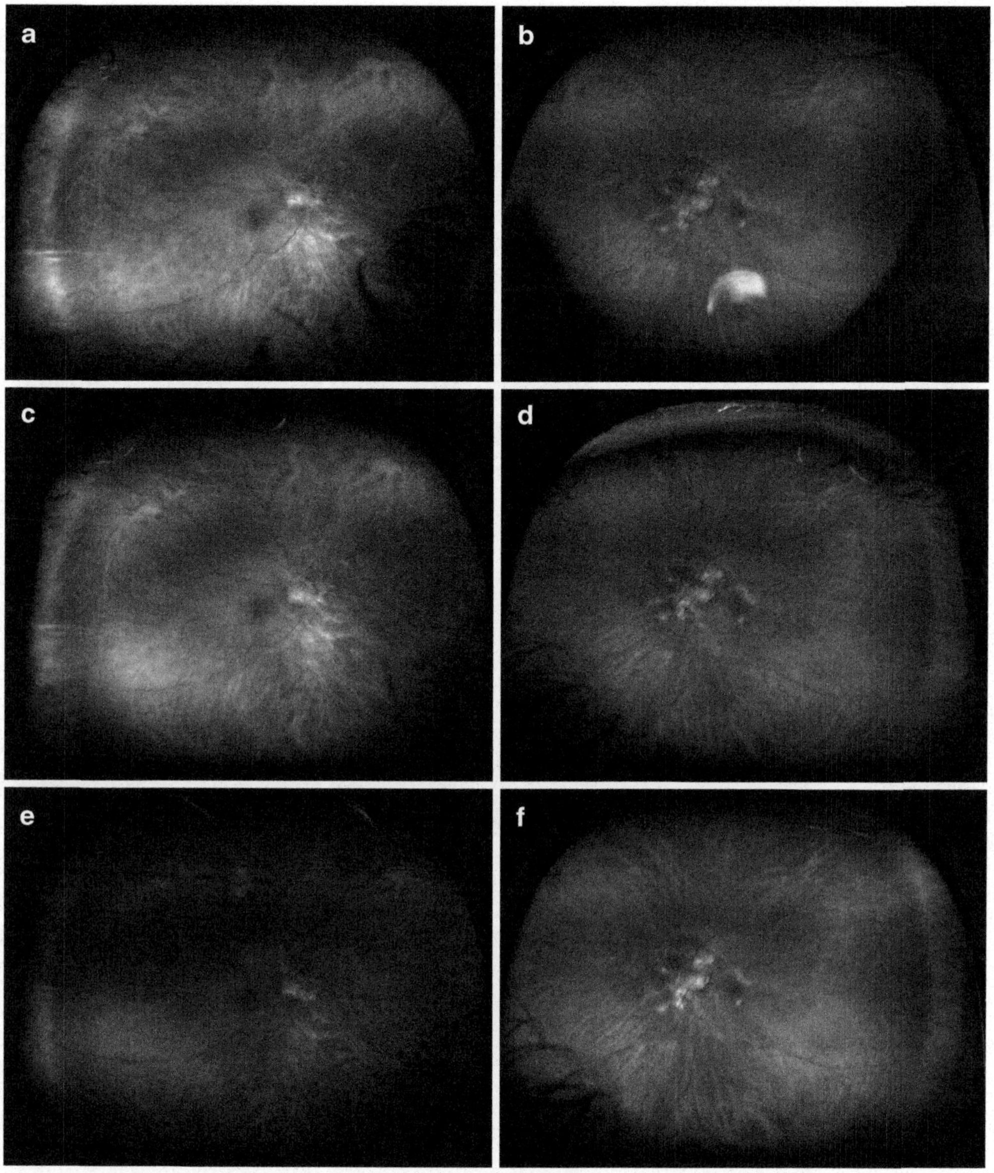

Fig. 25 UWF green-free retinography of the patient described in Fig. 22. Enhanced choroidal images (**a**, **b**) showed no changes in peripapillary and perifoveal old lesions at 1 month (**c**, **d**) and 2 months (**e**, **f**) of ATT and tapering oral prednisone doses. However, new serpiginous lesion in the left eye appeared less hyperreflective, indicating response to specific treatment (**b**, **d**, **f**)

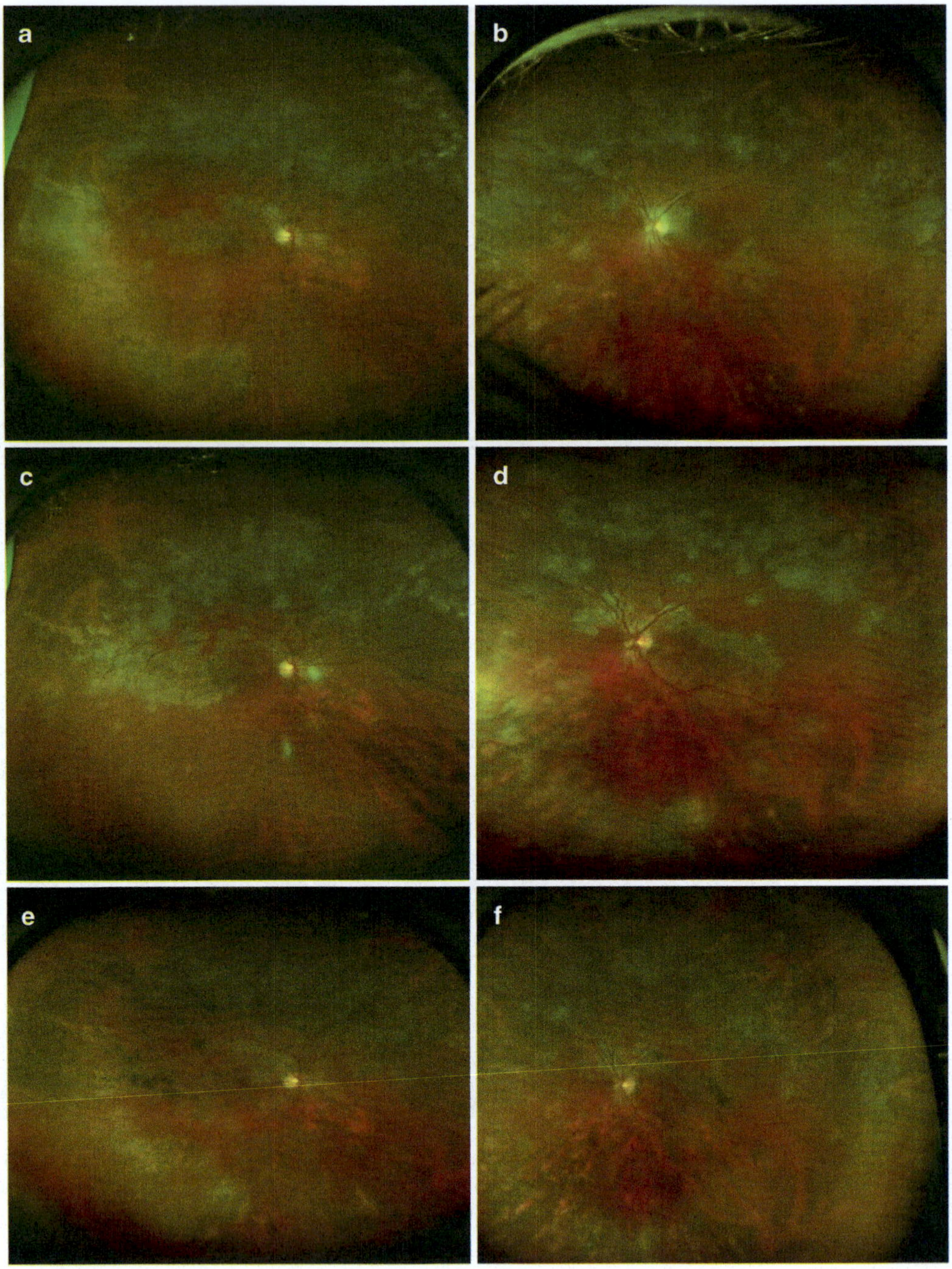

Fig. 26 The patient was a Caucasian man, 47 years old, who complained of bilateral visual loss (**a**, **b**). He had been treated with oral prednisone 1 mg/kg/day as well as peripheral retinal photocoagulation 3 weeks before. At baseline, central and peripheral multifocal choroiditis was observed in both eyes (**c**, **d**). Peripheral retinal hemorrhages were also observed in the inferior periphery of the left eye (**d**). Tuberculin skin test measured 20 mm at 48 h with necrosis and quantiFERON-TB also tested positive. Extensive extraocular investigations including chest x-ray were normal or negative. Presumed tuberculosis-related serpiginous-like choroiditis was diagnosed and full-course of standard ATT was then started along with 0.5 mg/kg/day of oral prednisone. Laser photocoagulation was also completed in the periphery of the left eye. Lesions started to heal after 4 weeks of treatment, progressively appearing more scattered and pigmented (**e**, **f**). Visual acuity improved from 20/60 and 20/30 in the right and left eyes, respectively, to 20/25 in both eyes after 9 months of ATT

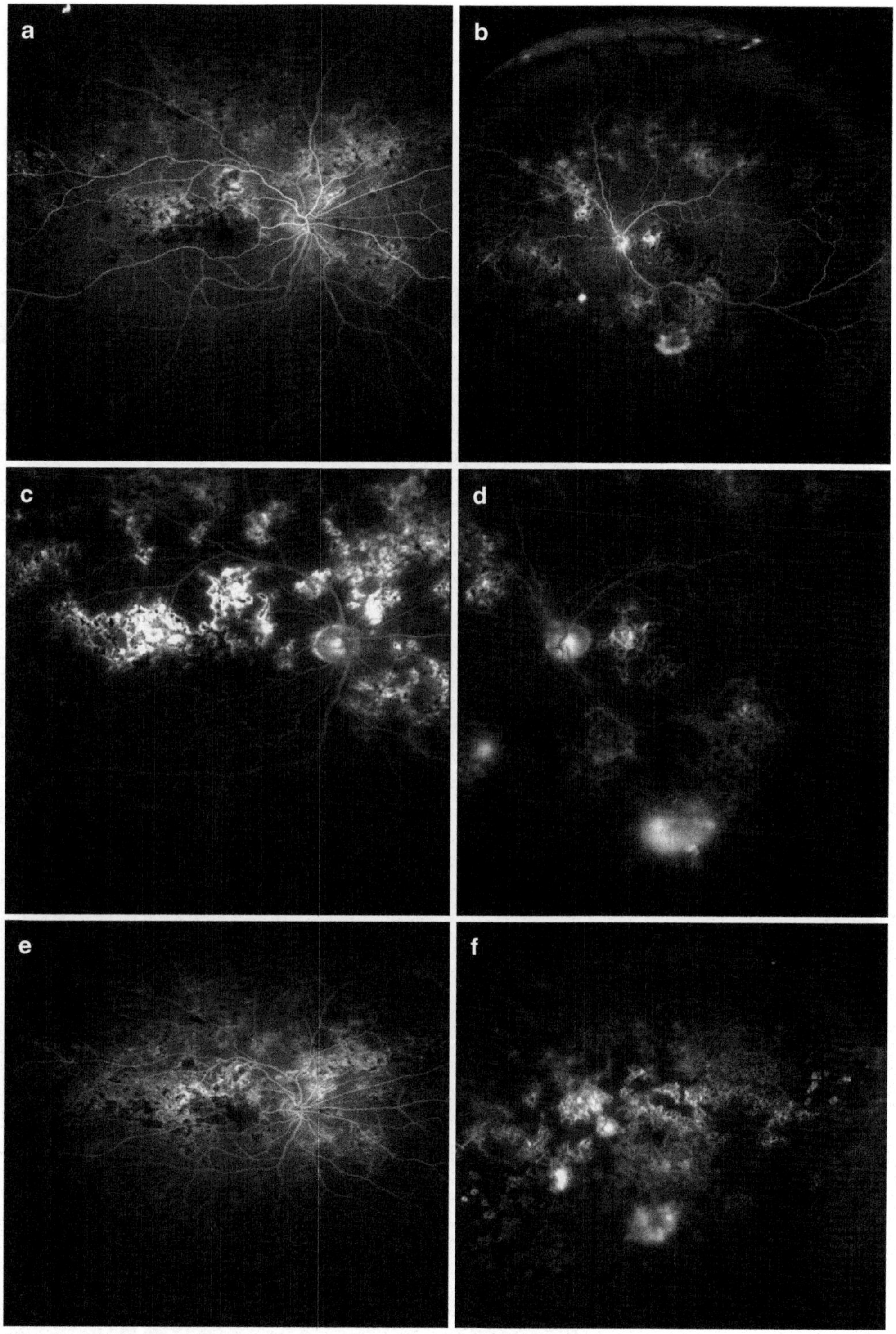

Fig. 27 UWF-FA of the same patient described in Fig. 26. New active foci of serpiginous-like choroiditis showed early hypofluorescence (**a, b**) and late hyperfluorescence (**c–f**) with surrounding leakage in later frames (**e, f**). Fibrotic lesions remained hyperfluorescent from early frames (**a, b**) and progressively enhanced (**c–f**). Importantly, a retinal neovascular fan was observed in the lower-temporal periphery of the left eye (**d**) and extensive areas of peripheral capillary nonperfusion in the left eye were demonstrated by wide-field angiography (**f**), leading to laser photocoagulation and regression of retinal new vessels

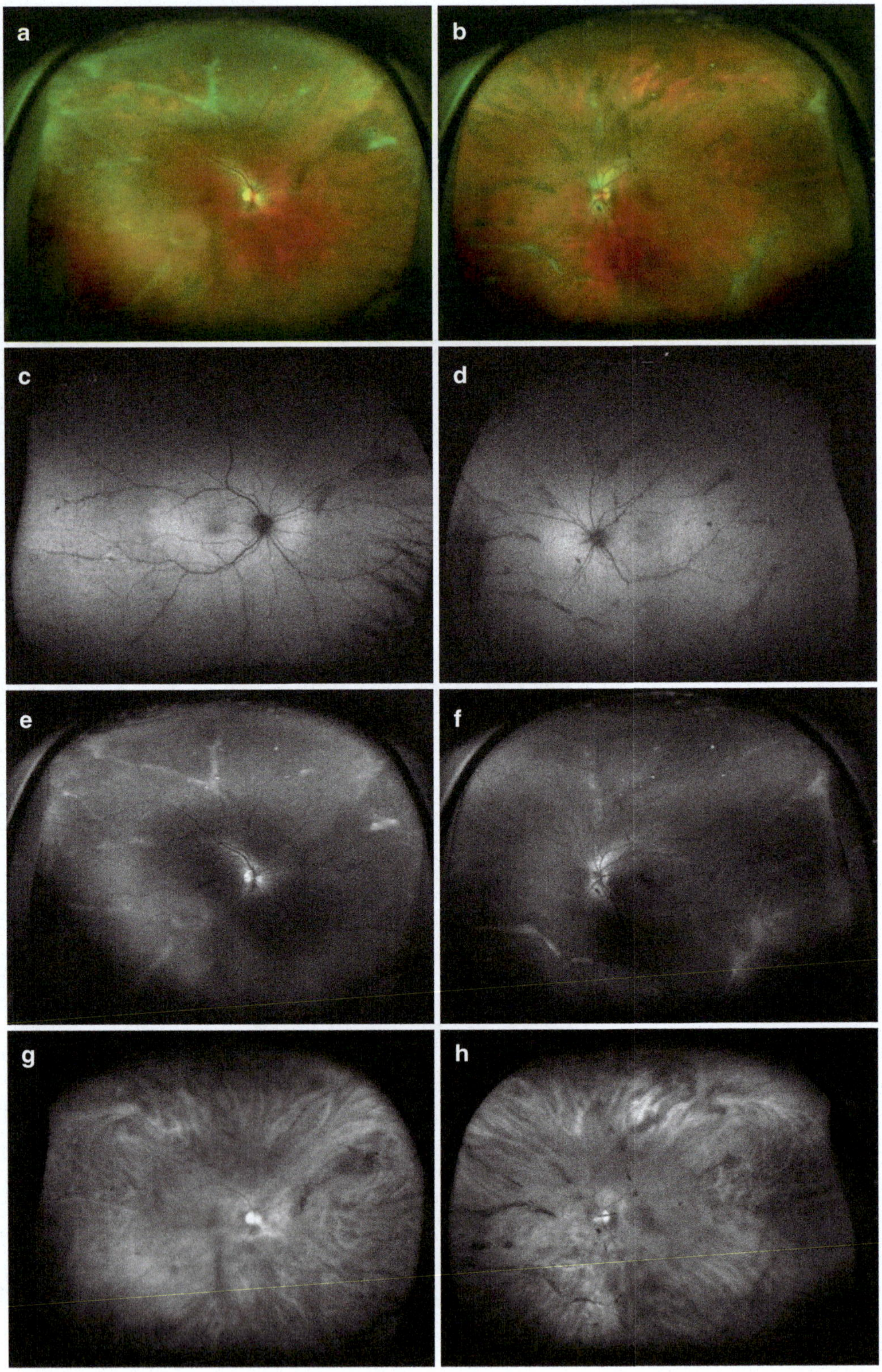

Fig. 28 Presumed tuberculosis-related vasculitis. Wide-field retinography performed in a 35-year-old man complaining of bilateral floaters for 9 months. Bilateral retinal vasculitis along with small chorioretinal scars near inflamed vessels and persistent vitreous opacities can be observed (**a**, **b**). Extensive studies resulted normal or negative, except a strong tuberculin skin test reaction. Wide-field fundus autofluorescence showed only a small hyperautofluorescent perivascular focus in the lower-temporal arcade of the right eye (**c**, **d**). Red-free imaging enhanced the visualization of peripheral vascular sheathing in both eyes (**e**, **f**). Green-free images look apparently normal, except the presence of vitreous opacities (**g**, **h**). A stability of lesions has been observed during follow-up (visual acuity 20/25 in both eyes)

Syphilitic Uveitis

Syphilitic uveitis can adopt a wide variety of different clinical patterns so it has won the appellative of "the great mimicker." Syphilitic retinitis may involve the peripheral retina in a not well-defined manner, affecting one retinal sector or appearing as multiple small round patches [17]. Intense vitritis is an important handicap for an appropriate fundus exploration, which may difficult the diagnosing process [18, 19]. UWF imaging is a helpful tool in syphilitic uveitis. Indeed, UWF retinography allows a good view of the peripheral retina in one click, so patches of syphilitic retinitis can be reached in spite of the presence of significant vitreous haze. Red-free UWF techniques are very useful to enhance retinitis areas when vitritis is present. UWF fundus autofluorescence is also helpful in monitoring peripheral retinitis lesions, becoming hypoautofluorescent after appropriate treatment and showing the retinal pigment epithelium migration and clumping after healing. This pattern has been named as a pseudoretinitis pigmentosa (Figs. 29 and 30).

UWF-FA is key to study the clinical signs associated to syphilitic uveitis. Slight to moderate peripheral vasculitis can be demonstrated, along with diffuse or well-defined foci of retinitis or retinochoroiditis [17–19]. The "salt-and-pepper" pattern is commonly seen in diffuse pattern, whereas the leopard-spots pattern can be appreciated in better-defined lesions. Optic disc leakage and persistent vitreous-hyaloid small round aggregates are also typical findings (Figs. 31 and 32) [20].

Other syphilitic uveitis forms such as posterior placoid forms or neuroretinitis are less frequent and are usually circumscribed to the posterior pole (Fig. 33) [17–19].

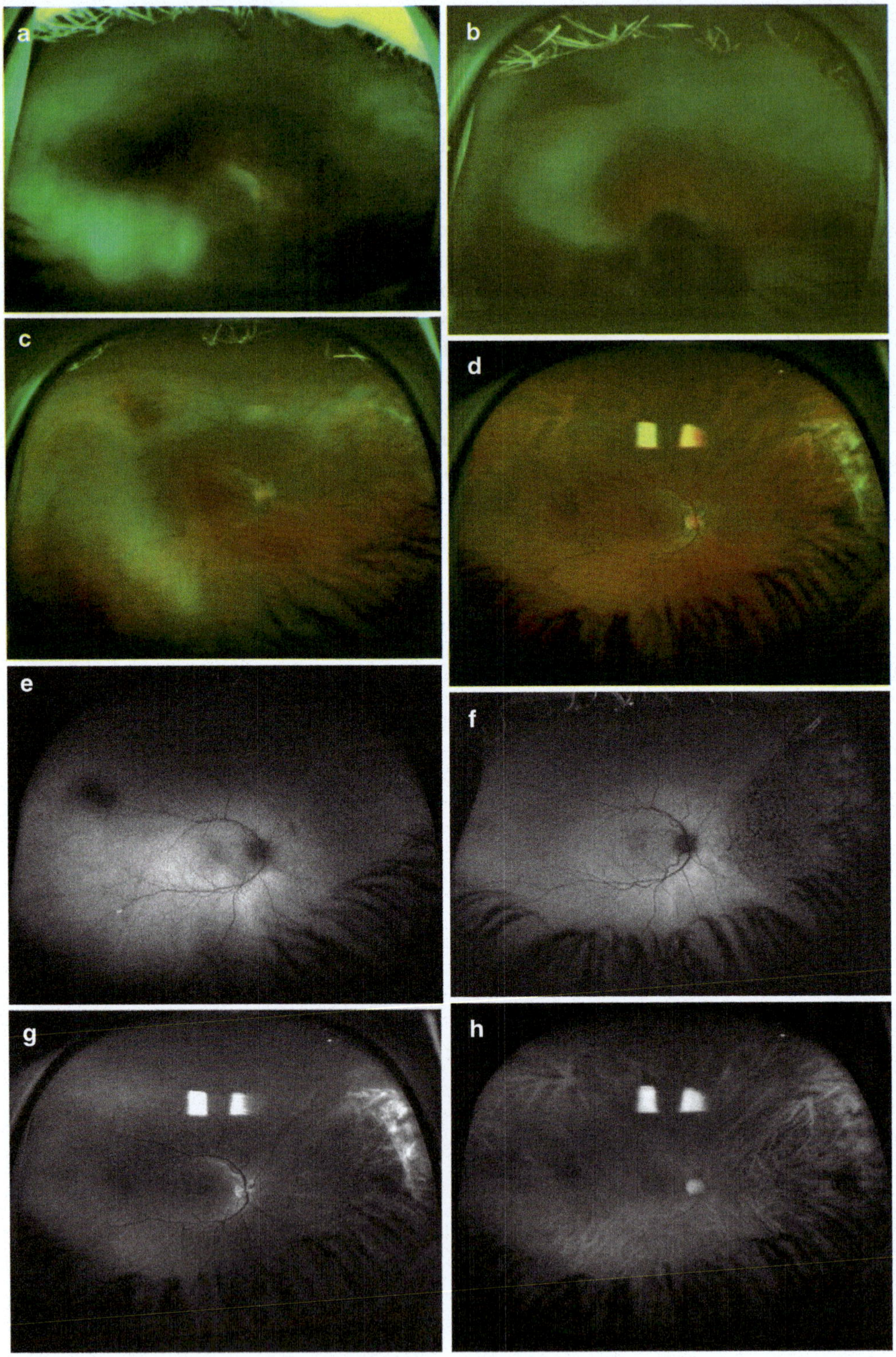

Fig. 29 Syphilitic uveitis. Wide-field retinography performed in a 42-year-old Caucasian patient. Significant vitreous haze disappeared after intravenous penicillin full-course treatment (**a–d**). Peripheral retinitis was discovered after vitreous haze resolution (**d**). After 3 weeks of antibiotic treatment, wide-field fundus autofluorescence did not disclose important lesions (**e**), but 2 months afterward, a round spotted hypoautofluorescent lesion appeared in the nasal area (**f**). Red-free image enhanced the retinal atrophic scar (**g**). Green-free images disclosed clear choroidal vessels along with retinal pigment epithelium hyperplasia (**h**)

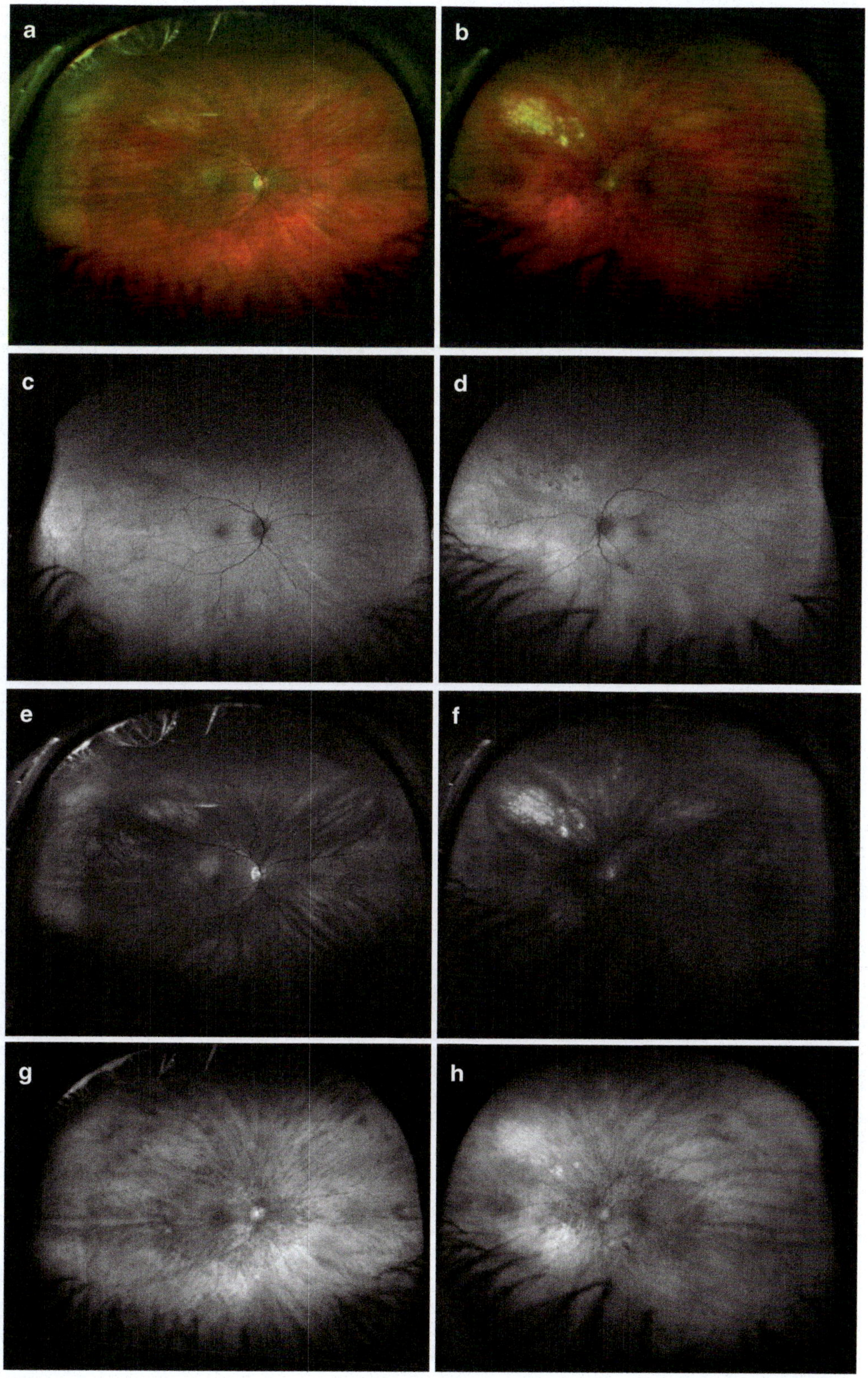

Fig. 30 Syphilitic retinitis. Wide-field retinography in a 25-year-old patient (**a**, **b**). After 4 weeks of intravenous penicillin therapy, remission was achieved and vitreous haze resolved. Healed retinitis foci can be seen in the upper-nasal part of the left eye (**b**). Wide-field fundus autofluorescence showed inactivation of the retinal lesions (hypoautofluorescence) (**c**, **d**). Red-free images enhanced retinal atrophy in the retinitis area (**e**, **f**). Green-free images enhanced pointed vitreous shadows and temporal choroidal folds in both eyes (probably unrelated to the uveitic process) (**g**, **h**)

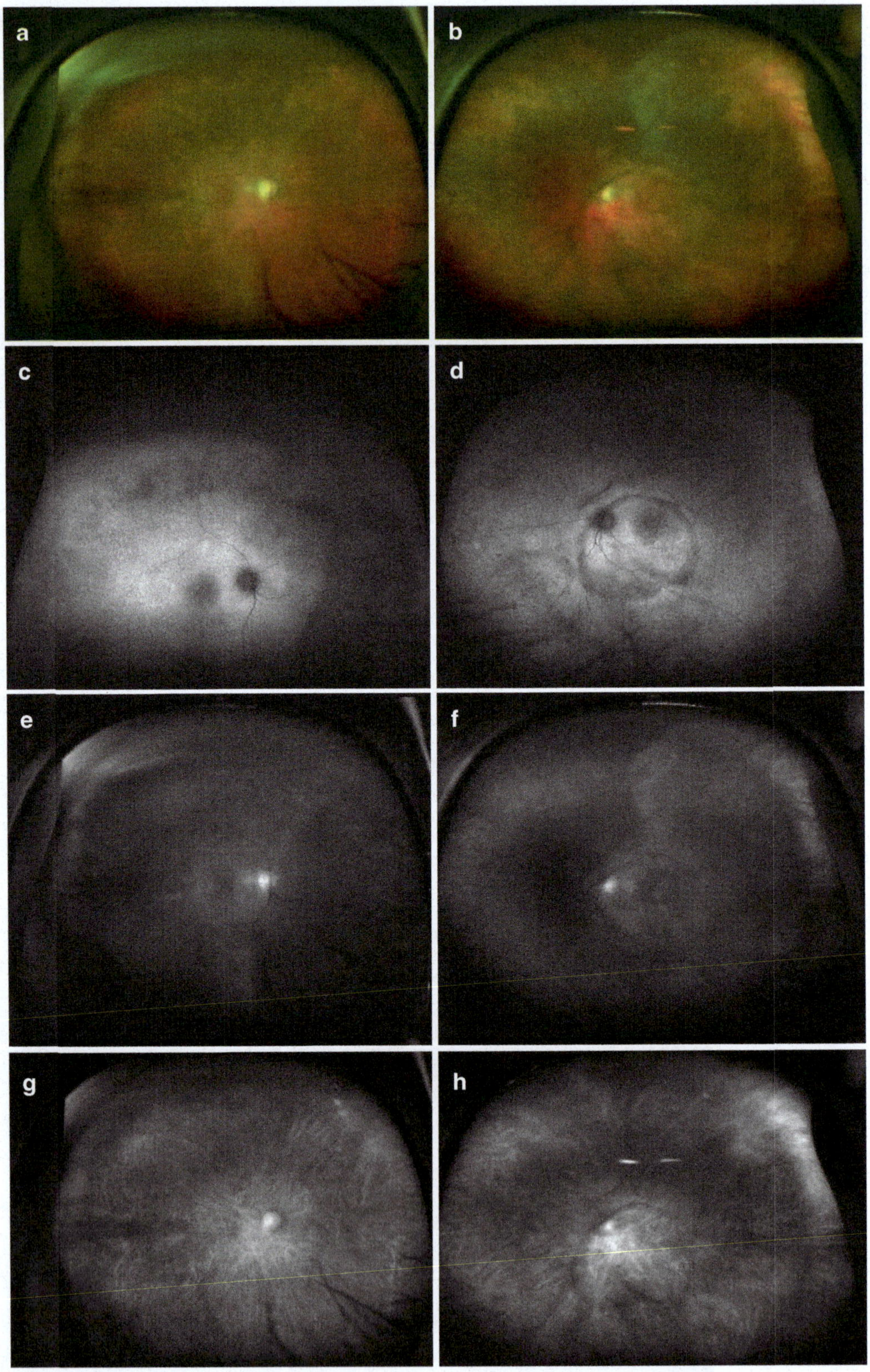

Fig. 31 Wide-field retinography in a 75-year-old patient with syphilitic uveitis (**a**, **b**). After 2 weeks of penicillin treatment, remission was achieved (**a**, **b**). Wide-field autofluorescence showed unspecific diffuse hyperautofluorescent lesions (**c**, **d**). Red-free images enhanced retinal scarring, atrophy, and peripheral vascular involvement (**e**, **f**). Green-free images enhanced pointed vitreous shadows in the left eye corresponding to small round aggregates (**g**, **h**)

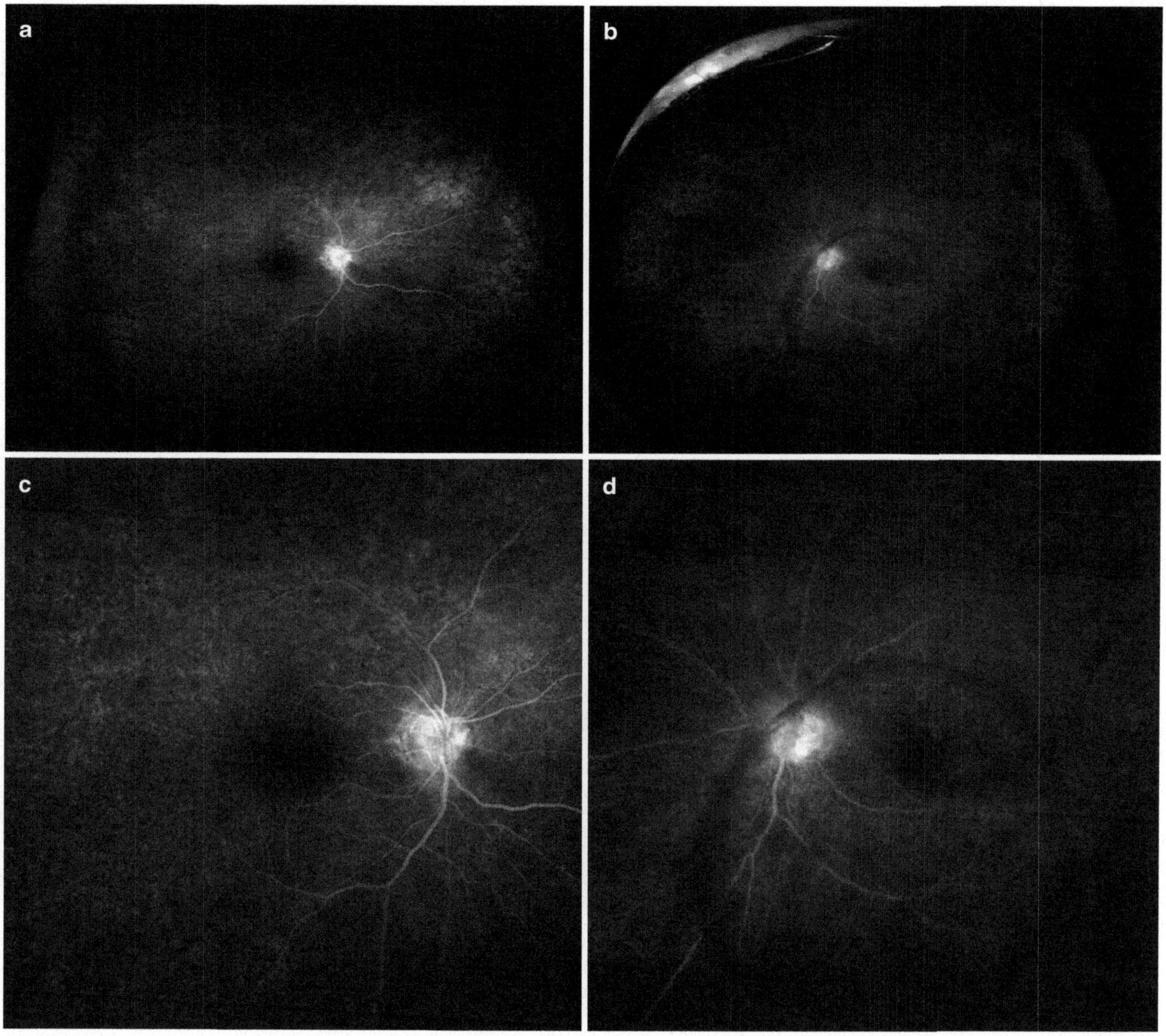

Fig. 32 Syphilitic uveitis. Wide-field angiography of the patient described in Fig. 31. Diffuse retinitis appeared in a "salt-and-pepper"–like pattern, more prominent in the periphery (**a–c**). Note vitreous shadows in the left eye corresponding to small round vitreous inflammatory aggregates (**d**). Visual acuity improved from counting fingers in both eyes to 20/25 and 20/30 in the right and left eyes, respectively

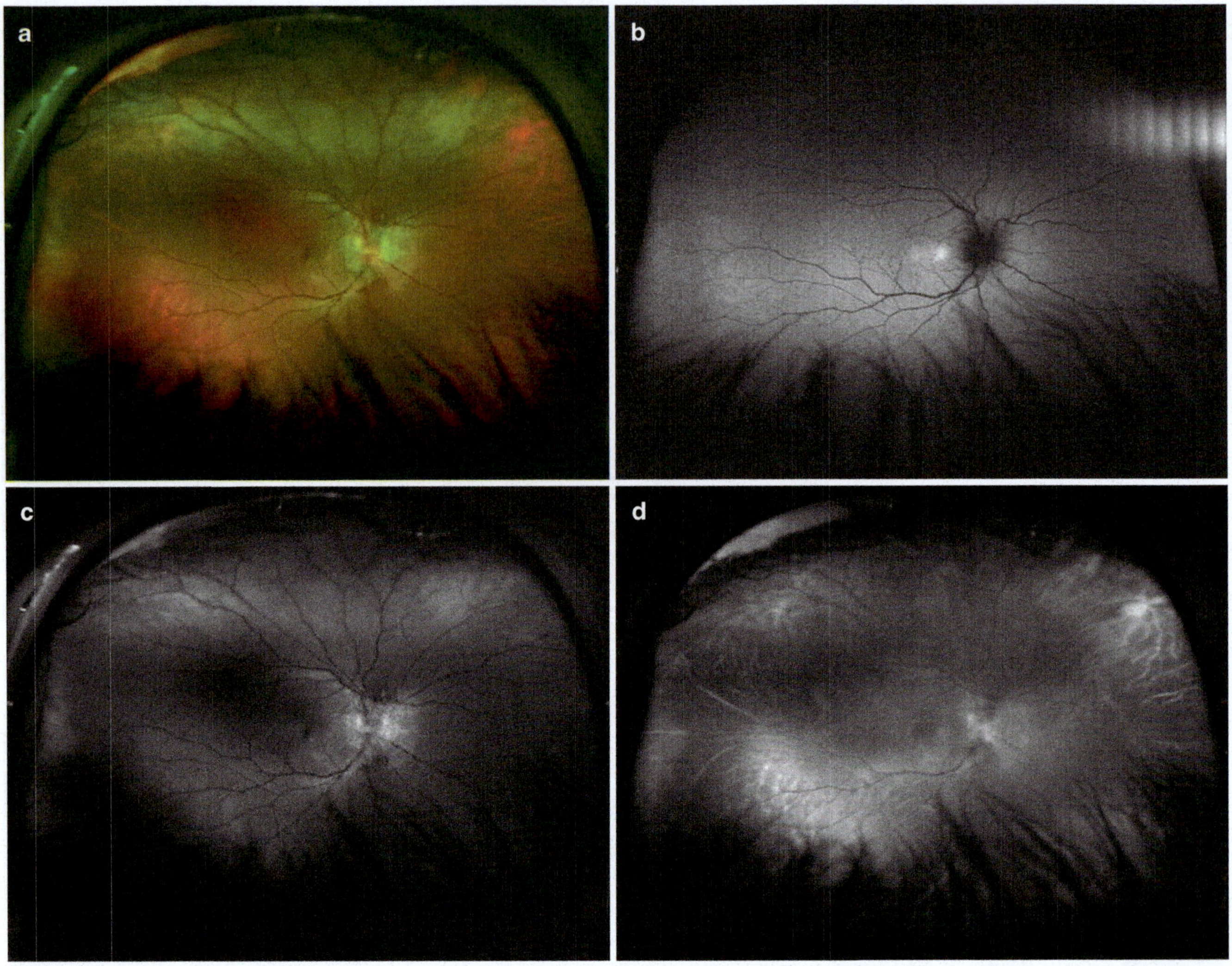

Fig. 33 Syphilitic neuroretinitis observed in a 24-year-old human immunodeficiency virus (HIV)–positive patient. Wide-field retinography showed optic disc infiltration in the right eye (**a**). A hyperautofluorescent area located between the macula and the optic disc can be identified in the wide-field autofluorescence, corresponding to exudation (**b**). Red- and green-free imaging ruled out further chorioretinal involvement (**c**, **d**)

Endophthalmitis

Imaging tests in the context of endophthalmitis may be limited by the intense vitritis present in some cases. However, UWF explorations may identify peripheral signs that can be the clue for the differential diagnosis. Peripheral hemorrhagic vasculitis and retinal necrosis are clinical features that may indicate the presence of an intraocular infection, prompting early antibiotic therapy [21]. Conversely, aseptic endophthalmitis is associated with vitritis that can be quite intense, but with no inflammatory infiltration of the peripheral retinal vessels (Fig. 34) [22, 23].

Fungal endogenous endophthalmitis can be sometimes difficult to diagnose. Whereas yeast intraocular infections tend to be easily identified by conventional ophthalmoscopy because they usually affect the posterior pole or extend to central vitreous cavity, mold endogenous endophthalmitis can be more difficult to diagnose because they can infiltrate the peripheral choroid and retina in a circumscribed lesion [24]. Wide-field imaging can allow early recognition of peripheral fungal lesions and specific therapy can be instituted early. Although the prognosis remains obscure in the vast majority of these cases, UWF imaging is useful in monitoring the progression of the infection and the necessity of additional antifungal therapies (Fig. 35).

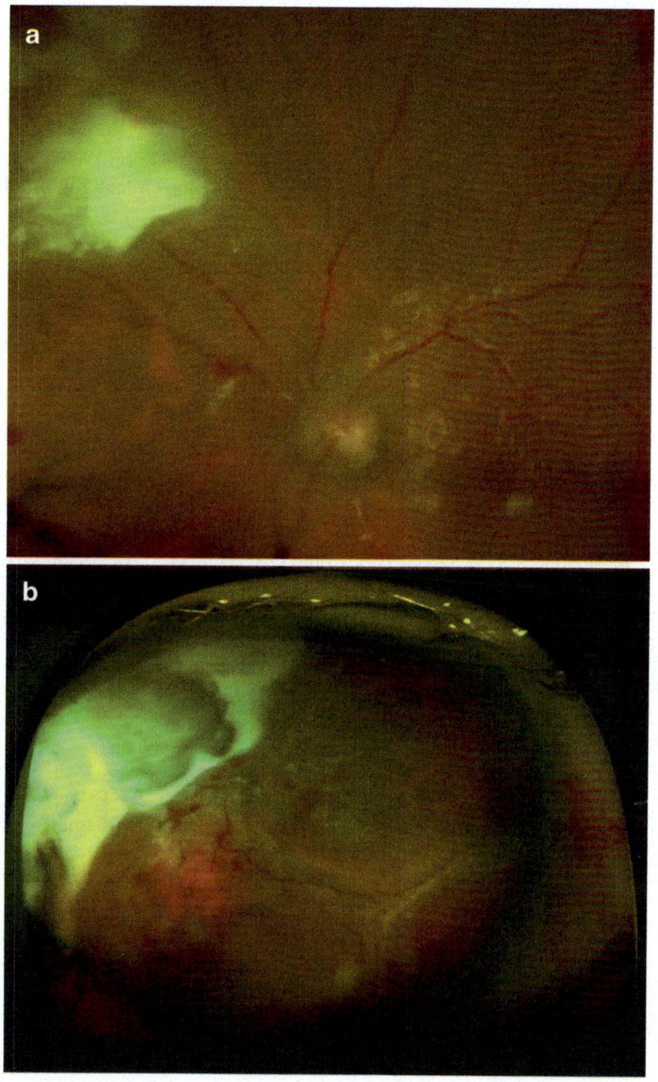

Fig. 35 Endogenous fungal endophthalmitis in a 79-year-old man under systemic immunosuppression owing to cutaneous pemphigoid (**a**). Prior retinal biopsy performed in another center was negative. Progression to subretinal abscess is clearly seen in wild-field retinography (**b**). A second vitreous biopsy disclosed an *Aspergillus fumigatus* etiology

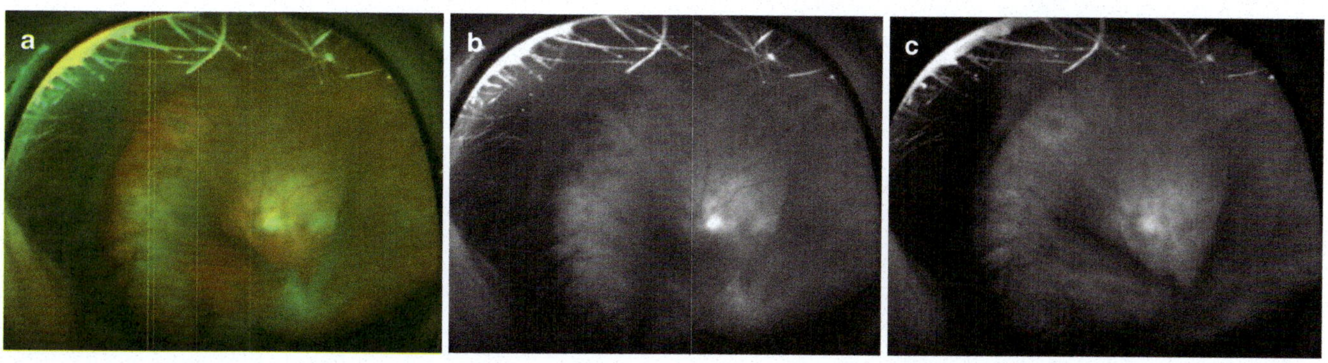

Fig. 34 Exogenous endophthalmitis in a 79-year-old woman diagnosed after intravitreal therapy with anti-VEGF. Aqueous tap culture was positive for *Staphylococcus hominis*. Wide-field retinography showed hemorrhagic peripheral vasculitis, indicating an infectious process (**a**). Red-free picture enhanced retinal involvement (**b**). Green-free picture showed intense vitreous inflammation (**c**)

References

1. Jabs DA. Cytomegalovirus retinitis and the acquired immunodeficiency syndrome—bench to bedside: LXVII. Edward Jackson Memorial Lecture. Am J Ophthalmol. 2011;151:198–216.e1.
2. Mudvari SS, Virasch VV, Singa RM, MacCumber MW. Ultra-wide-field imaging for cytomegalovirus retinitis. Ophthalmic Surg Lasers Imaging. 2010;41:311–5.
3. Urban B, Bakunowicz-Aazarczyk A, Michalczuk M. Immune recovery uveitis: pathogenesis, clinical symptoms, and treatment. Mediators Inflamm. 2014;2014:971417.
4. Wong RW, Jumper JM, McDonald HR, Johnson RN, Fu A, Lujan BJ, et al. Emerging concepts in the management of acute retinal necrosis. Postgrad Med J. 2013;97:478–85.
5. Roy R, Pal BP, Mathur G, Rao C, Das D, Biswas J. Acute retinal necrosis: clinical features, management and outcomes—a 10 year consecutive case series. Ocul Immunol Inflamm. 2014;22:170–4.
6. Pleyer U, Schlüter D, Mänz M. Ocular toxoplasmosis: recent aspects of pathophysiology and clinical implications. Ophthalmic Res. 2014;52:116–23.
7. Moshfeghi DM, Dodds EM, Couto CA, Santos CI, Nicholson DH, Lowder CY, et al. Diagnostic approaches to severe atypical toxoplasmosis mimicking acute retinal necrosis. Ophthalmology. 2004;111:716–25.
8. Adan A, Giralt J, Alvarez G, Alforja S, Burés-Jesltrup A, Casaroli-Marano RP, et al. Pars plana vitrectomy for vitreoretinal complications of ocular toxoplasmosis. Eur J Ophthalmol. 2009;19:1039–43.
9. Gupta V, Gupta A, Rao NA. Intraocular tuberculosis-an update. Surv Ophthalmol. 2007;52:561–87.
10. Llorenç V, González-Martin J, Keller J, Rey A, Pelegrín L, Mesquida M, et al. Indirect supportive evidence for diagnosis of tuberculosis-related uveitis: from the tuberculin skin test to the new interferon gamma release assays. Acta Ophthalmol. 2013;91:e99–107.
11. Nazari Khanamiri H, Rao NA. Serpiginous choroiditis and infectious multifocal serpiginoid choroiditis. Surv Ophthalmol. 2013;58:203–32.
12. Bansal R, Gupta A, Gupta V, Dogra MR, Sharma A, Bambery P. Tubercular serpiginous-like choroiditis presenting as multifocal serpiginoid choroiditis. Ophthalmology. 2012;119:2334–42.
13. Parchand S, Tandan M, Gupta V, Gupta A. Intermediate uveitis in Indian population. J Ophthalmic Inflamm Infect. 2011;1:65–70.
14. Tabbara KF. Tuberculosis. Curr Opin Ophthalmol. 2007;18:493–501.
15. Gupta A, Bansal R, Gupta V, Sharma A, Bambery P. Ocular signs predictive of tubercular uveitis. Am J Ophthalmol. 2010;149:562–70.
16. Singh R, Toor P, Parchand S, Sharma K, Gupta V, Gupta A. Quantitative polymerase chain reaction for Mycobacterium tuberculosis in so-called Eales' disease. Ocul Immunol Inflamm. 2012;20:153–7.
17. Davis JL. Ocular syphilis. Curr Opin Ophthalmol. 2014;25:513–8.
18. Fonollosa A, Martinez-Indart L, Artaraz J, Martinez-Berriotxoa A, Agirrebengoa K, Garcia M, et al. Clinical manifestations and outcomes of syphilis-associated uveitis in northern Spain. Ocul Immunol Inflamm. 2014;14:1–6.
19. Mathew RG, Goh BT, Westcott MC. British Ocular Syphilis Study (BOSS): 2-year national surveillance study of intraocular inflammation secondary to ocular syphilis. Invest Ophthalmol Vis Sci. 2014;55:5394–400.
20. Balaskas K, Sergentanis TN, Giulieri S, Guex-Crosier Y. Fluorescein and indocyanine-green angiography in ocular syphilis: an exploratory study. Graefes Arch Clin Exp Ophthalmol. 2012;250:721–30.
21. Davis JL. Diagnostic dilemmas in retinitis and endophthalmitis. Eye (Lond). 2012;26:194–201.
22. Hoevenaars NE, Gans D, Missotten T, van Rooij J, Lesaffre E, van Meurs JC. Suspected bacterial endophthalmitis following intravitreal anti-VEGF injection: case series and literature review. Ophthalmologica. 2012;228:143–7.
23. Jackson TL, Paraskevopoulos T, Georgalas I. Systematic review of 342 cases of endogenous bacterial endophthalmitis. Surv Ophthalmol. 2014;59:627–35.
24. Adam CR, Sigler EJ. Multimodal imaging findings in endogenous *Aspergillus* endophthalmitis. Retina. 2014;34:1914–5.

Wide-Field Retinal Imaging of Other Miscellaneous Retinal Diseases

15

J. Fernando Arevalo, Netan Choudhry, Igor Kozak, and The KKESH Collaborative Retina Study Group*

The peripheral retina is the site of pathology in many ocular diseases. Whereas careful clinical examination of a patient's peripheral retina with scleral indentation is of utmost importance in clinical decision making, there is a need for additional testing and an objective and reliable documentation of findings. Ultra-wide-field (UWF) imaging is one of the new technologies available to retinal specialists. Current UWF imaging modalities can provide several options for posterior segment documentation and evaluation, including options for color images, red-free images, fluorescein and indocyanine green angiography, and fundus autofluorescence [1, 2]. Information from these imaging devices has truly changed the ophthalmologist's clinical assessment and has led to more understanding of the role of the peripheral pathology in retinal diseases [3–6].

Previous chapters have discussed the use of wide-field fundus photography and fluorescein angiography in various common retinal diseases. This chapter is a collection of unusual presentations, rare retinal conditions, as well as the use of monitoring and documentation of surgical retinal cases (Figs. 1, 2, 3, 4, 5, 6, 7, 8, 9, 10, 11, 12, 13, 14, 15, 16, 17, 18, 19, 20, 21, 22, 23, 24, 25, 26, 27, 28, 29 and 30). UWF imaging can be a very useful tool for comparison of pre- and postoperative retinal findings in conditions such as retinal detachments. In addition, UWF autofluorescence may reveal abnormalities in rhegmatogenous retinal detachment that allow excellent demarcation of the extent of the retinal detachment and assist in preoperative characterization of the detachment and may help in postoperative counseling [7]. It may also be useful in documenting multiple foci of exudative detachment spread throughout the retinal periphery and response to treatment.

The KKESH Collaborative Retina Study Group

J.F. Arevalo, MD, FACS (✉)
Edmund F. and Virginia B. Ball Professor of Ophthalmology, Chairman, Department of Ophthalmology, Johns Hopkins Bayview Medical Center, Retina Division, Wilmer Eye Institute, The Johns Hopkins University School of Medicine, Baltimore, MD, USA
e-mail: arevalojf@jhmi.edu

N. Choudhry, MD
Vitreoretinal Surgery Division, Herzig Eye Institute, Toronto, ON, Canada
e-mail: netan.choudhry@gmail.com

I. Kozak, MD, PhD
Senior Academic Consultant, Vitreoretinal Division, King Khaled Eye Specialist Hospital, Riyadh, Kingdom of Saudi Arabia
e-mail: ikozak@kkesh.med.sa

I. Kozak, J.F. Arevalo (eds.), *Atlas of Wide-Field Retinal Angiography and Imaging*, DOI 10.1007/978-3-319-17864-6_15

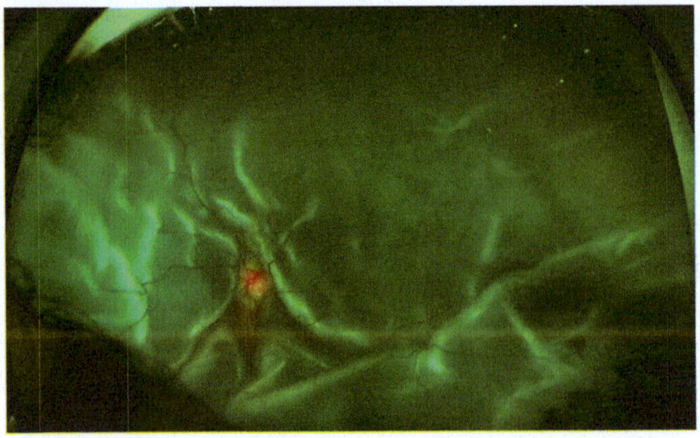

Fig. 1 Acute rhegmatogenous retinal detachment. A 36-year-old man presented to the emergency room with hand-motion vision. Wide-angle fundus photography shows total retinal detachment. Scleral indentation revealed a small break at 7 o'clock

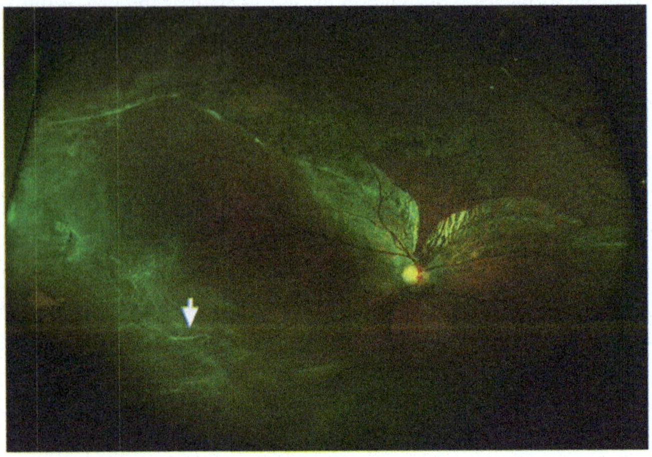

Fig. 2 Chronic retinal detachment. A 38-year-old man has had decrease in vision for over a year. Wide-angle fundus photography of his right eye shows subretinal fluid with sclerosed retinal vessels (*white arrow*) and pigmentary changes in the superior retina

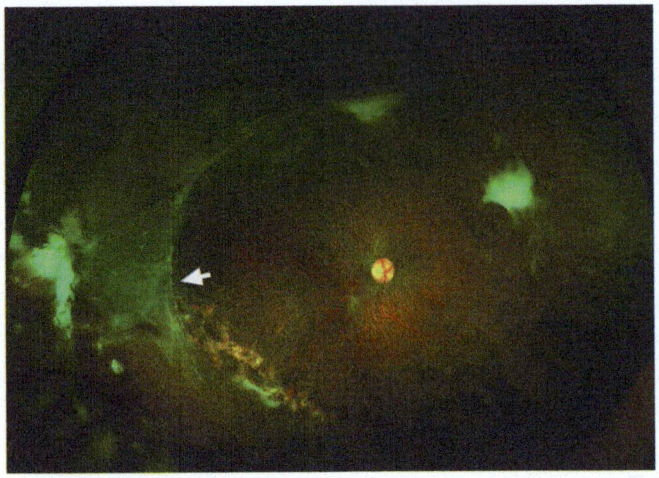

Fig. 3 Proliferative vitreoretinopathy in Stickler syndrome. A 22-year-old woman with Stickler syndrome after multiple retinal detachment surgeries in her right eye. Wide-angle fundus photography demonstrates peripheral fibrotic tissue and proliferative membranes (*white arrow*) with flat posterior retina

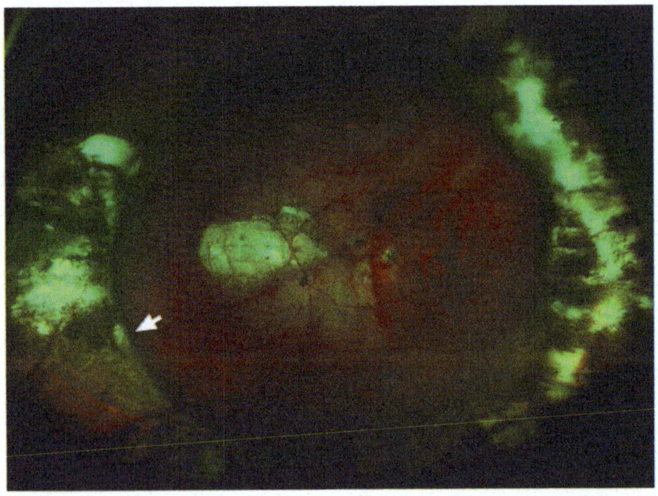

Fig. 4 Scleral buckle in high myopia. A 65-year-old man with high myopia, areas of peripapillary atrophy, and myopic maculopathy had scleral buckle surgery with cryotherapy for rhegmatogenous retinal detachment repair in his left eye. Wide-angle fundus photography demonstrates flat retina with buckle and cryotherapy scars in the retinal periphery (*white arrow*)

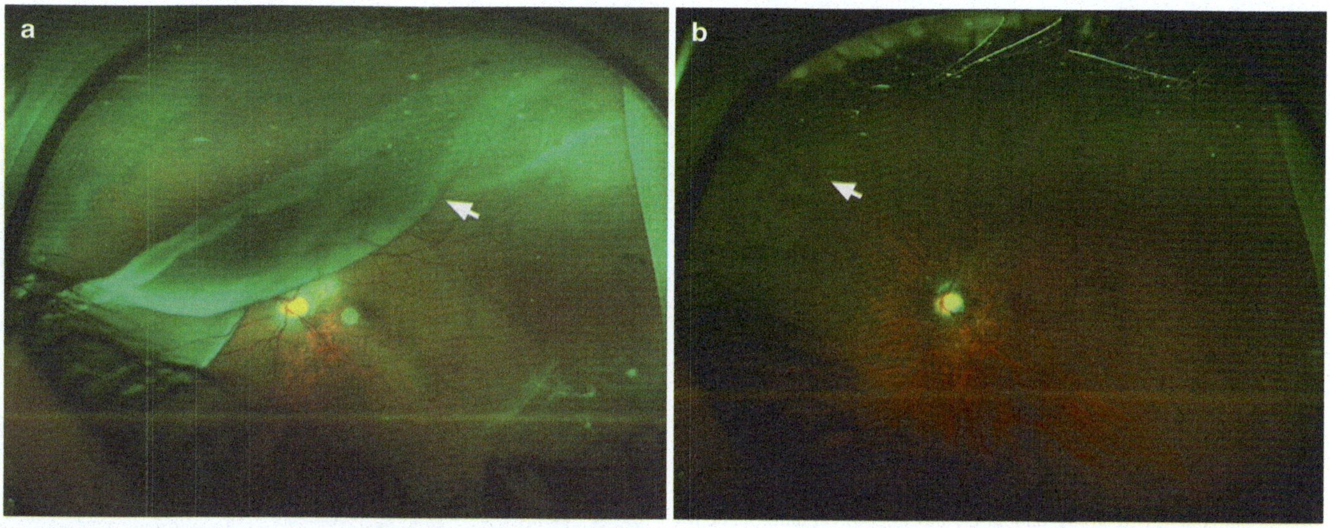

Fig. 5 (**a**) Giant retinal tear. A 45-year-old man presented with a "curtain" in his vision in the left eye. Clinical examination revealed a giant retinal tear from 8:30 to 13:30 clock hours and visual acuity of 20/20. Wide-angle fundus photography demonstrates macula-on detachment with an inverted anterior retinal flap (*white arrow*). (**b**) Postoperative finding in the same eye shows a completely flat retina with peripheral laser photocoagulation scars (*white arrow*) and visual acuity of 20/20

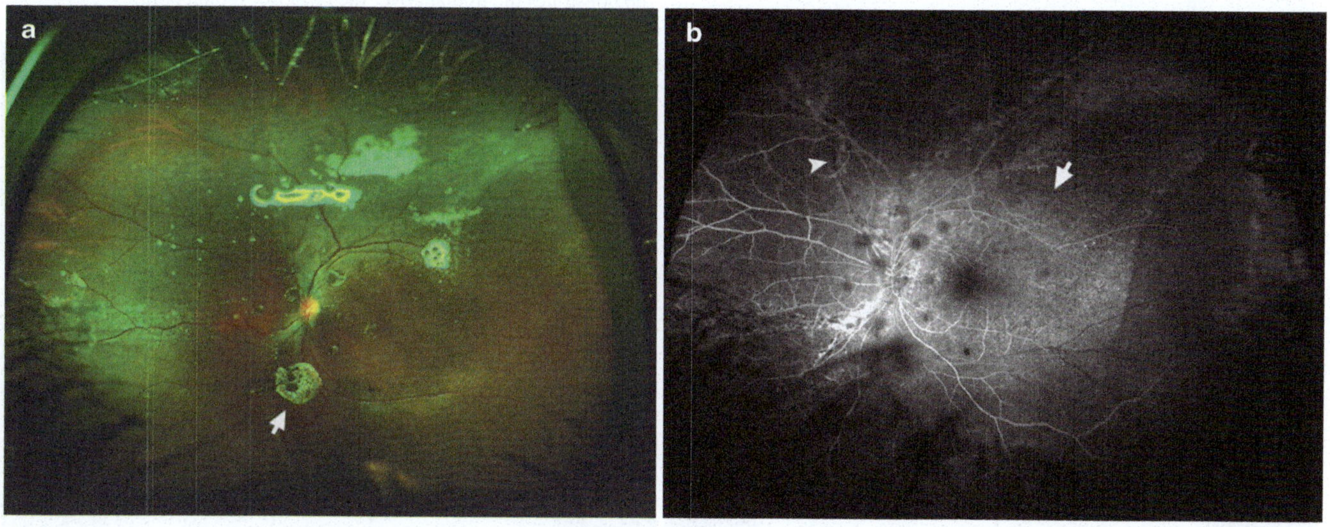

Fig. 6 (**a**) Retinal detachment surgery in Goldman-Favre syndrome. An 80-year-old man with autosomal recessive Goldman-Favre syndrome had retinal detachment repair with pars plana vitrectomy and silicone oil tamponade in left his eye. Wide-angle fundus photography demonstrates the flat retina under silicone oil with artifacts from oil emulsification (*white arrow*). (**b**) Wide-angle fluorescein angiogram of the same eye demonstrates subretinal pigmentary retinopathy (*white arrowhead*) with retinal blood vessel nonperfusion (*white arrow*) and RPE atrophy in the area of prior peripheral retinoschisis inferotemporally

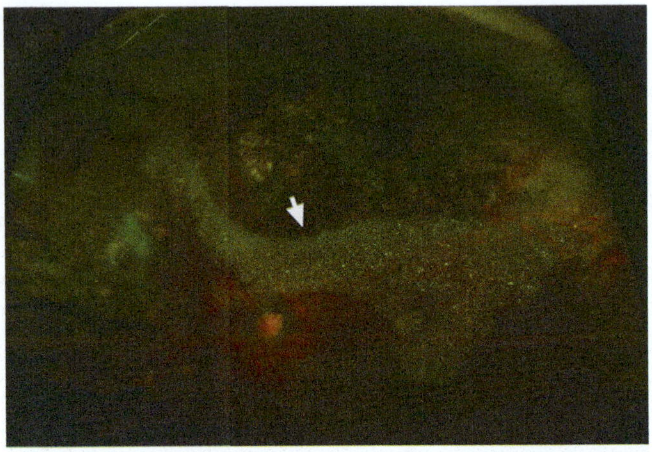

Fig. 7 Emulsified silicone oil. A 63-year-old diabetic man with a history of pars plana vitrectomy, endolaser, and silicone oil tamponade for traction retinal detachment in his left eye. Wide-angle fundus photography demonstrates the flat retina under silicone oil, which is emulsified (*white arrow*)

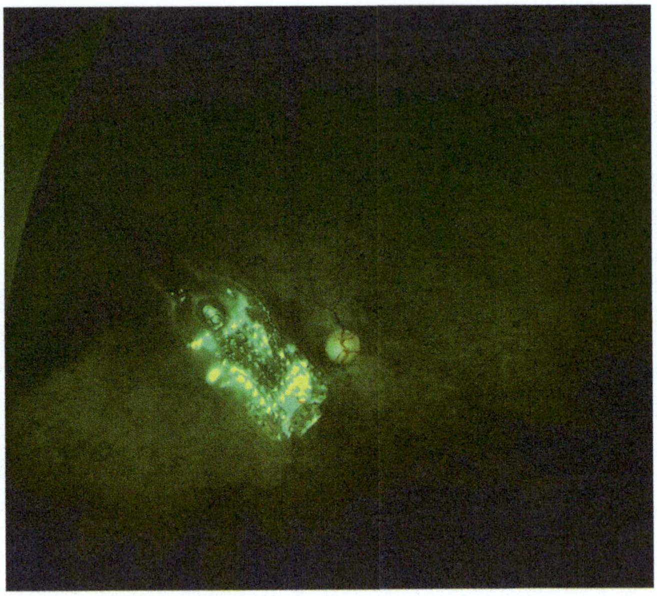

Fig. 8 Argus epiretinal implant. A 37-year-old man with retinitis pigmentosa post retinal implant surgery. Wide-angle fundus photography demonstrates the implant over the posterior retinal pole

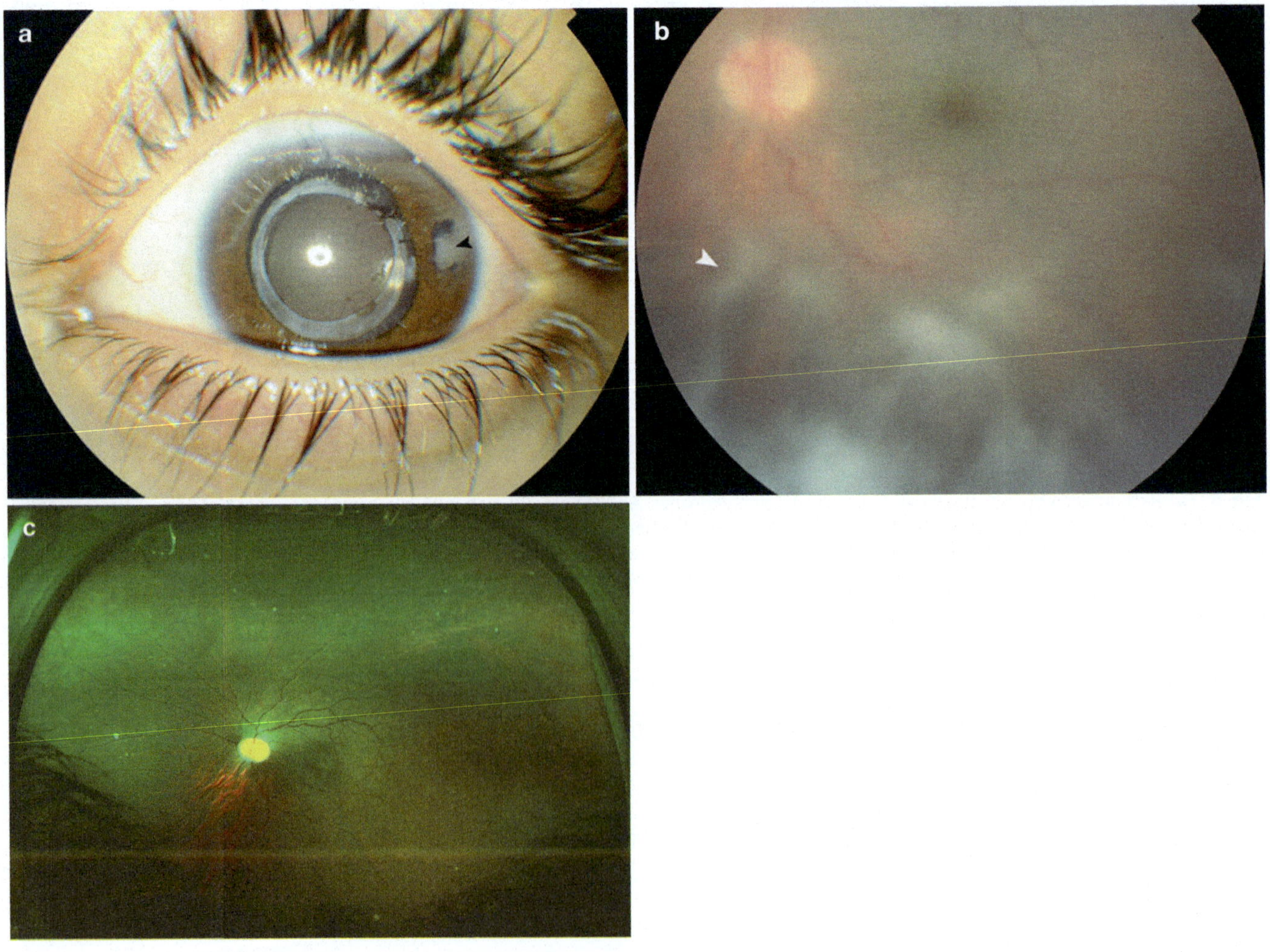

Fig. 9 (**a**) Bleb-related endophthalmitis. An 11-year-old boy with bilateral juvenile glaucoma had a history of cataract and glaucoma surgeries in his left eye. One year after the last surgery, he developed thin bleb and endophthalmitis with light-perception vision. Slit-lamp photography shows pus occluding the iridectomy. (**b**) Color fundus image of the same eye shows pus in the vitreous cavity (*white arrowhead*). (**c**) Wide-angle color fundus photography after vitreous tap, pars plana vitrectomy, and intravitreal antibiotic injection demonstrates the flat retina and clear vitreous cavity with enlarged optic disc. Vitreous culture showed multiple cocci. Vision after treatment improved to 20/60

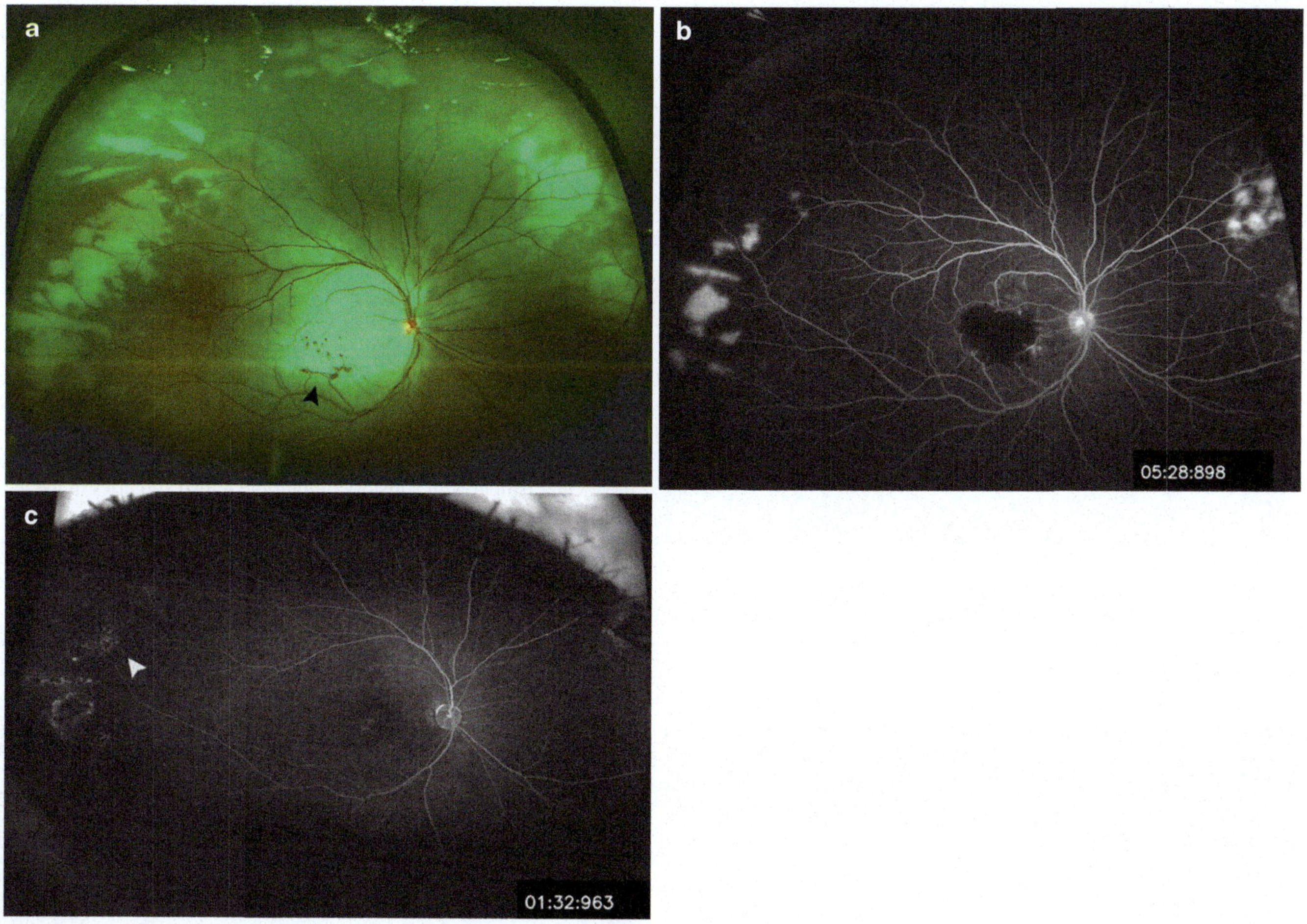

Fig. 10 (**a**) Retinal complication of endoscopic sinus surgery. A 40-year-old man underwent ethmoid sinus endoscopic surgery, which resulted in right eye exotropia and vision loss to hand motion. Orbital magnetic resonance imaging demonstrated transected medial rectus muscle and optic nerve damage. At presentation, the right eye demonstrated macular ischemia with hemorrhages (*black arrowhead*) and peripheral subretinal whitening. (**b**) Wide-angle fluorescein angiogram of the same eye shows macular hypofluorescence (absence of blood) and well-defined peripheral subretinal leakage. (**c**) Wide-angle fluorescein angiogram of the same eye 4 months later (with no intervention) shows macular staining and RPE atrophy with staining in the retinal periphery (*white arrowhead*). Vision improved to 20/300

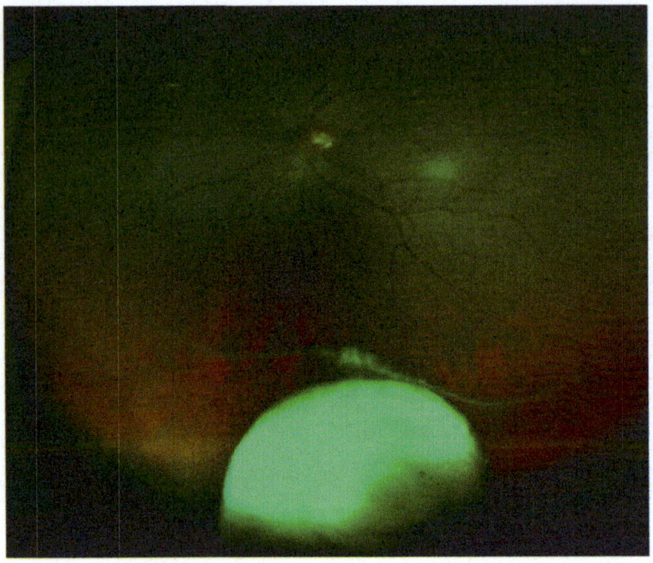

Fig. 11 Lens luxation in Marfan syndrome. A 24-year-old man with a history of Marfan syndrome presented with spontaneous luxation of the natural lens in his left eye. Wide-angle color fundus photography shows the dropped lens inferiorly

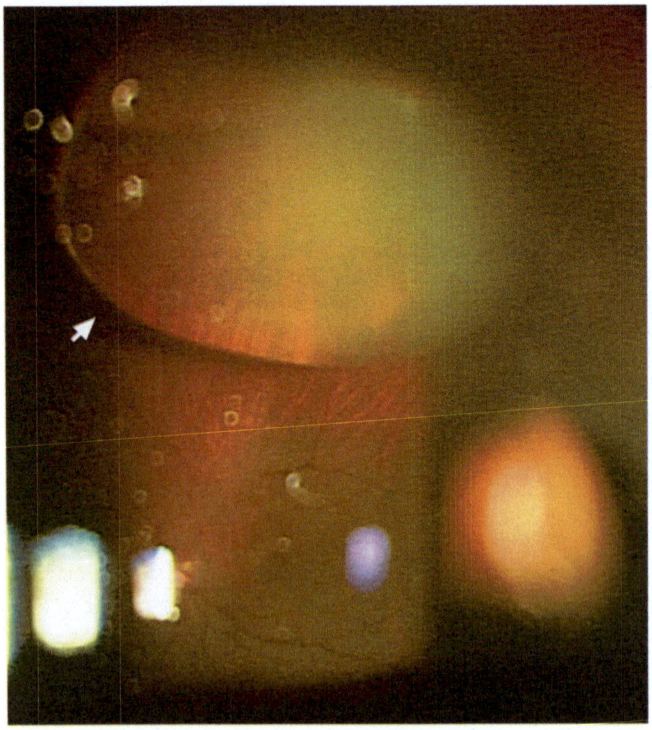

Fig. 12 Spontaneous lens luxation. A middle-aged woman presented with spontaneous natural lens luxation in her right eye. Wide-field biomicroscopic image shows the lens dislocated inferiorly (inverted image) (*white arrow*)

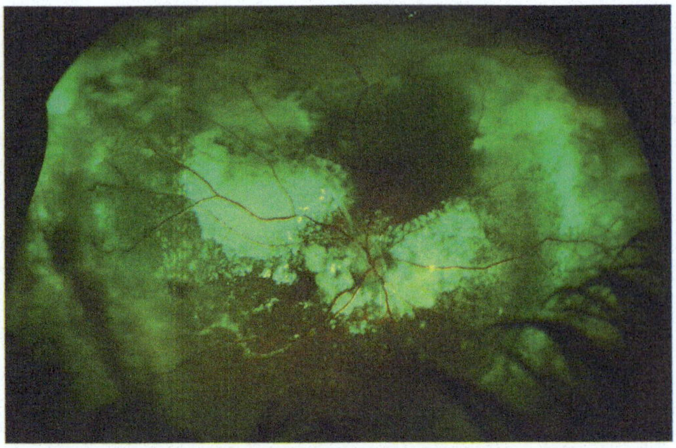

Fig. 13 Familial exudative vitreoretinopathy (FEVR). A 31-year-old monocular patient with a history of multiple retinal surgeries in the left eye and one pars plana vitrectomy in the right eye and Ozurdex implant has visual acuity of 20/100 in his right eye. Wide-angle color fundus photography shows subretinal crystalline deposits

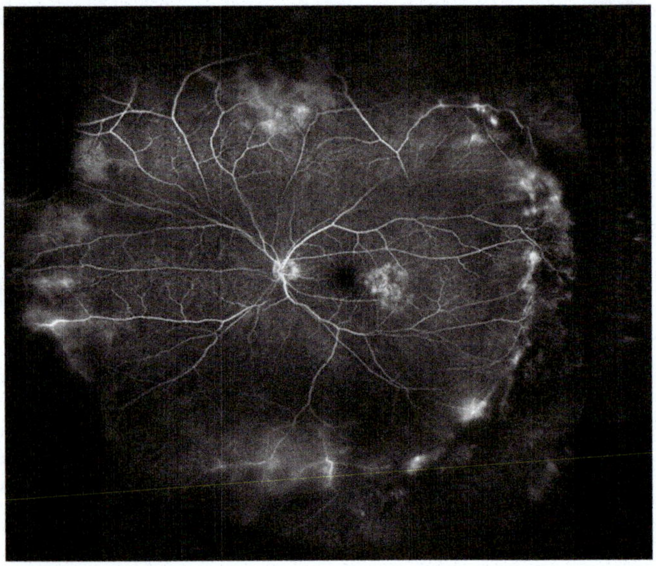

Fig. 14 FEVR. A 23-year-old woman with status post laser and pars plana vitrectomy/endolaser gas in her right eye (hand motion) has visual acuity of 20/32 in her left eye. Wide-angle fluorescein angiogram of her left eye shows perimacular staining, peripheral nonperfusion, and neovascularization

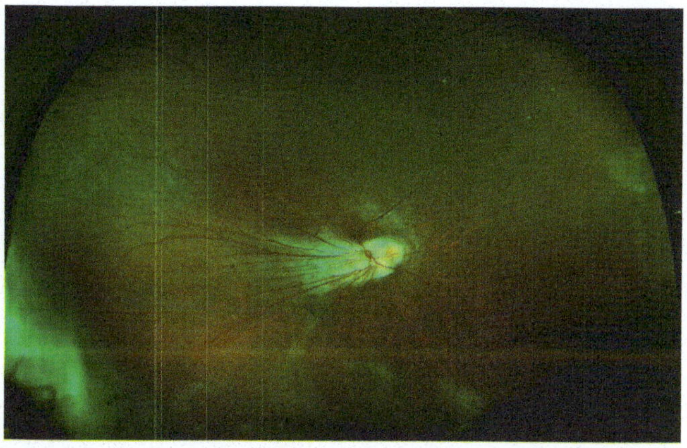

Fig. 15 History of retinopathy of prematurity. A 23-year-old man with monocular vision with a history of retinopathy of prematurity in both eyes and left prosthesis. Wide-angle color fundus photography of his right eye shows extensive macular dragging. Visual acuity is 20/70

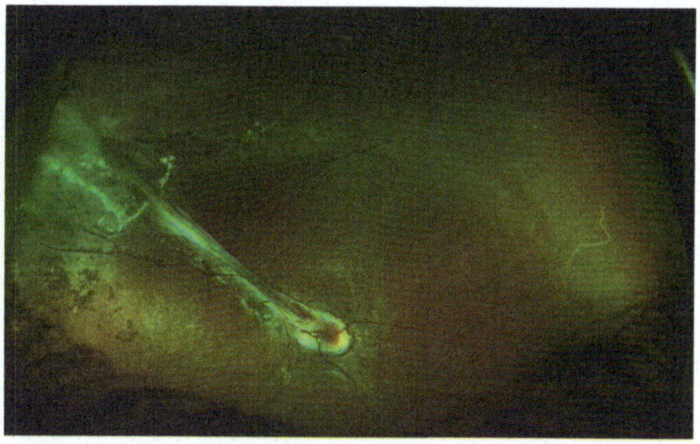

Fig. 16 History of retinopathy of prematurity. A 13-year-old boy with a history of retinopathy of prematurity post laser photocoagulation. Wide-angle color fundus photography of his right eye shows the flat retina with folded traction extending from the optic disc. Visual acuity is 20/200

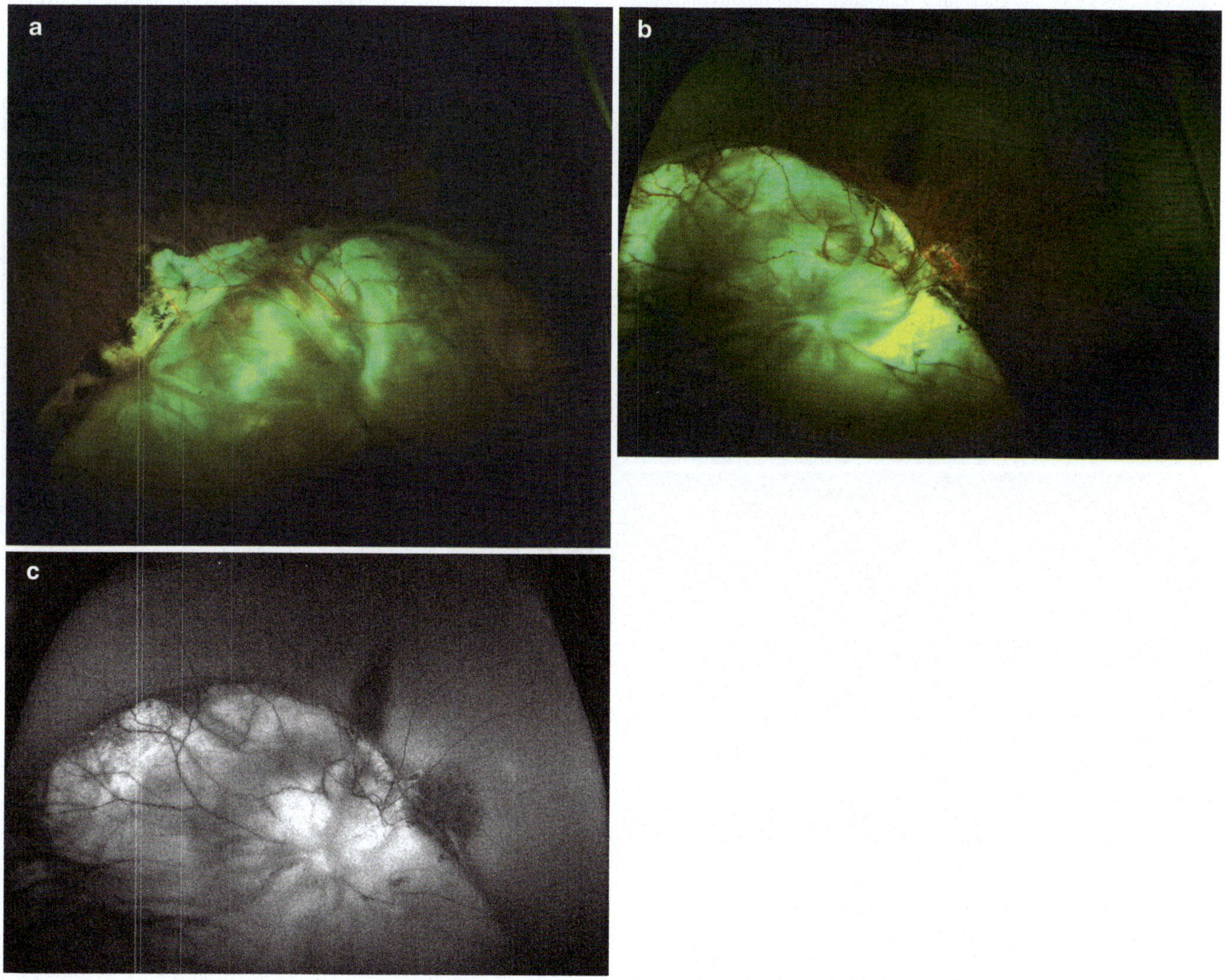

Fig. 17 (**a**) Chorioretinal/iris coloboma. A 32-year-old man with bilateral microcornea and a history of recurrent retinal detachment associated with chorioretinal and iris coloboma in his right eye. Wide-angle color fundus photography of his right eye shows the flat superior retina and inferior/nasal coloboma with underlying scleral tissue. Visual acuity is 4/200. (**b**) Wide-angle color fundus photography of the left eye of the same patient shows flat retina and inferior/nasal coloboma with underlying scleral tissue and peripapillary atrophy. Visual acuity is 6/200. (**c**) Wide-angle fundus autofluorescence of the left eye of the same patient shows absence of RPE in the area of the coloboma

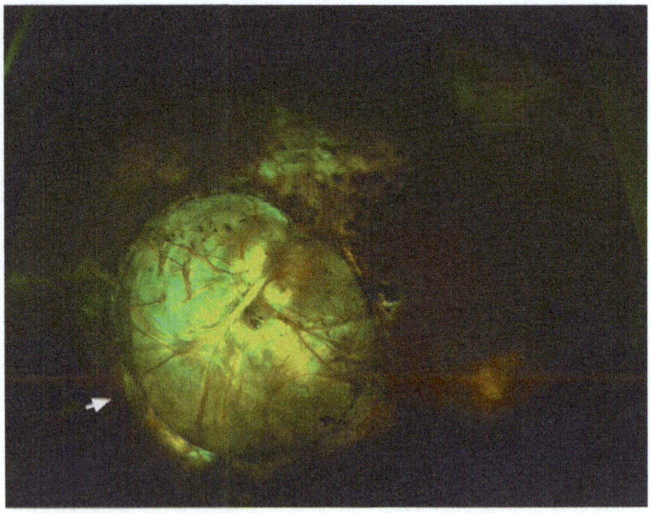

Fig. 18 Optic disc coloboma. A 29-year-old woman with a history of pars plana vitrectomy/endolaser for retinal detachment associated with optic disc coloboma and glaucoma. Wide-angle color fundus photography of her left eye shows a large coloboma (*white arrow*), flat retina, and laser photocoagulation spots. Visual acuity is 20/200

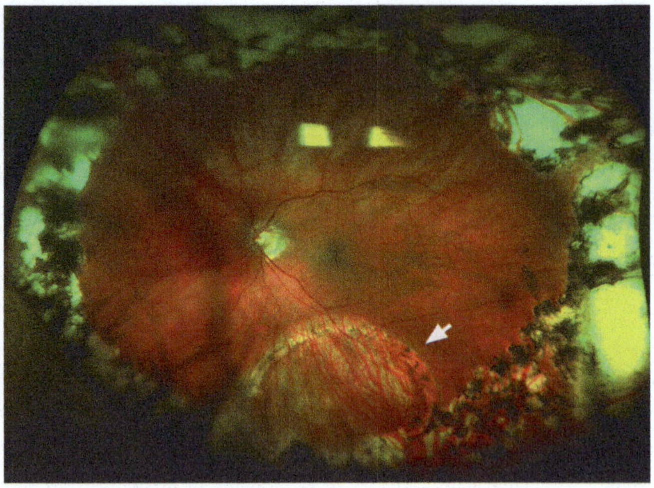

Fig. 20 Peripheral staphyloma. A 68-year-old myopic man has a history of recurrent retinal detachment. Wide-angle color fundus photography of his left eye shows flat retina, status post peripheral laser photocoagulation and cryotherapy, and a large peripheral staphyloma (*white arrow*). Visual acuity is 20/25

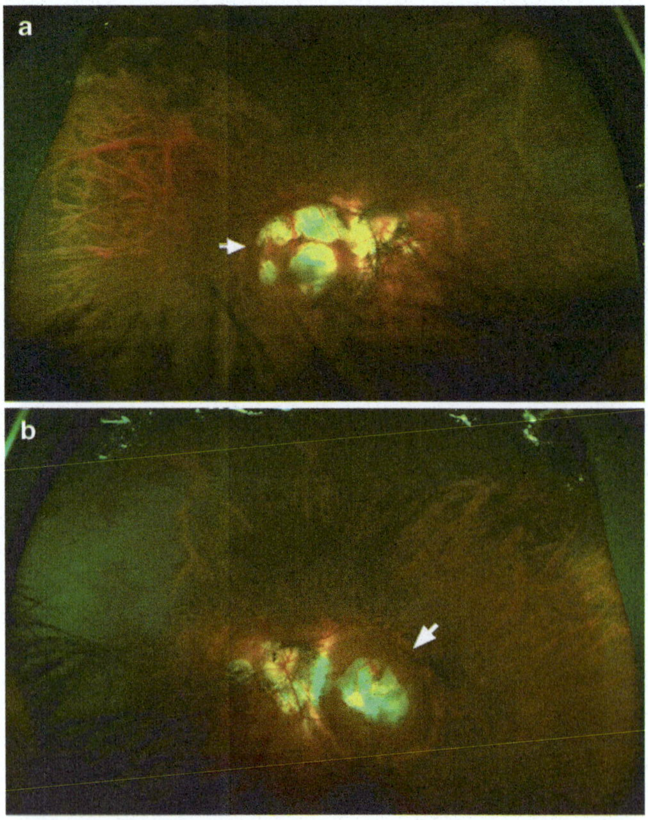

Fig. 19 (**a**) Bilateral central staphyloma. A 58-year-old man with high myopia and visual acuity decreased to 20/100. Wide-angle color fundus photography of his right eye shows large central staphyloma reaching to the vascular arcades (*white arrow*) with no choroidal neovascular membrane. (**b**) Wide-angle color fundus photography of the left eye (20/300) of the same patient shows peripapillary atrophy and a large central staphyloma reaching to the vascular arcades (*white arrow*) with no choroidal neovascular membrane

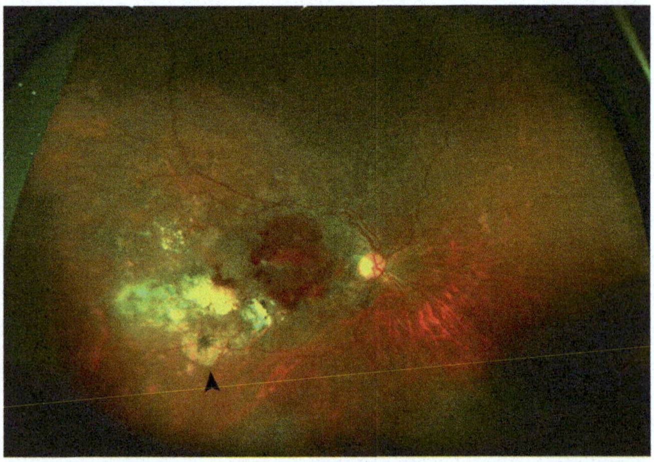

Fig. 21 Simultaneous exudative age-related macular degeneration and geographic atrophy. A 63-year-old woman has a history of bilateral age-related macular degeneration. Wide-angle color fundus photography of her right eye shows confluent drusen and subretinal fibrosis, areas of geographic atrophy (*black arrow*), and macular hemorrhage covering an area of geographic atrophy

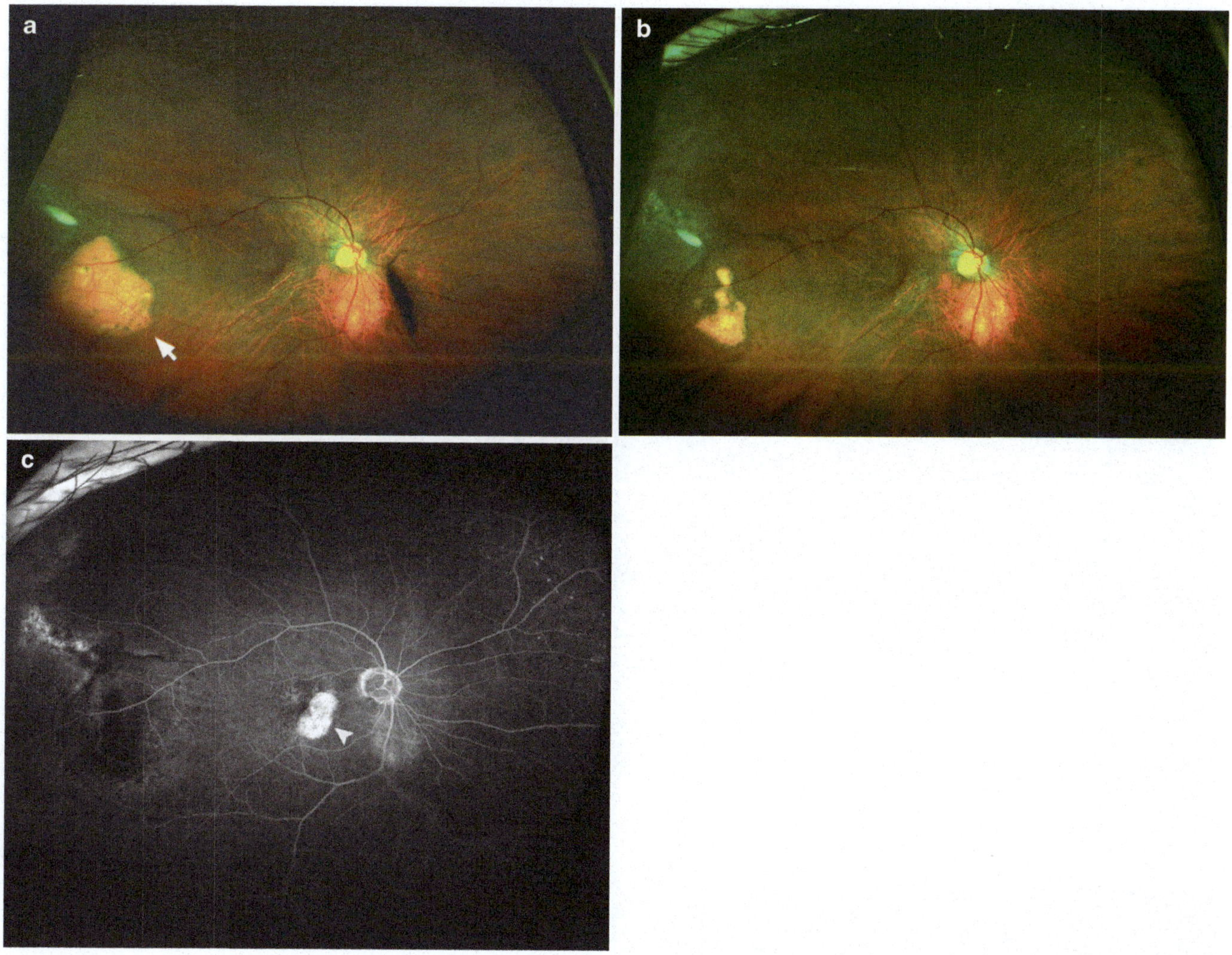

Fig. 22 (**a**) Peripheral subretinal hemorrhage in age-related macular degeneration. A 93-year-old woman has a history of bilateral age-related macular degeneration. Wide-angle color fundus photography of her right eye shows macular atrophy and an irregular peripheral subretinal mass (*white arrowhead*). There is no history of systemic malignancy. (**b**) Wide-angle color fundus photography of the same eye after 3 months of observation shows reduction in subretinal mass size. (**c**) Wide-angle fluorescein angiogram of the same eye demonstrates peripheral lesions with central hypofluorescence and adjacent RPE disturbance with staining. There is a window defect in the area of geographic atrophy (*white arrowhead*) and some peripheral drusen nasally

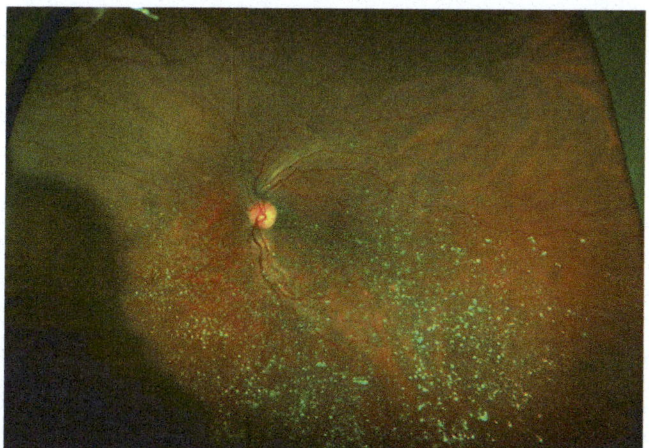

Fig. 23 Asteroid hyalosis. A 58-year-old man with no systemic disease complains of floaters in his left eye. Wide-angle color fundus photography shows refractile deposits in the vitreous. Visual acuity is 20/20

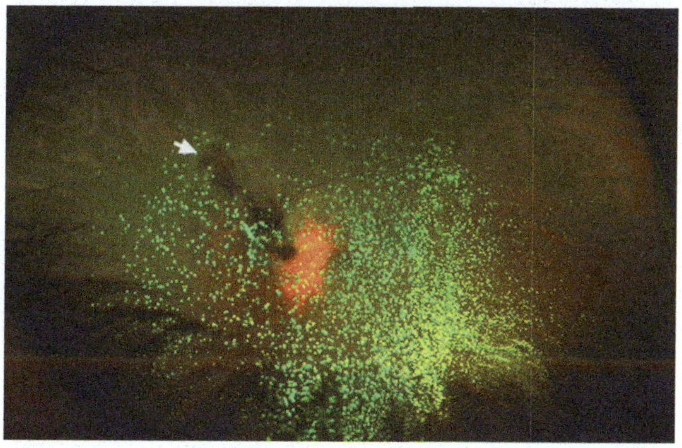

Fig. 24 Asteroid hyalosis in a diabetic eye. A 75-year-old man with diabetic retinopathy complains of floaters in his left eye. Wide-angle color fundus photography shows refractile deposits in the vitreous and preretinal hemorrhage (*white arrow*). Visual acuity is 20/30. The patient underwent pars plana vitrectomy with endolaser photocoagulation

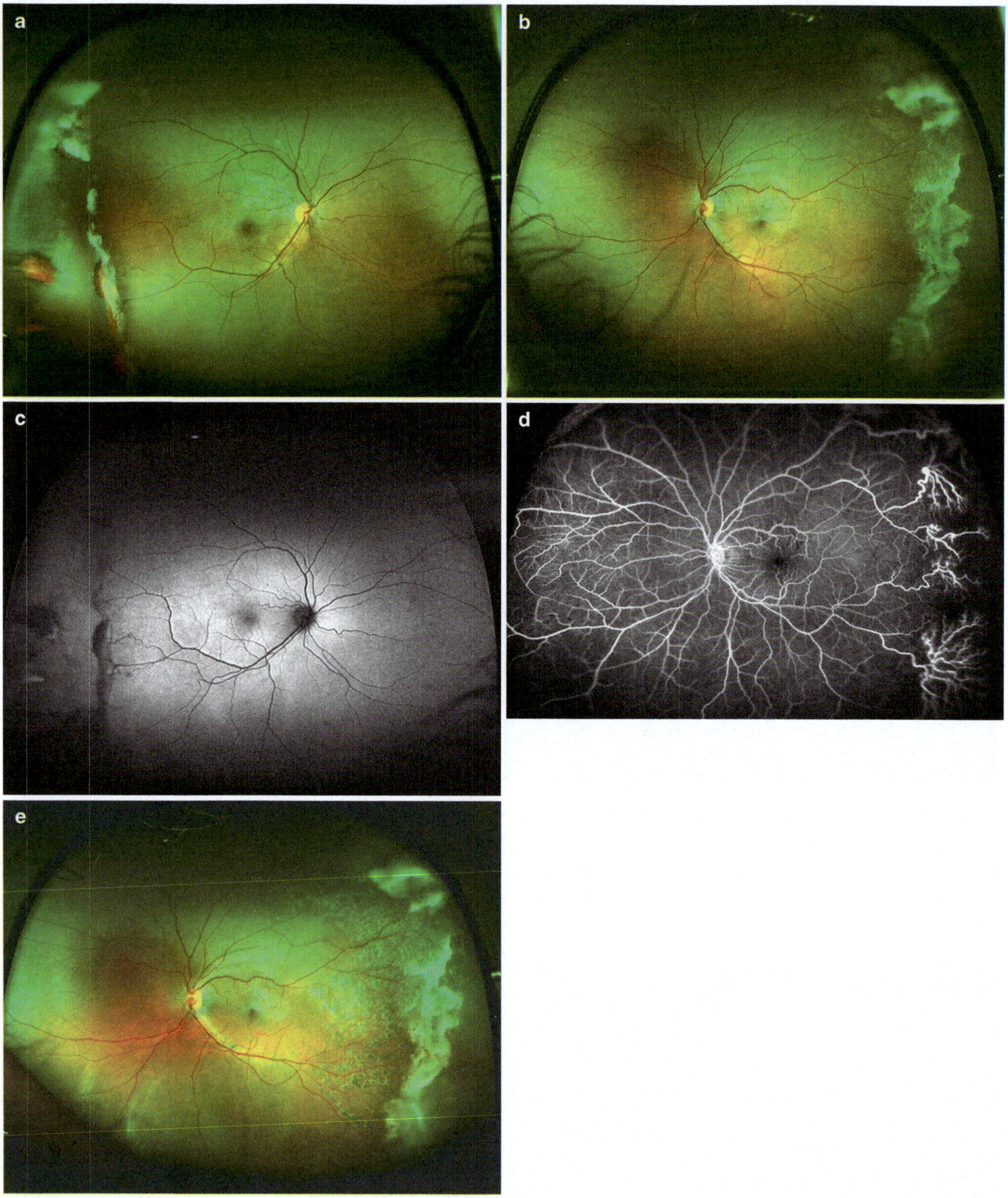

Fig. 25 (**a**) Sickle cell retinopathy. A 48-year-old man with newly diagnosed sickle cell disease (SC), without complaints, was referred for an epiretinal membrane. Visual acuity is 20/25 in both eyes. Wide-angle color fundus photography of his right eye shows peripheral sea fans of neovascularization. (**b**) Wide-angle color fundus photography of the left eye of the same patient shows prominent epimacular membrane and peripheral sea fans of neovascularization temporally. (**c**) Wide-angle fundus autofluorescence image of sea fans in sickle cell retinopathy. (**d**) Wide-angle fluorescein angiogram of the left eye of the same patient shows peripheral sea fans of neovascularization and nonperfusion in the retinal periphery. The patient underwent retinal laser photocoagulation in both eyes. (**e**) Wide-angle color fundus photography of the left eye of the same patient after retinal photocoagulation shows peripheral laser spots

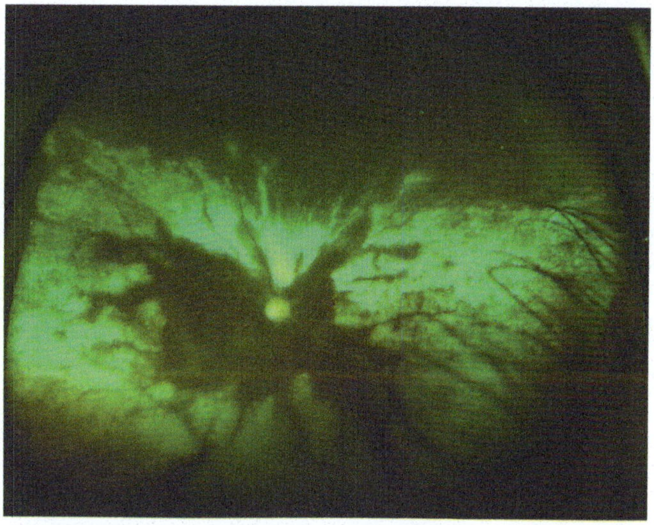

Fig. 26 Acute retinal necrosis. A 31-year-old man with severe pancytopenia and immunocompromised lost his vision in right eye (no light perception). Wide-angle color fundus photography of his right eye shows a pale optic disc and widespread areas of retinitis

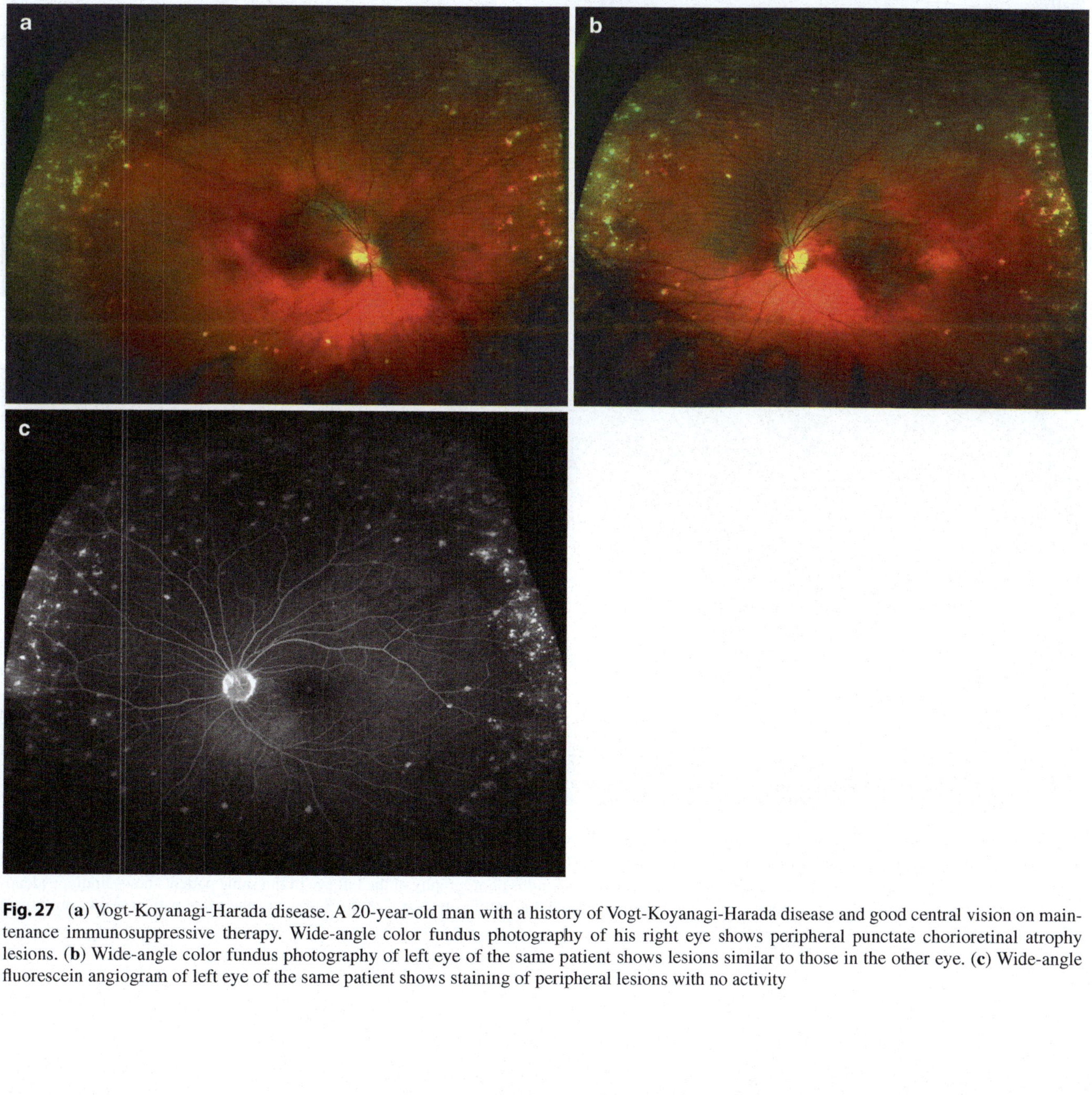

Fig. 27 (**a**) Vogt-Koyanagi-Harada disease. A 20-year-old man with a history of Vogt-Koyanagi-Harada disease and good central vision on maintenance immunosuppressive therapy. Wide-angle color fundus photography of his right eye shows peripheral punctate chorioretinal atrophy lesions. (**b**) Wide-angle color fundus photography of left eye of the same patient shows lesions similar to those in the other eye. (**c**) Wide-angle fluorescein angiogram of left eye of the same patient shows staining of peripheral lesions with no activity

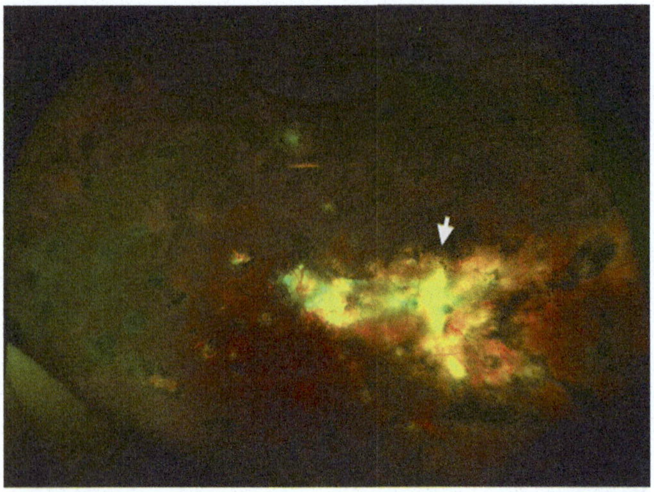

Fig. 28 Multifocal choroiditis/subretinal fibrosis syndrome. A 57-year old man with a history of posterior uveitis and vision loss. Wide-angle color fundus photography of his left eye shows clear vitreous, multiple subretinal lesions, and submacular fibrosis (*white arrow*). Visual acuity is hand motion

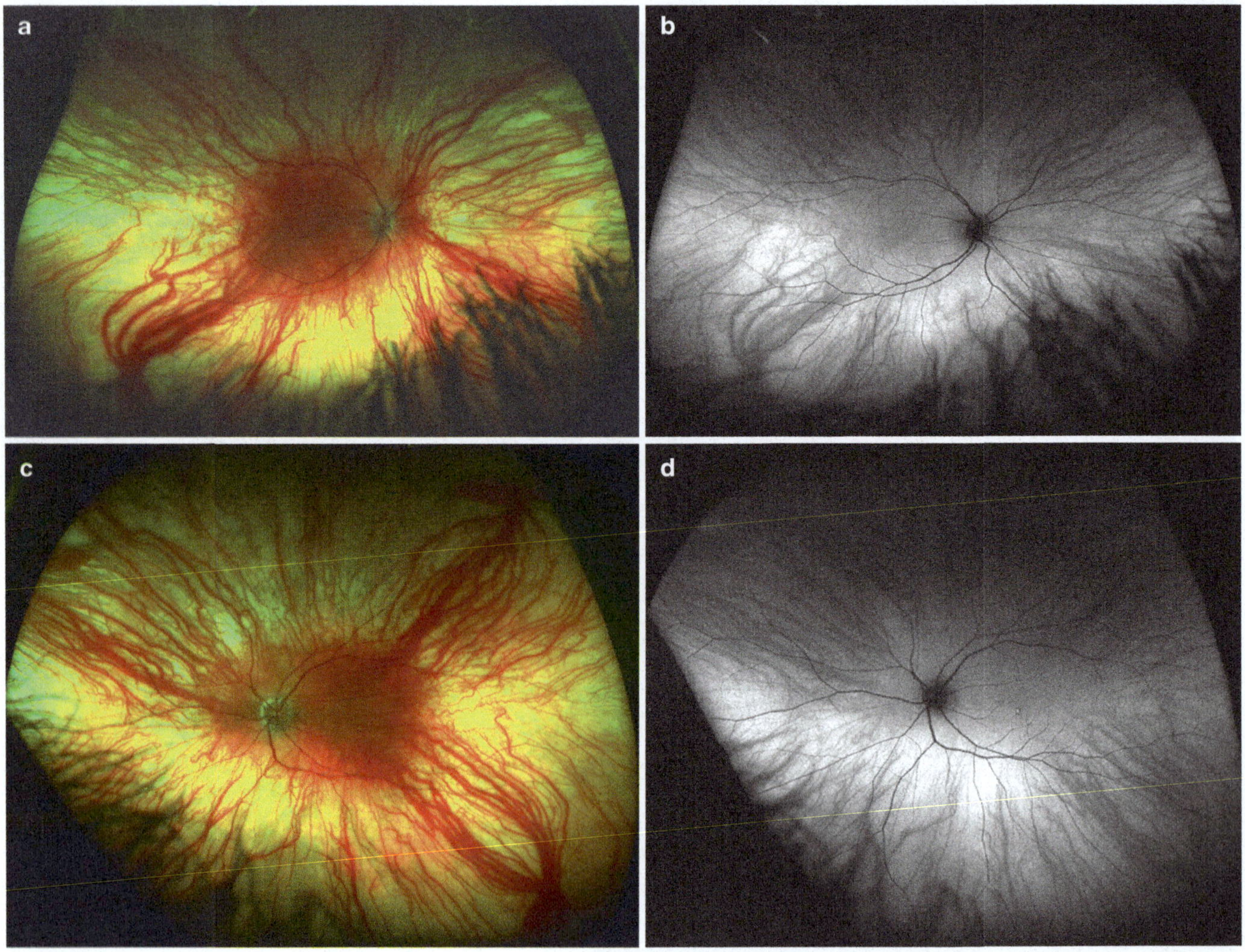

Fig. 29 (**a**) Ocular albinism. A 25-year-old woman with tyrosinase-negative ocular albinism. Visual acuity is 20/200. Wide-angle color fundus photography of her right eye shows absent RPE, prominent choroidal vessels, and hypoplastic fovea. (**b**) Wide-angle fundus autofluorescence of the same eye shows prominent choroidal vessels. (**c**) Wide-angle color fundus photography of the left eye of the same patient shows findings identical to those in the other eye. Visual acuity is 20/160. (**d**) Wide-angle fundus autofluorescence of the left eye of the same patient shows prominent choroidal vessels

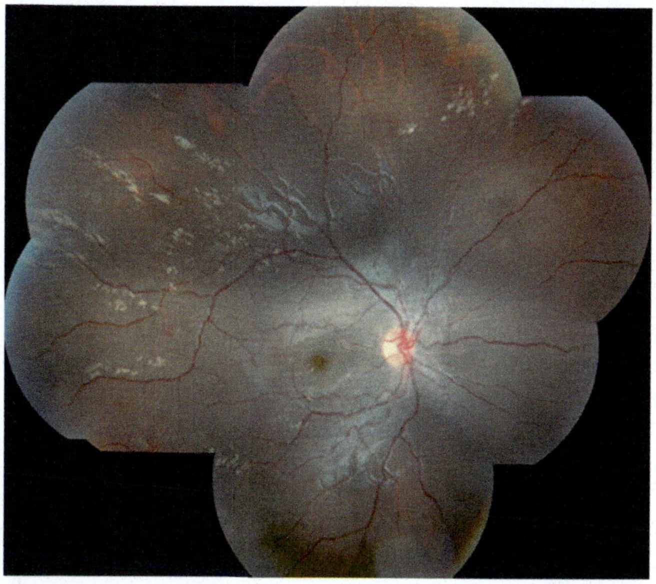

Fig. 30 Polar bear tracks. Color fundus photo montage of the right eye of an 8-year-old Hispanic girl shows yellowish-white silent flecks. Optical coherence tomography located lesions at the level of the RPE. Visual acuity is 20/20. The clinical picture has been stable for 5 years

Future Directions

Wide-field technology has become important clinically with regards to early diagnosis, effective treatment, and monitoring of most sight-threatening retinal diseases. In the future, wide-field imaging will have significant utility as a research tool, particularly for evaluating new treatment approaches. Advancements in telemedicine methods and the development of portable fundus cameras have increased the accessibility of retinal imaging, but most of these approaches rely on separate computers for viewing and transmission of fundus images. Recently, a novel portable handheld smartphone-based retinal camera capable of capturing high-quality, wide-field fundus images was developed. The use of the mobile phone platform creates a fully embedded system capable of acquisition, storage, and analysis of fundus images that can be directly transmitted from the phone via wireless telecommunication system for remote evaluation [8]. Telemedicine programs have shown that nonphysician operators can be trained to obtain images for remote expert interpretation [9]. Photographic documentation can also be a valuable asset for medicolegal and medical training educational purposes [10].

Acknowledgment *The following investigators belong to The King Khaled Eye Specialist Hospital (KKESH) Collaborative Retina Study Group: J. Fernando Arevalo, MD, FACS (PI), Saba Al Rashaed, MD, Eman Al Kahtani, MD, Sawsan Nowilaty, MD, Hassan A. Al-Dhibi, MD, Yahya A. Al-Zahrani, MD, Igor Kozak, MD, PhD, Sulaiman Al-Sulaiman, MD, Patrik Schatz, MD, Abdulelah Al-Abdullah, MD, Khalid Al Rubaie, MD, Yousef Al Dhafiri, MD, Badr Al Ahmadi, MD, Abdulaziz Al Hadlaq, MD, Majed Al Harbi, MD, Abdulaziz Al Oreany, MD, Adel Al-Akeely, MD, Mohammad Hazzazi, MD, Mohammed Talea, MD, Ghazai Al-Thobaiti, MD.

References

1. Tan CS, Sadda SR, Hariprasad SM. Ultra-widefield retinal imaging in the management of diabetic eye diseases. Ophthalmic Surg Lasers Imaging Retina. 2014;45:363–6.
2. Pang CE, Shah VP, Sarraf D, Freund KB. Ultra-widefield imaging with autofluorescence and indocyanine green angiography in central serous chorioretinopathy. Am J Ophthalmol. 2014;158:362–371.e2.
3. Manivannan A, Plskova J, Farrow A, Mckay S, Sharp PF, Forrester JV. Ultra-wide-field fluorescein angiography of the ocular fundus. Am J Ophthalmol. 2005;140:525–7.
4. Patel M, Kiss S. Ultra-wide-field fluorescein angiography in retinal disease. Curr Opin Ophthalmol. 2014;25:213–20.
5. Oliver SC, Schwartz SD. Peripheral vessel leakage (PVL): a new angiographic finding in diabetic retinopathy identified with ultra wide-field fluorescein angiography. Semin Ophthalmol. 2010;25:27–33.
6. Wessel MM, Aaker GD, Parlitsis G, Cho M, D'Amico DJ, Kiss S. Ultra-wide-field angiography improves the detection and classification of diabetic retinopathy. Retina. 2012;32:785–91.
7. Witmer MT, Cho M, Favarone G, Chan RV, D'Amico DJ, Kiss S. Ultra-wide-field autofluorescence imaging in non-traumatic rhegmatogenous retinal detachment. Eye (Lond). 2012;26:1209–16.
8. Maamari RN, Keenan JD, Fletcher DA, Margolis TP. A mobile phone-based retinal camera for portable wide field imaging. Br J Ophthalmol. 2014;98:438–41.
9. Fijalkowski N, Zheng LL, Henderson MT, Wang SK, Wallenstein MB, Leng T, et al. Stanford University Network for Diagnosis of Retinopathy of Prematurity (SUNDROP): five years of screening with telemedicine. Ophthalmic Surg Lasers Imaging Retina. 2014;45:106–13.
10. Chan PRV, Williams SL, Yonekawa Y, Weissgold DJ, Lee TC, Chiang MF. Accuracy of retinopathy of prematurity diagnosis by retinal fellows. Retina. 2010;30:958–65.

Index

I. Kozak, J.F. Arevalo (eds.), *Atlas of Wide-Field Retinal Angiography and Imaging*, DOI 10.1007/978-3-319-17864-6

The manufacturer's authorised representative in the EU is Springer Nature Customer Service Centre GmbH, Europaplatz 3, 69115 Heidelberg, Germany. If you have any concerns regarding our products, please contact ProductSafety@springernature.com

Printed and bound by CPI Group (UK) Ltd, Croydon, CR0 4YY
22/09/2026
02221078-0001